A
Pocket Guide
for
Medical-Surgical Nursing

Saint Francis Medical Center
Home Health Care Agency
2620 W. Faidley   P.O. Box 2118
Grand Island, Nebraska 68802

A
Pocket Guide
for
Medical-Surgical Nursing

Carol J. Neel, R.N., B.S.N
Mark B. Wallerstein, R.N., B.S.N., MICN

Brady Communications Company, Inc.
A Prentice-Hall Publishing Company
Bowie, MD 20715

A Pocket Guide for Medical-Surgical Nursing

Library of Congress Cataloging in Publication Data

Neel, Carol, 1952-
   A pocket guide for medical-surgical nursing.

   Includes index.
   1. Nursing—Handbooks, manuals, etc. 2. Diagnosis—Handbooks, manuals, etc. 3. Surgical Nursing—Handbooks, manuals, etc. I. Wallerstein, Mark, 1956-   II. Title. [DNLM: 1. Nursing—handbooks. 2. Nursing—outlines. 3. Surgical Nursing—handbooks. 4. Surgical Nursing—outlines. WY 39 N378c]
   RT51.N374   1985   610.73   84–23071

ISBN 0-89303-772-9

Prentice-Hall of Australia, Pty., Ltd., *Sydney*
Prentice-Hall Canada, Inc., Scarborough, *Ontario*
Prentice-Hall Hispanoamericana, S.A., *Mexico*
Prentice-Hall of India Private Limited, *New Delhi*
Prentice-Hall International (UK) Limited, *London*
Prentice-Hall of Japan, Inc., *Tokyo*
Prentice-Hall of Southeast Asia Pte. Ltd., *Singapore*
Editora Prentice-Hall Do Brasil LTDA., *Rio de Janeiro*
Whitehall Books, Limited, Petone, *New Zealand*

Printed in the United States of America

85 86 87 88 89 90 91 92 93 94 95   1 2 3 4 5 6 7 8 9 10

Publishing Director: David Culverwell
Acquisitions Editor: Richard Weimer
Production Editor: Deborah Corson
Copy Editor/Text Designer: Lisa G. Kolman
Art Director/Cover Design: Don Sellers, AMI
Assistant Art Director: Bernard Vervin
Manufacturing Director: John Komsa

Indexer: Leah Kramer
Typesetter: Hodges Typographers, Silver Spring, Md.
Printer: Edwards Brothers, Ann Arbor, Mich.
Typefaces: Times Roman (text) and Optima (display)

CONTENTS

PREFACE

During the process of going to nursing school and later working on a medical-surgical unit, we found that some of our colleagues, as well as ourselves, developed pocket-sized notebooks filled with a collection of useful information. After surveying available resource material, we found a need for a comprehensive pocket-sized text for use in the medical-surgical area.

This book is designed as such a pocket reference book for nurses working in hospital medical or surgical units. Although primarily intended to assist students and graduate and returning nurses, this book is an invaluable resource for experienced nurses and practitioners.

This book attempts to answer nurses' questions regarding assessment and interventions in patient care at the time those questions arise. Hospital reference material is frequently located in obscure places and requires valuable nursing time to locate. Since this book can be carried in your pocket, it serves as a quick reference guide when and where you need it. It is also the purpose of this book to focus nurses' attention on the assessment and intervention aspects of the nursing process. We have provided guidelines for collecting the data necessary to formulate nursing diagnoses.

It is not within the scope of this book, however, to guide nurses in the interpretation and organization of that data. The key points pertaining to patient assessment and nursing interventions are presented simply and directly for easy referral. Because the content is structured in an outlined, step-by-step format that excludes detailed rationale for key interventions, the nurse must refer to textbooks for supplemental information. Nurses are, therefore, referred to texts that deal with nursing diagnosis in greater depth. A list of approved nursing diagnoses is provided in Appendix E for reference purposes.

A basic review of anatomy and physiology precedes each system assessment. This review will help the nurse to understand the disease process and treatment modalities involved. The nurse will also find it helpful for patient and family teaching.

The assessment sections contain a guide to a complete physical examination of each system. The entire process may be rather time-consuming and will not always be necessary. The nurse must be judicious in determining the extent of the exam.

Potential problems for each condition are listed to indicate what should be observed when assessing the patient. Although the focus of the medical plan is in resolving the patient's "actual" problem, much of the nursing focus is on preventing potential problems from occurring secondary to the actual problem.

The key nursing interventions are presented under the heading of "medical" diagnoses rather than "nursing" diagnoses. The structure and organization of this book is based on the medical model which is a body system approach. Within each medical diagnosis a variety of nursing diagnoses may be made on the basis of each individual's response to illness and hospitalization. Although the key nursing interventions are specific to the medical diagnosis, they should be integrated into the patient care plan appropriately as determined by the nursing diagnosis. The general goal of the key nursing interventions is to accelerate the recovery process and prevent potential problems from occurring.

Patient and family teaching are essential aspects of nursing practice and are, therefore, addressed in each condition. Here again, the "key" points relative to the medical condition are emphasized for direct and simple reference.

We want to stress that this book is not meant to replace policy and procedure manuals. Each hospital is distinct, and it is the nurse's legal responsibility to know and follow hospital procedure at all times.

We hope you will carry this book and use it daily when providing and planning patient care. Nothing would please us more than if our book increases the quality of care, decreases anxiety, makes practical use of theoretical knowledge, and makes your contribution to nursing rewarding.

—Carol J. Neel
  Nursing Instructor
  Kaiser Foundation Hospital
  Panorama City, California

—Mark B. Wallerstein
  MICN—Emergency Room
  Holy Cross Hospital
  Mission Hills, California

Acknowledgments

We would like to thank Estella Campos for her editorial and typing skills, encouragement, and support; Anna Archambeau, R.N., for her patience, support, and understanding; Harriet Goldware-Sorkin for her friendship, counsel, and manuscript preparation; Val Castle, R.N.; Judy Child, R.N.; Karen Downing, R.N.; Gordon Hagerman, M.D.; Carol Mears, R.N.; Sue Neel; Lyn Thornton, R.N.; Dot Walker; and our families, friends, and colleagues for their faith and encouragement.

THE NURSING HISTORY

The nursing history and physical assessment are the beginning steps for formulating nursing diagnoses and initiating a plan of care for the patient. This section is a guide for obtaining a nursing history. Guidelines for physical assessment of each body system follow in subsequent chapters. A list of approved nursing diagnoses from the Fifth National Conference on Classification of Nursing Diagnosis is provided in Appendix E for reference purposes. After collecting the data from the nursing history and physical exam, the nurse must use her/his knowledge of nursing theory to interpret and organize the data and finally, formulate nursing diagnoses.

Biographical Data

1. To obtain the nursing history, identify if the patient is alert and oriented. If the patient is unable to participate in the interview, attempt to contact a family member or significant other for assistance.
2. Identify the following data:

   a) Patient's name
   b) Sex
   c) Race
   d) Nationality
   e) Marital status
   f) Occupation
   g) Age

Chief Complaint

What led you to seek medical care?

History of Present Illness

1. When was the onset of this problem? Time? Date?
2. What were you doing and what were the circumstances when the problem first occurred?
3. What was the manner of the onset? Gradual? Sudden?

4. Where (in the body) is the problem located? Does it radiate to other areas? Where?

5. Describe the problem. What do you feel or experience?

6. Is the problem mild, moderate, or severe?

7. Is there anything which aggravates or relieves the problem?

8. Do you experience any other symptoms?

9. How frequently have you been experiencing the symptom since it first began? (Was it a single occurrence? Does it happen intermittently? Is it a chronic problem?)

Past Medical History

1. What immunizations have you had? When?

2. What illnesses have you had in the past (i.e., childhood illnesses, polio, tuberculosis, hepatitis, rheumatic fever, stroke, heart attack, etc.)?

3. Have you ever been in the hospital before? Reason? Date? Name of hospital?

4. What surgeries have you had? When?

5. Do you have disabilities as a result of these illnesses or surgeries?

6. Do you presently have any chronic illnesses or conditions (i.e., lung, kidney, liver, heart disease; diabetes; hypertension; blood dyscrasias; etc.)?

7. Have you ever had blood transfusions? When?

8. Have you traveled out of the country? Have you had any illnesses as a result?

Family History

1. Who are the living members of your family? What are their ages?

2. What is the health status of the living members of your family?

3. Does anyone in your family have any illnesses or health related conditions at this time (i.e., cancer, heart disease, kidney disease, arthritis, diabetes, hypertension, etc.)?

4. What diseases have your family members had in the past?

5. What was the cause of death for deceased members?

Psychosocial

1. What do you do for a living?

2. Describe your work environment.

3. Do you like your job? Is it stressful?

4. Where are you originally from?

5. Where do you live now?

6. What are your living arrangements or who do you live with (i.e., alone, roommate(s), family, extended family, retirement home, nursing home)?

7. Do you have any difficulties with the people you live with? Specify. Is your home environment stable?

8. Who are the people most important in your life?

9. What language do you best communicate in?

10. What is your cultural background?

11. Will this hospitalization disrupt your religious practices? Do you think your religious beliefs will help you cope with your illness? Would you like your spiritual advisor contacted (i.e., priest, rabbi, pastor, elder, etc.)?

12. Will this hospitalization create a financial burden for you or your family?

13. How do you feel about yourself most of the time?

14. Do you ever feel depressed, anxious, suicidal, or angry? Do you have sudden changes in mood, episodes of crying, hear voices, etc.? Are these feelings ever a problem for you?

15. Have you experienced any recent losses (i.e., deaths, job, social status, financial status, physical losses)?

16. Have you had any recent lifestyle changes (i.e., marriage, divorce, home relocation, job changes, children, development of a chronic illness, etc.)?

17. Attempt to identify major roles that the patient occupies (i.e., father, wife, breadwinner, occupation, social roles, etc.).

18. How might this hospitalization affect these roles?

Medications

1. What prescribed medications are you taking? Why?

2. What over-the-counter or home remedies are you taking (brand names)?

Allergies

Do you have any allergies (i.e., medications, foods, contrast dyes, iodine, tapes, soaps, flowers, pollen, etc.)? Describe your reaction.

Sensory

1. Do you have any visual problems? Have you had any changes in your vision?
2. Do you wear glasses, contact lenses, or have an eye prosthesis? What is the length of time worn?
3. Do you have a hearing problem? Describe in detail.
4. Which ear do you hear better out of? Do you wear a hearing aid? What is the length of time worn?

Skin Integrity

Do you have any problems with your skin? Describe.

Sleep/Rest

1. Do you have any of the following problems: Difficulty in falling asleep, difficulty in awakening, insomnia, frequent waking, not feeling rested after sleep, sleepwalking, nightmares?
2. What time do you usually go to bed?
3. How many hours do you sleep per day?
4. Do you require a nap? What time of the day do you usually take a nap?
5. Do you use any aids in falling asleep (i.e., medications, alcohol, television, radio)?

Activity

1. Do you have any of the following problems: Range of motion limitations, problems with walking or running, painful joints, tremors, spasticity, weakness after activity?
2. Do you need assistance when walking or moving about (i.e., use of crutches, braces, canes, walkers, wheelchairs)?
3. How much activity do you do at work?
4. Do you exercise daily? If so, what type?
5. Are you able to perform activities of daily living (i.e., brush teeth, comb hair, bathe, dress, etc.)?

Nutrition

1. How much do you weigh?
2. How tall are you?
3. Describe a typical day in terms of what you eat.
4. Do you have any problems in obtaining or preparing food?

5. Will the hospital food conflict with your cultural or religious beliefs?

6. Do you have any dentures or partial plates? Do they interfere with your eating?

7. What are your likes and dislikes?

8. Do you have any of the following problems: Recent weight gain or loss, poor appetite, nausea, vomiting, abdominal pain, food intolerances, trouble with swallowing?

Elimination

1. Has there been a recent change in your urinary or bowel habits?

2. Do you have any of the following urinary problems: Painful urination, change in color, frequency, urgency, hesitation, chills, incontinence, retention, blood in the urine, absence of urine?

3. Do you have any of the following bowel problems: Diarrhea, constipation, cramping, incontinence, hemorrhoids, straining, black or red stools, flatulence?

4. Do you use any laxatives, suppositories, or enemas?

5. Identify the presence of ostomies or urinary catheteters.

Habits

1. Do you smoke cigarettes or other tobacco? If so, how many packs per day? How many years? What brand?

2. Do you drink alcohol? If so, how much per day? How many years? Type consumed?

3. Do you use any recreational drugs or do you have any drug habits? How often are these drugs used?

Valuables

1. Did you bring any jewelry, money, or other valuables to the hospital?

2. Would you like to keep them in the hospital safe? Send them home?

3. Document patient valuables brought to the hospital. State the disposition of these valuables (i.e., to safe, with patient, sent home with family, etc.). Describe jewelry in terms of *color* of metal and stones (i.e., yellow metal ring with a clear stone).

Review of Systems

1. Neurological (see page 43)

2. Respiratory (see page 81)

3. Cardiovascular (see page 113)

 4. Circulatory (see page 152)
 5. Gastrointestinal (see page 186)
 6. Endocrine (see page 231)
 7. Renal (see page 268)
 8. Reproductive (see page 311)
 9. Sensory (see page 333)
10. Integumentary (see page 344)
11. Musculoskeletal (see page 365)

II

VITAL SIGNS ASSESSMENT

I. TEMPERATURE

A. Oral

1. Obtain an oral temperature on cooperative and oriented patients.

2. Wait 15 minutes if patient has just swallowed liquids or smoked.

3. Do not take oral temperatures on confused patients, those with nasogastric tubes, patients receiving oxygen, those with endotracheal tubes, or patients who are on seizure precautions.

4. Place thermometer under patient's tongue. Have patient keep lips closed.

5. If using glass thermometer, leave in place 3–5 minutes.

B. Rectal

1. Obtain a rectal temperature on the following patients:

   a) disoriented.

   b) uncooperative.

   c) comatose.

   d) those with seizure disorders.

   e) those with nasogastric tubes.

   f) those receiving continual oxygen therapy.

   g) those who are orally intubated.

   h) those with wired jaws.

   i) facial fractures.

2. Do not take rectal temperatures on those who have had peritoneal or rectal surgery.

3. Insert thermometer 1½ inches into rectum.

4. Leave glass thermometer in place for 2 to 3 minutes.

C. Axillary

1. Attempt to obtain either an oral or rectal temperature when at all possible. Axillary temperature should only be taken when the other methods are not possible since it is an unreliable method.

2. If patient's axilla has just been washed, delay obtaining temperature.

3. Leave glass thermometer in place for 5 to 8 minutes.

D. Normal Body Temperature

1. Normal oral temperature is:
   97.7–99.5° F.
   36.5–37.5° C.

2. Normal rectal temperature is approximately one degree (F.) or 0.28 to 0.56 degrees (C.) higher than oral temperature:
   98.7–100.5° F.
   37.5–38.5° C.

3. Normal axillary temperature is approximately 0.5 degree (F.) or 0.28 degree (C.) lower than oral temperature:
   97.2–99.0° F.
   36.1–37.1° C.

4. Temperature may vary according to time of day. Both rectal and oral temperatures are usually 1–2 degrees (F.) lower in the early morning.

5. Environmental temperature, age (infants and children usually have higher temperatures than adults), and exercise also influence body temperature.

E. Elevated Body Temperature

1. Terms
   a) *Onset:* The time when pyrexia or fever began.
   b) *Intermittent Temperature:* Alternating between normal temperature and pyrexia.
   c) *Remittent:* Fluctuating temperature above normal that does not reach normal between fluctuations.
   d) *Continued:* Consistently elevated temperature with minimal fluctuation.

2. Associated Symptoms

   a) Tachypnea.

   b) Tachycardia.

   c) Anorexia.

   d) Headache.

   e) General malaise.

   f) Occasional delirium (hyperpyrexia).

   g) Flushed face.

3. Normal Pyrexia
   A slight elevation in temperature is not abnormal for one to two days following surgery, after a myocardial infarction, or after a cerebrovascular accident.

4. Abnormal Pyrexia
   Suspect the following etiologies:

   a) Pulmonary postoperative complications (pneumonia, bronchitis, pneumonitis, etc.).

   b) Wound infection.

   c) Urinary tract infection.

   d) Thrombophlebitis.

   e. Septic shock (sudden fever above 101° (F.), chills, malaise, confusion, tachypnea, tachycardia, systolic blood pressure below 80 mm Hg).

   f) Cerebral edema.

   g) Cerebrovascular accident.

   h) Neurosurgery.

   i) Brain trauma.

   j) Brain tumor.

   Obtain temperature at frequent intervals when elevation exists. In severe cases insert a rectal probe for continuous monitoring.

F. Hypothermia

1. Medically-induced hypothermia.
   Patients undergoing cardiac, neurological, vascular, or gastrointestinal hemorrhage surgery may have their temperature intentionally lowered to reduce oxygen requirements.

2. Accidental exposure.
   Body temperature below 34 degrees (C.) or 93.2 degrees
   (F.) usually results in death.

3. Patients with hypothermia should have their temperature
   checked at frequent intervals or have a rectal probe inserted
   for continuous monitoring.

II. PULSE

A. Pulse Rate

1. Use first, second, and third fingers to obtain radial pulse
   rate.

2. Count rate for 30 seconds and multiply by 2 to obtain rate for
   one minute.

3. Take pulse for a full minute if irregularities are noted.

4. Normal rate in the average adult is 60–80 beats per minute.

5. Check pulse whenever patient's condition changes.

B. Abnormal Pulse Rates

1. Tachycardia

   a) Rate is greater than 100 beats per minute.

   b) Etiologies include the following: Pain, fear, anger, sur-
      prise, anxiety, exercise, fever, anemia, congestive heart
      failure, shock, hypoxia, decreased blood pressure, pul-
      monary emboli, drugs, thyrotoxicosis, decreased blood
      volume.

2. Bradycardia

   a) Rate is less than 60 beats per minute.

   b) Etiologies include the following: Increased blood pres-
      sure, athletes, Valsalva maneuver, carotid sinus mas-
      sage, sinus node ischemia, hypothyroidism, increased
      intracranial pressure, increased intraocular pressure,
      hyperkalemia, Stokes-Adams disease, drugs.

C. Pulse Rhythm

1. Normally, pulse rhythm is regular with equal time intervals
   between beats.

2. Irregular pulse rhythms are called arrhythmias.

3. There are two normal arrhythmias:

   a) Sinus arrhythmias occurring in young adults and in children. Pulse rate speeds up at the end of inspiration and slows down with expiration.

   b) Occasional premature beats.

4. When irregularities are noted during a radial pulse, auscultate apical pulse for one full minute while palpating radial pulse.

   a) Place stethoscope over apex of heart, located in the fifth intercostal space on the left midclavicular line.

   b) Pulse deficit exists when the apical rate differs from the radial rate. This is usually found in atrial fibrillation or with premature contractions.

D. Abnormal Pulse Rhythm

See Cardiac Assessment for abnormal arrhythmia evaluation.

E. Pulse Amplitude

1. Pulse amplitude is the force of the pulse or pulse strength.

2. Evaluate quality of pulse on the following three-point scale:

   $3+$ = bounding pulse
   $2+$ = normal pulse
   $1+$ = weak, thready pulse
   0 = absent pulse

F. Abnormal Pulse Amplitude

1. Bounding pulse

   a) Usually implies a widened pulse pressure (difference between systolic and diastolic pressures).

   b) This is produced by the following: Increased stroke volume (anxiety, complete heart block, aortic regurgitation), by increased cardiac output (fever, anemia, thyrotoxicosis, arteriovenous fistula, Paget's disease, beriberi, cirrhosis of the liver), lowered peripheral resistance.

2. Paradoxical pulse (pulses paradoxus)

   a) Force of pulse decreases with inspiration.

b) This is produced by cardiac tamponade, constrictive pericarditis, chronic obstructive pulmonary disease, cardiomyopathy, shock.

3. Weak, thready pulse

a) This implies a narrowed pulse pressure.

b) This is produced by the following: Decreased cardiac output (congestive heart failure, shock, hypovolemia, acute myocardial infarction, cardiac tamponade, constrictive pericarditis, cardiomyopathy, myocarditis), peripheral vasoconstriction (shock, hypovolemia, valvular disease, aortic disease.

G. Pulse Points

1. Obtain peripheral pulses in patients going to surgery for cardiac and peripheral vascular surgeries.

2. Peripheral pulses include the following:

a) Radial.

b) Ulnar.

c) Brachial.

d) Femoral.

e) Popliteal.

f) Dorsalis pedis.

g) Posterior tibialis.

3. Other pulse points include the following:

a) Temporal.

b) External maxillary.

c) Carotid.

III. RESPIRATIONS

A. Respiratory Rate

1. Observe chest rise and fall for 30 seconds and multiply by 2 for respiratory rate for one minute.

2. Count respirations for a full minute on patients with cardiac or respiratory problems.

3. Normal respiratory rate in average adults is 16–20 per minute.

B. Abnormal Respiratory Rate

1. Tachypnea

   a) Rate of more than 25 per minute.

   b) Etiologies include the following: Pneumonia, bronchiectasis, advanced pulmonary tuberculosis, consolidation of lung, asthma, emphysema, abscess, tumors, aneurysms, partial airway obstruction, chest wall diseases, anemia, kidney disease, fever, cardiac diseases, drugs, anxiety.

2. Bradypnea

   a) Rate of less than 12 per minute.

   b) Etiologies include the following: Brain compression and hemorrhage, uremia, coma, carbon monoxide poisoning, opium and its derivatives, high flow oxygen levels in patients with C.O.P.D.

C. Quality of Respirations

See Respiratory Assessment for quality evaluation.

IV. BLOOD PRESSURE

A. Normal Blood Pressure

1. Use cuff size 12–14 cm for average adult arm, 18–20 cm for obese arm, and pediatric cuff for children, infants, and adults with thin arms.

2. Apply cuff 2 cm above antecubital space.

3. Place center of bladder over brachial artery.

4. Place stethoscope over brachial artery.

5. Release inflated cuff slowly.

6. Check blood pressure in both arms on initial patient assessment. Normally, the difference is not greater than 5 mm Hg.

7. If it is necessary to recheck blood pressure, completely deflate cuff and wait awhile before reinflating.

8. Normal blood pressure in the average adult is 100/60 to 140/90 mm Hg.

B. Abnormal Blood Pressure

1. Hypertension

   a) Blood pressure consistently greater than 140/90 mm Hg.

   b) Etiologies include the following: Atherosclerosis, fever, anemia, thyrotoxicosis, anxiety, beriberi, aortic insufficiency, coarctation of the aorta, aldosteronism, pheochromocytoma, Cushing's syndrome, hyperparathyroidism, renal disease, polycythemia, central nervous system lesions, lead poisoning, burns.

2. Hypotension

   a) Systolic less than 90 mm Hg.

   b) Etiologies include the following: Shock, hemorrhage, infections, fevers, cancer, anemia, neurasthenia, Addison's disease, wasting diseases, hypovolemia, metabolic acidosis, heat exhaustion.

III

ASSESSMENT/INTERVENTION GUIDELINES

PREOPERATIVE CARE

POTENTIAL PROBLEMS

Pain   Psychosocial Problems

KEY NURSING INTERVENTIONS

- Obtain a complete nursing history on admission.

- Create a relaxed environment conducive to open communication during initial interview (see Interviewing Guidelines and Nursing History).

- Identify patient's nursing needs on care plan and describe appropriate nursing interventions.

- Contact spiritual advisor if desired by patient.

- Document preoperative teaching in progress notes.

- Assess and support patient's psychosocial needs. Many of these can be resolved with the teaching process. Recognize that patient's fears may inhibit learning or make the patient resistive to discussion.

- Several hours before scheduled surgery, prepare patient in the following manner:

  - Be sure that operative consent form reads correctly and is signed by the patient and other responsible parties per hospital policy.

  - Check physician orders to be sure that preoperative procedures have been completed regarding skin preparation, catheter insertions, enemas, etc.

  - Provide patient with hospital gown.

  - Remove all undergarments.

  - Remove all jewelry and hair pins. Rings may be taped per hospital policy if unable to remove. Give jewelry to relatives or place in safe.

- Remove artificial articles (contact lenses, dentures, partials, hair-pieces, prosthetic limbs, eyeballs, etc.).
- Have patient void prior to premedication.
- Keep side-rails upright after giving premedication.
- Keep call light within reach.

- Check chart for presence of laboratory, x-ray, and electrocardiogram reports.
- Document preoperative vital signs.

PATIENT AND FAMILY TEACHING

- See Patient Education for teaching guidelines.
- Determine what patient knows about illness and proposed surgery.
- Teach patient through conversation, audiovisual aids, demonstrations and return demonstrations.
- Encourage patient to ask questions and express concerns and feelings. Clarify questions.
- Explain preoperative preparations.
- Inform patient and family of when surgery is to occur, approximate length of surgery, and recovery room stay.
- Emphasize that the patient plays an important role in the recovery process postoperatively.
- Inform patient and family of recovery room procedures:
  - Verbal coaching in arousal, coughing, deep breathing, and reorientation.
  - The use of oxygen masks.
  - Length of stay.
  - Possible equipment to be used for specified surgery.
- Explain that placement of an intravenous line is part of surgical routine and may stay in postoperatively.
- Describe the presurgical interventions outlined in Key Nursing Interventions.
- Explain the importance of remaining in bed after premedication is given to prevent falls.
- Explain the purpose of premedication and mode of transportation to the operating room.

- Inform family of location of surgical waiting areas and the importance of remaining there to speak to the surgeon.
- Teach diaphragmatic breathing technique:

  - With patient in semi-Fowler's position, have patient place hands on abdomen or lower rib cage and exhale.
  - Inhale deeply through nose and mouth, allowing abdomen to rise.
  - Hold breath for 5 seconds.
  - Exhale completely.

  Encourage patient to practice this preoperatively.

- Demonstrate coughing technique. Provide a pillow for patients having abdominal or thoracic surgery to use for splinting wound. Following a diaphragmatic breath, have the patient cough four quick times during exhalation. In the following exhalation, have patient cough with greater force one or two times.
  NOTE: Coughing is contraindicated in eye surgeries and some neurosurgeries.
- Stress the importance of deep breathing, coughing and turning from side to side postoperatively to prevent respiratory problems.
- Demonstrate foot and leg exercises:

  - Patient is to be supine.
  - Have patient bend knee, keeping foot on bed.
  - With knee bent, have patient raise lower leg off bed.
  - Hold for 3 seconds or as tolerated.
  - Lower leg to bed.
  - Trace an imaginary circle with great toe.

  Encourage patient to practice these with each leg preoperatively.

- Stress the importance of frequently doing leg exercises postoperatively to prevent thromboembolism.

POSTOPERATIVE CARE

POTENTIAL PROBLEMS

Airway Obstruction
Respiratory Insufficiency
Aspiration
Pulmonary Embolism
Shock
Renal Failure
Atelectasis
Thromboembolism
Thrombophlebitis
Hemorrhage
Hypothermia
Bronchitis
Pneumonia
Pleurisy
Vomiting

Paralytic Ileus
Intestinal Obstruction
Fecal Impaction
Acidosis
Wound Infection
Wound Dehiscence
Evisceration
Urinary Retention
Pain
Disorientation
Thirst
Constipation
Nausea
Psychosocial Problems

KEY NURSING INTERVENTIONS

- Observe respirations for patent airway and adequate ventilations. Abnormal respiratory patterns are the following: Rapid and dyspneic (indicative of anoxia, shock, or hypoxemia); shallow, slow (indicative of respiratory center depression); shallow respirations with use of diaphragm and accessory muscles (indicative of paralysis from anesthesia). Normally, respirations are slow, deep and regular with a rate about 12.

- Position patient in semi-Fowler's position or laterally with neck extended, unless contraindicated, to promote good air exchange.

- Verbally coach patient to take deep breaths and cough frequently (see Preoperative Care).

- Suction excessive secretions as needed using aseptic technique.

- Assess patient for signs of respiratory distress: Restlessness; fast, thready pulse; confusion; shallow, rapid breathing; snoring; stridor; wheezing; apprehension.

- Notify physician immediately if respiratory distress or abnormal breathing patterns are noted. Prepare to insert oral or nasal airways, assist with intubation and mechanical ventilation, administer oxygen and respiratory drugs (bronchodilators, expectorants, respiratory stimulants).

- Observe blood pressure for good cardiac output. Compare postoperative values with preoperative values. Abnormal blood pressure values are the following: Systolic below 90 mm Hg, or more than 20 mm Hg drop in blood pressure.
  NOTE: A stable low blood pressure as compared to preoperative blood pressure may be a sign of pain.

- Assess pulse for rate and rhythm. Usually pulse is more rapid immediately postoperatively as compared to preoperative values. Abnormal pulse values are as follows: Less than 60 or more than 110; irregularities not previously observed.

- Monitor patient for signs and symptoms of shock: Cool extremities; decreased urinary output; narrowing pulse pressure (difference between systolic and diastolic pressures): rapid, thready pulse; falling blood pressure; pale, clammy skin; cyanosis of lips and mucous membranes; apprehension; apathy.

- If signs of shock are noted, obtain an accurate temperature as well as other vital signs and notify physician immediately.

- Assist physician in identifying type of shock by reporting appropriate observations:

  - *For Hematogenic Shock:* Visible bleeding, low hemoglobin and hematocrit, subnormal temperature, complaints of ringing in ears and visual "spots."
    NOTE: Hemorrhage may be concealed. Therefore, a thorough assessment of the involved surgical area must be performed.

  - *For Septic Shock:* Fever; warm, flushed, diaphoretic skin.

  - *For Cardiogenic Shock:* Distended neck veins, chest pain.

  - *For Neurogenic Shock:* Hypotension with slow pulse and warm extremities.

- *FOR SHOCK:*

  - Maintain patent airway and adequate ventilation.
  - Elevate legs and feet, keeping trunk and head flat.
  - Maintain patent IV.

- Record vital signs every 15 mins.
- Prepare to transfer to Intensive Care Unit if shock is severe.

- Observe for signs and symptoms of respiratory acidosis and report to physician: Disorientation, stupor, hypoventilation, somnolence, pH less than 7.35, pCO_2, greater than 45.

- Prevent urinary tract infections by avoiding catheterization if possible. If patient has difficulty voiding, try stimulation techniques such as the following: Providing privacy, warming bedpan, placing patient in sitting position if allowed, running water in sink, pouring warm water over perineum. Notify physician if these measures fail.

- If Foley catheter is to be inserted, use strict aseptic technique.

- Prevent complications associated with immobility such as pneumonia, atelectasis, thrombophlebitis, osteoporosis, urinary retention, and renal calculi. Encourage turning, coughing, and deep breathing frequently. Have patient do foot and leg exercises every 30 mins. to 1 hr. Assist with these exercises if patient is weak. Assist and encourage ambulation as soon as permissible (see Preoperative Care).

- Instruct patient not to cross legs or sit for long periods.

- Pain control measures include the following: Administration of analgesics as ordered before pain becomes severe, changing position in bed, giving back rubs.

- Control nausea and vomiting with the following: Antiemetics as ordered, NPO or small pieces of ice chips if allowed, nasogastric tube to intermittent suction as ordered.

- Promote patient safety by keeping side-rails up after analgesic or sedative administration.

- Keep call light within reach. Check patient frequently when bed rest is ordered.

- Assess patient for evidence of paralytic ileus: Absent bowel sounds, no flatus passed, abdominal distention. Report to physician and pass nasogastric tube as ordered (see Nasogastric Tubes).

- Monitor accurate intake and output and report output of less than 30 to 50 cc/hr. for adults.

- Moisten lips and assist with rinsing mouth while on NPO.

- When NPO is discontinued, encourage PO fluids to 3 to 4 liters unless restricted.

- When advancing diet from NPO to regular, start with clear liquids in small amounts. If tolerated, advance to full liquids, and then to regular diet.

- Observe wound for signs and symptoms of infection: Redness, tenderness, heat, drainage.
- Use aseptic technique to change dressings.
- Observe temperature for sign of infection. Slight elevation is normal 1 to 2 days postoperatively. Persistence of temperatures over 37.7 degrees Centigrade should be reported to the physician.
- Assess and support patient's psychosocial needs. Surgery has different meanings to each individual based on previous experiences and the preoperative diagnosis. If cancer is suspected, the patient may be extremely frightened and nervous. Provide as many comfort measures as possible. Convey empathy in all aspects of care. Spend time with patient to allow verbalization of feelings and questions. Use interviewing techniques to prompt discussion (see Interviewing). Accept patient's feelings. Give as much information as possible about treatments without overwhelming the patient (see Preoperative Care).

PATIENT AND FAMILY TEACHING

- Reinforce teaching given preoperatively (see Preoperative Care).
- Stress the importance of measures to prevent complications:
  - Turning, coughing and deep breathing.
  - Early ambulation (as ordered).
  - Foot and leg exercises.
  - Adequate fluid intake (when PO fluids are allowed).
- Instruct patient in special equipment used postoperatively.
- Advise a diet high in protein and carbohydrates to promote healing and prevent negative nitrogen balance.
- Utilize audiovisuals and other teaching aids pertinent to postoperative diagnosis.

THE IMMOBILIZED PATIENT

POTENTIAL PROBLEMS

Respiratory Acidosis
Pneumonia
Tracheitis
Bronchitis
Thrombus Formation
Orthostatic Hypotension
Tachycardia
Fluid and Electrolyte
   Imbalance
Decubitus Ulcers
Urinary Retention
Urinary Tract Infection

Renal Calculi
Negative Nitrogen Balance
Anorexia
Constipation
Diarrhea
Fecal Impaction
Dyspepsia
Osteoporosis
Contractures
Fatigue
Psychosocial Problems

KEY NURSING INTERVENTIONS

- Encourage and assist patient in turning, coughing and deep breathing every hour. Have patient expectorate secretions.

- If patient is unable to cough effectively, consult physician for IPPB and incentive spirometry orders.

- Suction secretions if patient is unable to expectorate. Maintain aseptic technique for nasotracheal suctioning.

- Assess patient for signs and symptoms of pneumonia: Pleuritic chest pain, fever, chills, purulent sputum, increased tactile and vocal fremitus, decreased breath sounds and fine rales over affected area, tachypnea, tachycardia.

- Encourage regular respirations during position changes. The Valsalva maneuver tends to be used when changing positions; this causes bradycardia, followed by tachycardia.

- Prevent thrombus formation. Remove antiembolism hose for 30 mins. and reapply BID. Encourage hourly foot and leg exercises (see Preoperative Care). Assist with passive range of motion exercises to legs and feet every hour if patient is unable to do effective exercises.

- Assess patient for signs and symptoms of thrombophlebitis: Tenderness and redness over affected vein, edema, cyanosis, mottling, diminished pulses, positive Homans' sign (calf pain with dorsiflexion of foot) in affected extremity.

- Prevent contractures. Encourage and assist with active and/or passive range of motion exercises to all joints QID. Change position from lateral to supine to prone if possible.

- Assist patient with resistive muscle exercises QID.

- Maintain good body alignment. Avoid knee and hip flexion for long periods. Maintain foot board or anti-foot drop devices firmly against dorsum of foot.

- Assess skin over entire body for signs of decubitus formation. Observe the following closely: Occipital region, rims of ears, side of head, shoulders, scapulae, dorsal thoracic area, elbows, spinal column, sacrum, coccyx, hips, ischial tuberosities, trochanters, patellae, lateral malleoli, medial malleoli, heels. Inspect skin for redness, edema and tenderness with each position change.

- Prevent decubitus formation. Use pull sheets to prevent shearing of the epidermidis. Use pillows or foam pads to prevent extremities from touching. Maintain a wrinkle-free, *dry* bed. Avoid direct skin contact with linen savers. Use protective skin devices over pressure areas. Use mattress devices (eggcrates, water mattress, sheepskin, alternating air mattress, etc.). Gently massage bony prominences and reddened areas to increase circulation.

- Keep body clean and dry. Wash patient after each incident of incontinence. Avoid excessive use of lotions and powders. Avoid overuse of soap.

- Assist patient with oral hygiene BID.

- Shampoo hair PRN as ordered.

- Keep enough covers on patient to prevent chilling, but keep at a minimum to prevent excessive heat production.

- Encourage fluids to 3000 cc/day unless contraindicated.

- Observe for urinary retention: Absent voiding, bladder distention, voiding 25–50 cc more than one time per hour, complaints of fullness and discomfort, restlessness.

- Assess urine for inadequate fluid intake: Dark amber color, decreased output, strong smelling.

- Observe for signs and symptoms of urinary tract infections: Frequency, urgency, dysuria, low-grade fever, cloudy urine.

- Encourage acid residue foods such as cereals, meat, poultry, and fish if diet allows to help maintain an acidic urine pH.

- Initiate a bowel management program to be followed daily to prevent constipation and fecal impaction.

  - Obtain an elimination history from patient.
  - Incorporate patient's daily habits into bowel program.
  - Stress the importance of responding immediately to defecation stimuli.
  - Provide the bedpan after breakfast.
  - Allow 10–15 mins. minimum for defecation.
  - Provide privacy.
  - Assist patient to a sitting position, if possible.
  - Provide air fresheners PRN.
  - Use cathartics and enemas cautiously.

- Encourage a high-protein diet with sufficient carbohydrates and fats to prevent negative nitrogen balance.
- If anorexic, give 6 small feedings per day.
- To prevent osteoporosis, use a tilt table or position mechanical beds in reverse Trendelenburg position with foot support to allow weight-bearing unless contraindicated.
- Assess and support patient's psychosocial needs. Allow as much independence as possible in self-care activities and care planning. If orientation is a problem, provide a calendar and clock. Work with family in providing diversional activities. Check on patient at frequent intervals to communicate availability for help and concern for patient. Recognize that frustration from role disturbance and forced dependency may make the patient irritable at times.

PATIENT AND FAMILY TEACHING

- Instruct patient in diaphragmatic breathing and coughing exercises (see Preoperative Care). Emphasize the importance of expectorating secretions.
- Instruct patient in leg and foot exercises (see Preoperative Care).
- Instruct patient in doing isometric exercises to all muscle groups several times a day.
- Emphasize the importance of responding to defecation stimuli by explaining *basic* physiology of defecation.

- Inform patient of foods with laxative properties (prune juice, fruit juices, fresh fruit, high-fiber foods). Have dietician discuss diet with patient.
- Stress the importance of liberal fluid intake in preventing renal calculi formation.

THE CANCER PATIENT

NOTE: The authors recognize that the medical approach to the treatment of cancer varies and is determined by the type of cancer as well as the individual physician. It is their viewpoint that the needs of the patient with cancer are generally the same irrespective of the "type" of cancer.

POTENTIAL PROBLEMS

Weight Loss
Malnutrition
Nausea
Vomiting
Diarrhea
Constipation
Pathological Fractures

FOR RADIATION THERAPY

Radiation Sickness
Skin Irritation
Bone Marrow Depression
Alopecia
Radiation Cataracts
Leukemia
Lung Fibrosis

FOR IMMUNOTHERAPY

Allergic Reaction
Liver Dysfunction

Bowel Obstruction
Generalized Weakness
Ascites
Pleural Effusion
Pain
Psychosocial Problems

FOR CHEMOTHERAPY

Bone Marrow Depression
Thrombocytopenia
Leukopenia
Anemia
Alopecia
Nausea
Vomiting
Diarrhea
Stomatitis
Colonic Mucosa Sloughing
Renal Toxicity
Neurotoxicity
Skin Reactions
Malaise
Lethargy
Hemorrhagic Cystitis

KEY NURSING INTERVENTIONS

- Observe patients receiving cancer treatment for weight loss. Obtain weight several times per week.

- If no dietary restrictions are ordered, have family bring in patient's favorite foods.

- Offer small, frequent meals.

- Medicate with antiemetics as ordered prior to meals.

- Have dietician consult patient regarding foods which are easy to chew, appealing, high in protein and calories.

- Keep liquids within patient's reach. Provide non-irritating juices, milk shakes, protein beverages, eggnogs, etc., for calories. Assist patient as needed and at frequent intervals.

- Discuss analgesics and mouth rinses with physician which may reduce discomfort from stomatitis. Administer prior to meals.

- Observe for signs and symptoms of stomatitis: Burning sensation around lips when taking juices, erythema, vesicles, small oral ulcers.

- Keep prescribed oral rinsing solution within patient's reach if bed-bound. (Usually saline/hydrogen peroxide mix is ordered.) Encourage frequent mouth rinsing.

- Keep emesis basin in close reach if patient is vomiting.

- Observe for fluid and electrolyte imbalances, especially if patient has diarrhea or is vomiting (see Fluids and Electrolytes).

- Maintain accurate intake and output on patients with diarrhea and vomiting as ordered.

- Observe stools for presence of blood or test for occult blood.

- Have dietician consult patients with diarrhea regarding low roughage and constipating foods.

- Discuss sitz bath order with physician if rectum is irritated and sore.

- Initiate a bowel program if patient is constipated (see The Immobilized Patient).

- Assess patient for signs and symptoms of bowel obstruction: Vomiting, fever, abdominal distention, hyperactive, high-pitched bowel sounds above obstruction site; abdominal pain; hypotension; fecal emesis (see Nasogastric Tubes, if indicated).

- Prevent complications of bed rest (see The Immobilized Patient).

- Encourage ambulation as tolerated and ordered. Obtain assistive devices as needed (walker, cane, etc.). Protect patient from falling (see Safety).

- Assist patient in obtaining adequate rest. Medicate for pain as needed. Give back rubs, change linen or offer usual bedtime snacks to help relax the patient.

- Cancer pain tends to be continuous and chronic. Discuss other methods of pain control with physician. Create a calm environment which will help patient to relax. Move, touch, and talk to patient calmly and gently. Notify physician when analgesics lose their effectiveness. (Usual analgesics ordered include: Oral analgesics, Brompton cocktail, IV morphine sulfate, and methadone. Compazine or thorazine are frequently given with analgesics to potentiate their action.)

- Assess patient for signs and symptoms of pleural effusion: Dyspnea, pallor, pleural pain, dry cough, diminished chest expansion on affected side, absent or diminished breath sounds on affected side.

- See Thoracentesis or Abdominal Paracentesis, if indicated.

- See Total Parenteral Nutrition, if indicated.

- *FOR CHEMOTHERAPY:*

  - Observe lab reports for electrolyte imbalance, thrombocytopenia, leukopenia, anemia. Notify physician of all abnormalities.

  - Protect patient from bleeding (see Anticoagulant Therapy).

  - Protect patient from infection. All people entering patient's room must wash their hands before entering. No one with respiratory infections, cold, flu, or other communicable disease should enter patient's room. Frequently, fresh fruits, vegetables, and fresh fruit juices and potted plants are prohibited.

  - Monitor intake and output.

- Observe for complications specific to particular chemotherapeutic agent. (Refer to the *Physician's Desk Reference*).

- See Steroid Therapy, if indicated.

- Assure IV medication compatibility before administering multiple IV piggybacks. Flush IV line after each administration.

- Keep extravasation tray available. Observe IV site frequently for infiltration. Know hospital policy and procedure for extravasation.

- Protect yourself from exposure to chemotherapeutic drugs. Filter medications when reconstituting to prevent aerosolization. Wear gowns and gloves when solution contact is likely. Wear mask when aerosolization is likely.

- Bag and label chemotherapy bottles, tubing, and linen per hospital guidelines. (Usually, these items are handled the same as infective items for other isolation precautions.)

- *FOR RADIOTHERAPY:*

  - Observe skin in area of radiotherapy for redness, desquamation or telangiectasis (hyperemic spot similar to a birthmark) and notify physician.

  - Provide gentle skin care to affected area. Use only water to cleanse. Avoid powder, lotions and ointments unless prescribed. Avoid shaving and rubbing of area.

  - Do not remove marks applied by radiologist.

  - Observe lab data for bone marrow depression (see Chemotherapy Interventions).

  - See Safety for radiation implant precautions.

- *FOR IMMUNOTHERAPY:*

  - Observe patient for allergic reaction: Swelling of lymph nodes, fever, malaise, local abscesses.

- Assess and support patient's psychosocial needs. Patients with newly diagnosed cancer will experience the different stages of grieving: Denial, anger, bargaining, depression, and finally acceptance. Fear of pain, dependency, body mutilation, and death are major problems the patient is forced to cope with. Psychological support is probably the greatest and most difficult intervention. The nurse can be most therapeutic by listening to the patient. Recognize that at different times the patient may not be ready to discuss his/her feelings. Be available to listen when the patient is ready to talk. It is important that the patient not lose hope even when the prognosis is poor. Contact social service, spiritual advisor or psychologist for consult as needed. Involve family in hospital support groups when possible. Reinforce explanation of pathology to both family and patient to clarify misconceptions. Include patient, family, and all health care team members in all aspects of the care plan. Allow patient as much control as possible. Refer patient to American Cancer Society and local agencies specific for patient's type of cancer.

PATIENT AND FAMILY TEACHING

- Instruct patients with stomatitis to avoid traumatizing tissues. Arrange for family to bring in a soft toothbrush. Advise patient to avoid hard foods, hot and spicy foods, alcohol and smoking.

- Teach patient the importance of gentle rectal wiping after defecation to prevent perirectal abscess formation.

- Help the patient with chronic pain to realize that pain may not be abolished but controlled to tolerable levels. Discuss coping mechanisms the patient has used in the past to help control pain.

- If alopecia exists, stress that this is a temporary side effect of therapy and that hair growth will resume when therapy is finished.

NERVOUS SYSTEM

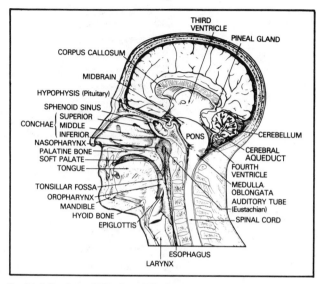

Sagittal Section of Head and Neck

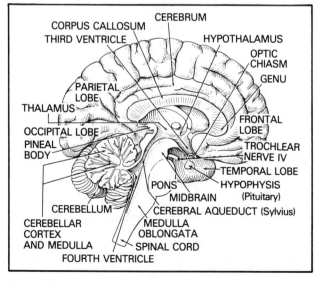

Sagittal Section of the Brain

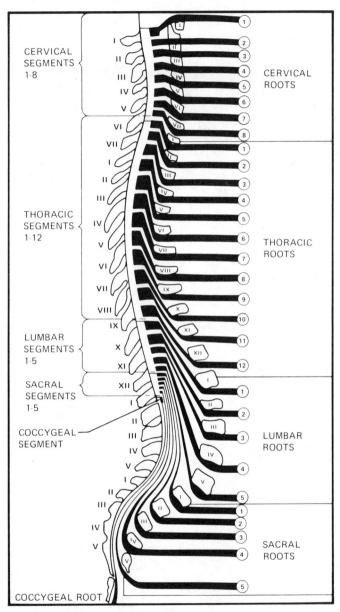

Vertebrae and Nerve Roots

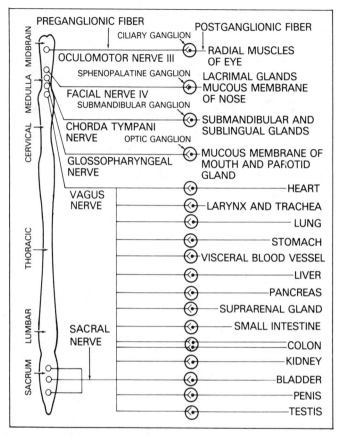

Parasympathetic Nervous System

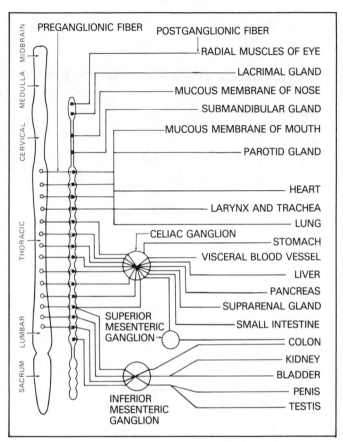

Sympathetic Nervous System

NERVOUS SYSTEM—PHYSIOLOGY SUMMARY

I. THE BRAIN

A. The Forebrain

1. The Cerebrum—is composed of an outer, grey matter, the cerebral cortex, and a core of white matter. It is divided into right and left hemispheres, each of which is divided into four lobes: Frontal, parietal, temporal, and occipital. The projection areas of the cortex are: (1) Motor—voluntary muscle movement, (2) Sensory—sensory interpretation (smell, taste, sight, hearing, equilibrium, touch), (3) Association—emotional and intellectual processes, memory, reasoning and judgment.

   a) Frontal lobe functions: Memories, emotions, voluntary movements, foresight, personality traits.

   b) Parietal lobe functions: General sensations (compare, evaluate, integrate), taste, sensory memories.

   c) Temporal lobe functions: Memories, emotions, hearing, smell, auditory memories.

   d) Occipital lobe functions: Vision, visual memories.

2. The Thalamus—is a sensory relay center to the cortex, integrates sensory impulses (pain, temperature, touch), interrelates with the motor centers of the cortex, cerebellum and basal ganglia, relays impulses from the hypothalamus to the prefrontal lobe, and contributes to arousal and reflex functions.

3. The Hypothalamus—coordinates and controls autonomic functions by inhibition and stimulation, synthesizes and regulates the release of hormones secreted by the posterior pituitary, relays between the cortex and lower autonomic centers, regulates temperature, is involved in productive mechanisms, appetite control, arousal and anterior pituitary hormone secretion.

B. The Midbrain

The midbrain functions as a communication tract between the spinal cord and the cortex, is involved with visual reflexes (blinking, pupillary response, lens focus), hearing (volume), and motor coordination.

C. The Hindbrain

1. The Cerebellum—serves to maintain equilibrium and posture, interrelates with the cortex in the integration of synergistic movements, and visual and auditory functions.

2. The Pons—serves as a relay center between the medulla and higher cortical centers, regulates respirations, contains motor nuclei of the facial, abducens and trigeminal nerves, and contains the sensory nucleus for the trigeminal nerve.

3. The Medulla—serves as a reflex center for respirations, cardiac activity, vasomotor functions, and nonvital mechanisms (swallow, hiccough, vomit, sneeze, cough). It is also involved in motor and sensory functions.

4. The Reticular Formation—serves to maintain consciousness by arousing the cortex and is involved in motor functions.

D. The Ventricles

The ventricles are the cavities in the brain and are divided into the right and left lateral, and the third and the fourth ventricles. Cerebrospinal fluid is formed in the ventricles and serves to cushion the brain from blows. It is also found in the cisterns around the brain and in the subarachnoid space around the brain and spinal cord.

E. The Cranial Nerves

The cranial nerves originate in the brain and are divided into twelve pairs.

I   Olfactory—smell.

II   Optic—vision.

III   Oculomotor—eye motor functions (accommodation, pupillary reactions, eye movements).

IV   Trochlear—eye movements.

V   Trigeminal—mastication, sensations of the head and face.

VI   Abducens—eye abduction.

VII   Facial—facial movements, taste, saliva, secretion.

VIII   Acoustic—hearing and equilibrium.

IX Glossopharyngeal—swallowing, saliva, secretion, taste, tongue sensations.

X Vagus—sensory and motor functions of pharynx and larynx muscles; innervates smooth muscles of the esophagus, stomach, and intestine; depresses cardiac activity; constricts the bronchi.

XI Spinal accessory—motor functions of shoulder, head, viscera, larynx and pharynx.

XII Hypoglossal—motor functions of the tongue.

II. THE SPINAL CORD

The spinal cord performs three main functions: Motor, sensory, and reflex. It is composed of two types of tracts, ascending and descending.

A. The Ascending Tracts

The ascending tracts conduct from peripheral nerves to the brain and are sensory. They transmit sensations of touch, pain, temperature, pressure, conscious position sense and unconscious position sense.

B. The Descending Tracts

The descending tracts conduct from the brain to skeletal muscle and are motor. They can be classified as pyramidal or extrapyramidal. Pyramidal tract impulses are associated with voluntary movements, especially refined movements. Extrapyramidal tract impulses are associated with muscle tone, automatic movements, and emotional expressions. The descending extrapyramidal tracts are also composed of facilatory and inhibitory tracts which receive impulses from the cortex, the cerebellum and the basal ganglia. Damage to pyramidal tracts leads to flaccid paralysis, whereas damage to extrapyramidal tracts leads to spastic paralysis.

C. Reflexes

Reflexes are nerve impulses which follow a reflex arc and are a function of the spinal cord (the cranial nerves are an exception).

1. Autonomic Reflex—smooth muscle and glandular contraction.

    2. Somatic Reflex—skeletal muscle contraction.

       a) Knee Jerk—tests L2, L3, L4, and femoral nerves.

       b) Ankle Jerk—tests L5, S1, and sciatic nerves.

       c) Babinski—tests pyramidal tract nerves.

       d) Corneal—tests 5th and 7th cranial nerves.

       e) Abdominal (upper)—tests T6 through 9 nerves.
               (lower)—tests T10 through 12 nerves.

III. NERVE IMPULSE TRANSMISSION

Nerve impulse conduction can occur in any of the following ways:
(1) Reflex arc (receptor-to-CNS-to-effectors), (2) without completing a reflex arc, (3) originating in the brain.

A. Depolarization

   1. The sending neuron releases a chemical transmitter (acetylcholine, serotonin, norephinephrine, glutamine, gamma-aminobutyric acid) into the synapse.

   2. The neurotransmitter combines with reactive sites of the postsynaptic neuron which initiates depolarization of the neuron.

   3. Depolarization occurs as the permeability of the cell membrane changes to allow an influx of sodium ions into the cell.

B. Repolarization

Repolarization occurs starting at the point of stimulation when the cell membrane's permeability changes to allow potassium into the cell and sodium to diffuse out.

C. Refractory Period

The time between depolarization and repolarization is the refractory period.

D. All-or-None Principle

Nerve impulse transmission will not occur unless the stimulus is of sufficient strength to meet its excitatory threshold (the all-or-none principle).

E. Excitation/Inhibition

1. Acidosis decreases excitability while alkalosis increases excitability.

2. Synapses may be excitatory or inhibitory. Excitatory synapses cause depolarization. Inhibitory synapses decrease the action potential of the postsynaptic neuron by increasing the cell membrane permeability to potassium and chloride causing postsynaptic inhibition. Inhibition also occurs when the amount of neurotransmitter is reduced causing presynaptic inhibition.

IV. THE AUTONOMIC NERVOUS SYSTEM

A. Functions

The autonomic nervous system:

1. Controls visceral functions.

2. Is an involuntary system.

3. Acts on internal effectors of smooth and cardiac muscle, exocrine glands, some endocrine glands.

4. Controls arterial pressure, gastrointestinal motility and secretion, urine output, temperature, etc.

B. Components

1. The autonomic nervous system is divided into sympathetic and parasympathetic systems.

2. The sympathetic system originates from the thoracic and Ll-3 segments of the spinal cord.

3. The parasympathetic system originates from cranial nerves 3, 7, 9, 10 and from S2-4.

V. AUTONOMIC NERVE IMPULSE TRANSMISSION

A. Stimulation

1. Preganglionic stimulation causes the release of acetylcholine in both sympathetic and parasympathetic systems.

2. Postganglionic stimulation of parasympathetic nerves causes the release of acetylcholine.

3. Postganglionic stimulation of sympathetic nerves causes a release of acetylcholine in some nerves and epinephrine in others.

4. All internal organs are innervated by both parasympathetic and sympathetic systems.

B. Cholinergic/Adrenergic Fibers

1. Nerves releasing acetylcholine are called cholinergic fibers and are generally inhibitory (except in the gastrointestinal tract).

2. Nerves releasing epinephrine are called adrenergic fibers and are generally excitatory (except in the gastrointestinal tract).

C. Alpha/Beta Receptors

1. Adrenergic receptors in muscles and glands are two types, alpha and beta.

2. Alpha receptors in smooth muscles respond by causing an excitatory response (constriction, contraction).

3. Beta receptors respond by causing an inhibitory response (relaxation, dilation).

4. Beta receptors in the heart respond by causing increased rate and strength of contractions.

5. After alpha and beta receptors have been stimulated, the catecholamines (norepinephrine and epinephrine) diffuse into the bloodstream where they are destroyed in the liver and other tissues by monamine oxidase (MAO) and catechol-O-methyl transferase (COMT). Excess molecules are excreted in the urine after being converted and inactivated.

6. Acetylcholine is destroyed at the synaptic junction by cholinesterase.

VI. AUTONOMIC CONTROLS

A. The Hypothalamus

The hypothalamus regulates and integrates parasympathetic and sympathetic systems.

B. The Adrenal Medulla

Stimulation of the adrenal medulla causes a release of nor-epinephrine and epinephrine which stimulates sympathetic tissues (vasoconstriction, increased heart rate, gastrointestinal tract inhibition).

VII. AUTONOMIC STIMULATION

SYSTEM/ORGAN	SYMPATHETIC	PARASYMPATHETIC
RESPIRATORY		
Bronchi	Dilation	Constriction
CARDIAC		
Heart	Increased rate Constriction	Decreased rate, contraction, and AV conduction
Coronary Vessels	Constriction Dilation	Dilation
PERIPHERAL VASCULAR		
Skin Vessels	Constriction	Dilation
Skeletal Muscle	Dilation (cholinergic)	Dilation
Vessels	Constriction (Adrenergic)	
Brain & Viscera	Constriction	Dilation
Genitalia	Dilation (cholinergic)	
GASTROINTESTINAL		
Smooth Muscle	Inhibition	Excitation
Sphincters	Contraction	Inhibition
Gastric & Salivary Glands	Inhibition	Excitation
Liver	Increased glycogenolysis	
Gallbladder	Relaxation	Contraction
ENDOCRINE		
Pancreas	Inhibition	Excitation
Adrenal Medulla	Increase secretion	
GENITOURINARY		
Bladder (detrusor)	Relaxation	Contraction
Urinary Sphincters	Contraction	Relaxation

SYSTEM/ORGAN	SYMPATHETIC	PARASYMPATHETIC
INTEGUMENTARY		
Sweat glands	Increased sweating	
Pilomotor Muscles	Constriction	
SENSORY		
Iris		
—circular fibers		Constriction
—radial fibers	Dilation	
Ciliary muscle	Relaxation (far vision)	Contraction (near vision)
Lacrimal Glands		Increased secretion

NEUROLOGICAL ASSESSMENT

The first six sections are of the greatest importance. They assess gross neurologic function. These areas should be included when doing hourly neurologic checks. The latter four sections are appropriate for a more detailed neurological assessment.

I. HISTORY

A. Past history of neurological problems

1. What type?
2. What therapy was utilized? Did it work?

B. Recent History

1. Syncope?

   a) Episodes of dizziness or fainting?
   b) How often?

2. Seizures?

   a) Type?
   b) Frequency?
   c) Duration?

3. Weakness or paralysis

   a) Unilateral or bilateral? How long?
   b) Difficulty in speech or swallowing?

4. Vertigo?

   a) Does the room feel like it is moving?
   b) Does the patient feel himself moving?

C. Pain

Use PQRST mnemonic.

P— Provokes.   What makes the pain worse or better? What was the patient doing prior to the onset of pain?

Q—Quality.   Subjective description of pain by the patient. Use the patient's own words, i.e., burning, stabbing, pressure.

R—Radiation.   Where is the pain located and does it radiate anywhere?

S—Severity.   Ask the patient to judge the pain on a scale of 1 to 10 with 10 being the worst pain ever felt.

T—Time.   How long has the patient had this pain? When did the pain begin and end?

D. Medications

1. List prescription medications.
2. List over-the-counter drugs.

E. Nutrition

Describe a typical:

1. Breakfast.
2. Lunch.
3. Dinner.
4. Snacks.

II. BACKGROUND INFORMATION

A. Lab Values

Check for abnormal values or worsening trends (cerebrospinal fluid for blood, color, cell count, differential, culture, glucose, cytology, VDRL).

B. Diagnostic Studies

Identify abnormal reports of diagnostic studies (x-rays, scans, angiography, electroencephalogram, lumbar punctures, electromyogram, echoencephalogram, myelogram).

C. Chart

Check old chart for past relevant information

III. LEVEL OF CONSCIOUSNESS

This is the single most important factor. It should be described in behavioral terms in response to the examiner's stimulus.

A. Awake

"Awake" implies some sort of awareness of self and environment. Determine whether the patient is awake by calling his name.

1. If the patient is awake, determine his orientation. The progression of disorientation occurs first to situation, then to time, place, and finally person. If the patient fails any one of these, he is said to be disoriented.

2. If the patient is disoriented, determine his response to verbal stimuli by asking him to open his eyes, move an extremity, or squeeze a hand. Check old chart for previous history of hemiparesis.

B. Unconsciousness

The patient who is not awake or aware of his environment is unconscious or comatose. Determine response to painful stimuli. Use proper and professional methods such as: The trapezius pinch, sternal rub, calf pressure, interdigital compression, or supraorbital compression. Two responses may be elicited:

1. Purposeful movement would be an obvious attempt to push away the painful stimulus.

2. Non-purposeful response would be a generalized body movement or no response at all. The patient may exhibit a brain stem posture, signifying serious brain damage.

    a) Decorticate Rigidity
    The elbows are flexed and close to the body with the wrists flexed over the chest. The feet are plantar flexed.

    b) Decerebrate Rigidity
    The elbows are extended and at the side with wrists flexed. The feet are plantar flexed. This is a more ominous sign than decorticate rigidity.

IV. PUPILS

A. Normal or PERL-A

1. Normally the pupils are equal in size and shape. Diameter is 2 mm to 3 mm.

2. Pupils react briskly to light. The room should be darkened. The opposite eye should be closed since the optic nerve can transmit to the other eye, causing a consensual reaction.

3. Pupils show accommodation, which is when the lens thickens and the pupil constricts when an object is brought from far to near.

B. Abnormal Pupil Changes

1. Aniscoria. Ten percent of the population has a congenital inequality of pupil diameter. This is not pathological.

2. Some people who are blind, have cataracts, or an eye prosthesis will have fixed or irregularly shaped pupils.

3. The pupils may be slow or sluggish to light.

4. Pinpoint pupils can no longer constrict but are still said to be reactive. They may be caused by myotic medications, localized pons involvement, or narcotics use.

5. Pupil dilation has numerous causes: Brain injury, third cranial nerve compression, anoxia as in cardiac arrest, atropine or scopalamine use, and barbiturate use.

V. RESPIRATIONS

Generally, the respiratory patterns listed below occur as a function of worsening brain damage as the coma deepens from thalamus to brainstem.

A. Eupnea

Normal breathing. May be present in the stuporous or semi-comatose patient.

B. Cheyne-Stokes Respirations

A gradual buildup and decline from hyperpnea to apnea. May be caused by deep diencephalic lesions, hypertensive encephalopathy, uremia, anoxia, or imminent transtentorial herniation.

C. Central Neurogenic Hyperventilation

Rapid regular breathing in a comatose patient. Caused by perceived metabolic acidosis in mid-brain lesions.

D. Biots Respirations

Similar to Cheyne-Stokes except that there are regular periods of hyperventilation followed by irregular periods of apnea. Only seen in neurologic conditions usually involving the pons and cerebellum.

E. Ataxic or Apneustic Breathing

Completely chaotic and irregular respiratory patterns. Caused by severe brain stem injury to the medulla.

VI. GLASGOW COMA SCALE

This can be utilized as an assessment tool. It can be included when performing neurologic checks. Use the total score as a relative value of improvement or decline in your patient's condition.

A. Eyes

1. Open spontaneously	4
2. Open to verbal command	3
3. Open to pain	2
4. No response	1

B. Best Motor Response

1. Obeys verbal command	6
2. Localizes pain from painful stimulus	5
3. Flexion—withdrawal	4
4. Decorticate posture	3
5. Decerebrate posture	2
6. No response	1

C. Best Verbal Response

1. Oriented and converses	5
2. Disoriented and converses	4
3. Inappropriate words	3
4. Incomprehensible sounds	2
5. No response	1
Total	____

VII. CRANIAL NERVE ASSESSMENT

This assessment is detailed, complex, and is best performed by an experienced practitioner.

A. Olfactory—I

1. Have the patient close his eyes and occlude one nostril. Ask him to identify common odors such as oranges, tobacco, soap, coffee, etc.

2. Alternate with the other nostril.

B. Optic—II

1. Test the patient's visual acuity by using a Snellen chart or newspaper print.

2. Inspect the fundus using an ophthalmoscope.

C. Oculomotor—III, Trochlear—IV, Abducens—VI

1. Check the pupils for size, shape, reaction to light and accommodation (PERL-A). This assesses the oculomotor nerve only.

2. Check the eyelids for equal movement and closure.

3. Test eye movement by asking the patient to follow your finger in different directions. Keep the head stationary. Observe for strabismus and nystagmus.

D. Trigeminal—V

1. Test corneal reflex by gently touching the cornea with a wisp of cotton. The eyelids should blink.

2. Check sensation of the entire face, ie: Forehead, cheeks, jaw, and chin. With the eyes closed, ask the patient to identify touch, temperature, and pain. Use a wisp of cotton, hot and cold test tubes, and a pin. (Use caution and avoid injury when using a hot test tube and a pin.)

3. Test the motor division of this nerve by asking the patient to open and close the jaw against resistance.

E. Facial—VII

1. Check the patient's ability to taste. Ask him to identify tastes that are sweet, sour, salty, and bitter. Use sugar, lemon juice, salt, and mustard. Be sure to occlude the nostrils to avoid confusion with the sense of smell.

2. Assess the patient's facial muscles. Ask the patient to smile, frown, tightly close the eyes, raise the eyebrows, puff out the cheeks, and show his teeth. Check for symmetry.

F. Acoustic—VIII

1. Check the patient's ability to hear. Ask him to identify a watch ticking, a whispered voice, and a tone from a tuning fork. Compare from side to side. Use an audiometer for a more precise assessment.

2. Test the oculovestibular reflex by utilizing the caloric test. Instill either cold or hot water into the external ear canal. Rotary type nystagmus should occur. This should be performed with caution to avoid injury to the canal.

G. Glossopharyngeal—IX, Vagus—X

1. Check the patient's ability to swallow. Ask him to swallow a small amount of water.

2. Check the gag reflex by gently touching the back of the throat with a tongue depressor.

3. Have the patient open his mouth and say ''ahh.'' Inspect the throat for deviation of the palate and uvula.

4. Assess the patient's ability to speak. Ask him to read aloud. Observe his speech during the assessment.

H. Spinal Accessory—XI

1. Test the sternocleidomastoid muscles. Ask the patient to shrug the shoulders with resistance from the examiner.

2. Without resistance from the examiner.

I. Hypoglossal—XII

1. Test tongue movements. Ask the patient to open his mouth and move his tongue in and out.

2. Ask the patient to move his tongue from side to side.

VIII. MOTOR

A. Speech

1. Normal
Should be appropriate in volume and choice of words.
Should be clearly articulated.

   2. Abnormal

     a) Aphasia: Inability to speak.

     b) Dysphasia: Difficulty in understanding or speaking.

     c) Dysarthria: Unclear articulation.

     d) Aphonia: Inability to speak due to laryngeal damage.

     e) Dysphonia: A raspy or hoarse voice due to laryngeal damage.

     f) Nasal Speech: Caused by palatal paralysis.

     g) Parkinsonian Speech: A monotonous, weak voice.

B. Gait

   1. Normal

     a) Gait should be upright, with steps equal, and movements smooth.

     b) Have the patient walk a few steps with eyes closed. Stay with the patient to protect him from falling.

   2. Abnormal

     a) Cerebellar Gait
       The patient walks with a wide base, the back is rigid, and the legs bend at the hips. Frequent falling may occur.

     b) Spastic Hemiparesis.
       The affected arm is flexed, the foot is circumducted, and the toes drag.

     c) Scissors Gait.
       A slow walk with the thighs crossing in front of each other.

     d) Steppage Gait.
       One or both feet are lifted high and then slapped on the floor.

     e) Parkinsonian Gait.
       A stooped, stiff posture with short, shuffling steps.

C. Muscle Tone

   1. Check for muscle rigidity. With the patient relaxed, flex and extend the upper and lower extremities. There should be no resistance.

2. Test muscles for strength and symmetry.

   a) Use resistance while the patient extends and flexes the arms.
   b) Attempt to depress an outstretched arm.
   c. Check finger spreading against resistance.
   d) Check hand grip.
   e) Have the patient touch the thumb to each one of the fingers.
   f) Check the trunk by having the patient flex, extend, and bend laterally.
   g) Check hip flexion by asking the patient to raise his knee while your hand applies resistance to the thigh.
   h) Test the hip abduction. Place your hands firmly on the outside of the knees. Ask the patient to spread the legs.
   i) Test for hip adduction. With the legs spread, place your hands firmly on the inside of the knees. Ask the patient to close the legs.
   j) Check flexion and extension of the knee against resistance.
   k) Check plantar and dorsiflexion of the foot against resistance.

D. Coordination

Have the patient do the following:

1. Touch his nose with the index finger of each hand, alternating, and with increasing speed.
2. Touch his nose, then your finger at a distance of eighteen inches, with increasing speed.
3. Run the heel of each foot down the opposite shin.
4. Do a knee bend without support.
5. Hop on one foot, then the other.
6. Stand with feet together, with eyes closed, for five seconds.
7. Walk a straight line with one foot in front of the other.

IX. SENSATION

Sensory assessment should be done randomly over the arms, legs and trunk. Distal areas are assessed first. If abnormalities are noted, a more proximal and detailed study over the dermatomes should be done.

A. Pain

Use a safety pin randomly alternating the sharp and dull sides.

B. Temperature

Use test tubes of hot and cold water.

C. Light Touch

Use a piece of cotton.

D. Vibration

Use a low pitched tuning fork over bony prominences.

E. Proprioception

Without the patient looking, move the big toe and ask the patient in which direction it was moved.

F. Discriminate Sensation

1. Place a familiar object such as a coin or a key in the patient's hand. Ask him to identify it.
2. With the blunt end of a pencil, draw a letter or number on the palm. Ask the patient to identify it.

X. REFLEXES

A. Deep Tendon Reflexes

This is done with a percussion hammer. There are five loctions. Note the grade of each reflex and symmetry from side to side.

Locations:
a) Biceps
b) Triceps
c) Brachioradialis
d) Patellar
e) Achilles tendon

Grades:

0   —No response
1 +—Diminished or below normal
2 +—Normal
3 +—Brisker than normal
4 +—Very brisk, hyperactive, or clonus

B. Cutaneous Reflexes

1. Abdominal Reflex
    Stroke the upper and lower abdomen separately towards the midline. The abdominal muscles should contract.

2. Cremasteric Reflex
    Elicited in males only. Stroking of the inner thigh causes elevation of the testicle on that side.

C. Pathologic Reflexes

1. Clonus
    A 4 + deep tendon reflex. This may indicate upper motor neuron disease.

2. Babinsky
    Stroke the sole of the foot from the heel, up the lateral aspect, over the ball of the foot. Dorsiflexion and fanning of the toes indicates upper motor neuron disease.

3. Meningeal Irritation Reflexes

    a) Nuchal Rigidity
       Stiff neck or inability to touch chin to sternum.

    b) Brudzinki's Sign
       While supine, the patient flexes his knees when the neck is flexed.

    c) Kernig's Sign
       Pain occurs when the leg is extended and the hip is flexed.

4. Oculocephalic or Doll's Eyes
    Elicited in unconscious patients only. When the head is rotated to the left, the eyes deviate to the right and vice versa. Be sure there is not a neck injury before performing this exam.

5. Oculovestibular Reflex
    Hot or cold water irrigation of the ear causes no nystagmus towards the opposite ear.

SUBARACHNOID HEMORRHAGE, HEAD TRAUMA, BRAIN TUMOR, CEREBRAL ANEURYSM, CRANIOTOMY

POTENTIAL PROBLEMS

Airway Obstruction	Stress Ulcer
Respiratory Insufficiency	Aphasia
Increased Intracranial Pressure	Nausea and Vomiting
	Specific Motor Problems
Seizures	Specific Sensory Problems
Pneumonia	Psychosocial Problems
Disorientation	
Vertigo	

KEY NURSING INTERVENTIONS

- See Preoperative and Postoperative Care.

- Assess neurological system by performing neurologic checks with vital signs and PRN. Neurologic checks should include the following: Level of consciousness, respiratory patterns, pupil size and reaction to light, and extremity movements (see Neurological Assessment).

- Observe for signs and symptoms of increased intracranial pressure: Decreased level of consciousness, bradycardia, increase in blood pressure, widening pulse pressure, respiratory pattern changes, increased or decreased respiratory rate, headache, nausea, vomiting, pupillary changes, seizures.

- Prevent increased intracranial pressure by the following: Maintaining head elevation of 20–40 degrees and avoiding Valsalva maneuver, rectal stimulation, straining, coughing, sneezing, vomiting, and rapid infusion of IV fluids.

- Assess patient for signs and symptoms of diabetes insipidus: Urinary output greater than 5 liters per 24 hours, urine specific gravity of 1.001–1.005, thirst.

- Maintain seizure precautions (see Seizure Disorders).

- Use hypothermia blanket or ice packs to control hyperthermia.

- Observe for signs and symptoms of stress ulcer: Abdominal pain, occult blood in stools, vomitus or nasogastric aspirate.

- Maintain patent airway and prevent aspiration. Use oral and nasal airways PRN. Position patient in lateral or semiprone positions. Avoid flexion of the head. Suction cautiously to avoid inducing coughing and vomiting which may increase intracranial pressure. Remove dentures or partial plates until full consciousness is present.

- Observe for partial airway obstruction: Noisy respirations, stridor, decreased inspiratory and expiratory volumes and restlessness, cyanosis.
  NOTE: Hypoxia increases intracranial pressure.

- Assess and support the patient's psychosocial needs. Orient the patient to person, place, time and situation as needed. Help the patient and family deal with losses, i.e., mental dysfunction, motor deficits, physical change, and personality changes. Encourage the family to touch and talk to the patient. Foster a hopeful atmosphere especially when the prognosis is uncertain. With assistance from the physician, help the family establish realistic goals and expectations for the patient.

PATIENT AND FAMILY TEACHING

- Involve family in patient care.

- Instruct patient's family to observe patient for signs of increased intracranial pressure after discharge: Severe headache, persistent vomiting, inability to arouse patient, altered mental status.

- Prepare patient and family for transfer to a rehabilitation center. Emphasize the difference in patient care from the acute facility and that a balance of independent and dependent behavior is encouraged. Point out that it may be a long-term program and to expect the patient to reach plateaus.

MENINGITIS

POTENTIAL PROBLEMS

Septic Shock	Disseminated Intravascular
Vasomotor Collapse	Coagulation
Hydrocephalus	Heart Failure
Convulsive Seizures	Pericarditis
Pneumonia	Psychosocial Problems

KEY NURSING INTERVENTIONS

- Assess neurological system by doing neurologic checks with vital signs and PRN. Neurologic checks should include the following: Level of consciousness, respiratory patterns, pupil size and reaction to light, and extremity movements (see Neurological Assessment).

- Observe for signs and symptoms of increased intracranial pressure: Decreased level of consciousness, bradycardia, increase in blood pressure, widening pulse pressure, respiratory pattern changes, decreased or increased respiratory rate, headache, nausea, vomiting, pupillary changes, seizures.

- Maintain seizure precautions (see Seizure Disorders).

- Observe for airway obstruction if altered level of consciousness is present: Noisy respirations, decreased inspiratory and expiratory volumes, restlessness.

- Monitor patient for signs and symptoms of fluid and electrolyte imbalance (see Fluids and Electrolytes).

- Assist the physician with a lumbar puncture. Send specimens to lab immediately. Keep head of patient flat for 6–12 hours to prevent headache (see Lumbar Puncture).

- Assess for signs and symptoms of septic shock: Fever, tachycardia, tachypnea, hot and dry or cool and clammy skin, cyanosis, oliguria, hypotension, heart failure, altered level of consciousness, lethargy, hallucinations, restlessness.

- Observe for signs and symptoms of disseminated intravascular coagulation: Petechiae, prolonged bleeding following venipuncture, oliguria, renal failure, convulsions, coma, prolonged prothrombin time and partial thromboplastin time, decreased platelet count and fibrinogen level, dyspnea, hemoptysis, rales, acrocyanosis.

- Monitor patient for signs and symptoms of heart failure: Increased CVP, distended neck veins, rales, wheezes, shortness of breath, tachycardia, edema in ankles and legs.

- Maintain appropriate isolation (see Isolation).

- Assess and support the patient's psychosocial needs. Provide a comfortable, low-stimulus environment, especially when the patient is acutely ill. Allow the patient and family to express their concern and ask questions. Explain the purpose of isolation if indicated. Encourage family and friends to visit. Stress that there is no danger if proper isolation technique is followed.

PATIENT AND FAMILY TEACHING

- Demonstrate proper isolation technique to all visitors if indicated. Stress its importance.

- Explain the procedure and purpose of lumbar puncture, if indicated.

- Discuss with the physician and family the possibility of antimicrobial prophylaxis for persons who were in close contact with the patient prior to admission.

THE UNCONSCIOUS PATIENT

POTENTIAL PROBLEMS

Respiratory Insufficiency
Airway Obstruction
Atelectasis
Aspiration
Corneal Irritation/Ulceration
Increased Intracranial
   Pressure
Fluid/Electrolyte Imbalance
Hyperglycemic
   Hyperosmolar Nonketotic
   Coma (HHNK)
Water Intoxication

Incontinence
Impaction
Skin Breakdown
Seizures
Hyper/Hypothermia
Paralytic Ileus
Urinary Tract Infection
Weight Loss
Dehydration

KEY NURSING INTERVENTIONS

- Maintain a patent airway and prevent aspiration. Use oral and nasal airways PRN. Position patient in lateral or semiprone positions. Avoid flexion of the head. Suction secretions PRN. Remove dentures or partial plates until full consciousness is present.

- Observe for signs and symptoms of partial airway obstruction: Noisy respirations, stridor, decreased inspiratory and expiratory volumes, restlessness, cyanosis.

- Monitor patient closely for signs and symptoms of respiratory failure: Irritability, anxiety, restlessness, tachypnea, shallow respirations, flaring nares, decreased tidal volume and vital capacity, increasing blood pressure and pulse, diaphoresis, cyanosis, stridor, Cheyne-Stokes respirations.

- Assess neurological system by doing neurologic checks with vital signs PRN. Neurologic checks should include: Level of consciousness, respiratory patterns, pupil size and reaction to light, extremity movement (see Neurological Assessment).

- Observe for signs and symptoms of increasing intracranial pressure: Decreased level of consciousness, bradycardia, widening pulse pressure, respiratory pattern changes, decreased or increased respiratory rate, headache, nausea, vomiting, pupillary changes and seizures.

- Monitor rectal temperature for hyper/hypothermia.
- Maintain seizure precautions (see Seizure Disorders).
- Observe for signs and symptoms of fluid and electrolyte imbalance. Dehydration and water intoxication are the most common problems in the unconscious patient (see Fluids and Electrolytes).
- Monitor arterial blood gases, blood urea nitrogen and blood glucose values.
- Prevent fluid overload and dehydration by monitoring IV infusion and nasogastric tube feeding rates closely. Maintain accurate intake and output.
- Prevent complications of tube feedings. Elevate head 45 degrees during feeding. Check for residual gastric contents and proper tube placement prior to each feeding. Restrain patient if restless during feeding to prevent dislodgement. Flush tube after feeding and observe tracheal secretions for evidence of tracheoesophageal fistula.
- Prevent corneal irritation and ulceration by: Use of prescribed eye drops, avoiding trauma from pillow and linen, and use of protective eye shields.
- Prevent skin breakdown, muscle atrophy, contractures, and pressure sores (see The Immobilized Patient).
- Assess and support patient and family's psychosocial needs. Talk to patient while giving care. Encourage family to touch and talk to patient and include them in patient care whenever possible. When patient regains consciousness, explain what has happened and reorient the patient. With assistance from the physician, help the family establish realistic goals and expectations for the patient. Foster a hopeful atmosphere, especially when the prognosis is uncertain.

PATIENT AND FAMILY TEACHING

- Inform family of patient's daily condition and any improvements.
- Inform family members of procedures and tests.
- Prepare family for the possibility of transfer to an extended-care facility.
- Inform patient, even though he or she is unconscious, of all procedures to be performed.

SEIZURE DISORDERS

POTENTIAL PROBLEMS

Airway Obstruction   Head and Body Trauma
Aspiration   Psychosocial Problems
Hypoxia

KEY NURSING INTERVENTIONS

- Maintain seizure precautions. Keep oral airway, padded tongue blade, and working suction at bedside. Pad all side rails. Maintain bed in low position.

- Protect the patient during a seizure. If possible, insert oral airway or padded tongue blade and suction secretions. Do not force because injury to the jaw, tongue or teeth may result. Place the patient in a lateral position. Protect the head and body from injury. Do not restrain the patient. Loosen restrictive clothing. If Valium is given intravenously to calm muscle activity, observe the patient closely for respiratory depression.

- If a seizure occurs, observe for and document the following: Presence of aura, eye movements, pupil changes, local and general body movements, type of movements, respiratory patterns, presence of cyanosis, urine or fecal incontinence, level of consciousness, duration of seizure, postictal behavior (paralysis, weakness, inability to speak, level of consciousness, if patient sleeps vs. stays awake), possible injuries.

- Following a seizure, establish a patent airway, suction secretions, turn patient to side, administer oxygen as ordered, reorient patient, take vital signs.

- Observe patient for signs and symptoms of antiepileptic drug toxicity: Drowsiness, visual disturbances, incoordination, arrhythmias, blood dyscrasias, nervousness.

- Assess and support patient's psychosocial needs. Reorient the patient after each seizure. Approach the patient in a calm and gentle manner, especially if resistive and aggressive after the seizure. Help patient deal with anxiety due to disruptions in self concept. Involve the family in care and emphasize that seizures can be controlled with proper medications, a well-balanced diet, rest, and minimal emotional stress.

- Refer patient to the Epilepsy Foundation of America.

PATIENT AND FAMILY TEACHING

- Instruct patient and family to avoid situations that may precipitate a seizure: Lack of sleep, overactivity, emotional stress, not taking medications as prescribed.

- Demonstrate to the family what to do during a seizure. Explain that the patient cannot swallow the tongue. Instruct the family never to put fingers into the mouth of a person having a seizure.

- Stress the importance of the prescribed medication dose and frequency. Inform patient that a sudden cessation could cause a seizure or increase seizure frequency.

- Emphasize that prescribed medications *control* rather than cure seizure disorders.

- Advise patient and family to record and report to physician the duration, number, time of seizure and other surrounding circumstances of seizures.

- Antiepileptics should be taken with meals to prevent gastritis.

- Instruct patient to be alert for signs and symptoms of antiepileptic drug toxicity (specific for prescribed drug).

- Some antiepileptics suppress hematopoiesis. Therefore, regular followup physician visits are important. Patients should report easy bruising, bleeding (gums, rectum, etc.), fever or symptoms of infection.

- Advise the patient to wear a Medic Alert tag at all times.

- Instruct the patient to avoid activities which are dangerous, i.e., driving, flying, swimming, operating dangerous equipment.

PARKINSON'S DISEASE

POTENTIAL PROBLEMS

Parkinsonian Crisis	Pain
Adverse Medication Reactions	Incoordination/Falls
Dysphagia	Emotional Instability
Excess Perspiration	Excessive Salivation
Sensitivity to Heat	Incontinence
Constipation	Psychosocial Problems

KEY NURSING INTERVENTIONS

- Assess the patient for signs and symptoms of parkinsonian crisis. This is a medical emergency. It may be caused by emotional upset or sudden cessation of antiparkinsonian medications. Signs and symptoms are an exacerbation of Parkinson symptoms: Tremor, rigidity, akinesia, anxiety, diaphoresis, tachypnea, tachycardia. Treatment of a parkinsonian crisis includes administration of sedatives and antiparkinsonian medications along with support of the respiratory and cardiac systems.

- Observe patient for adverse reactions to antiparkinsonian medications:

  —Levodopa—Arrhythmias, postural hypotension, nausea, vomiting, anorexia, constipation, insomnia, confusion, hallucinations, agitation, anxiety, restlessness. Observe for signs and symptoms of gastrointestinal hemorrhage if active gastric ulcer disease is present or in patient's medical history.

  —Anticholinergic drugs (Artane, Kemadrin, Cogentin, Disipal, Parsidol)—Tachycardia, vertigo, urinary retention, impaired vision, dry mouth, constipation, confusion.

  —Bromocriptine (Parlodel)—Gastrointestinal disturbances, abnormal involuntary motor movements, mental confusion, hallucinations.

  —Amantadine (Symmetrel)—Emotional instability, mental changes, restlessness.

- Minimize adverse effects of levodopa by administering with meals and administering antiemetics as ordered.

- Avoid sudden cessation of anticholinergics. This may trigger onset of toxic symptoms.
- Never administer MAO inhibitors with levodopa.
- Observe for difficulty swallowing and, if present, hold food and fluids. Keep suction available during meals.
- Assess and support the patient's psychosocial needs. Improve lowered self-esteem by encouraging independent activities. Include the patient in the formation of a care plan. Set realistic and attainable goals. Help the patient and family deal with the troublesome symptoms. Provide communication aids as needed. Refer the patient to the American Parkinson's Disease Foundation.

PATIENT AND FAMILY TEACHING

- Instruct the patient not to take Vitamin B6 with levodopa since it may negate its effectiveness.
- Point out that side effects of levodopa frequently disappear with continued use.
- Advise patients with postural hypotension to make gradual position changes until condition improves with dosage adjustments. Elastic hose may be helpful.
- Teach patient to do diaphragmatic breathing, range of motion exercises and speech improvement techniques such as holding a musical note for several seconds, scale singing and tongue exercises.
- Instruct patient to follow a daily bowel routine to avoid constipation, (Attempt to defecate 10–15 minutes after breakfast or according to patient's bowel history.) Drink three liters of fluid per day, and include high-fiber foods and juices in diet.

GUILLAIN-BARRE SYNDROME, INFECTIOUS POLYNEURITIS

POTENTIAL PROBLEMS

Airway Obstruction	Urinary Tract Infection
Aspiration	Dysphagia
Pneumonia	Skin Breakdown
Respiratory Failure	Fever
Paralysis	Weight Loss
Communication Problems	Psychosocial Problems

KEY NURSING INTERVENTIONS

- Muscle weakness usually begins in the lower extremities and ascends up the body over several days (10–14 days). In severe cases, the respiratory muscles are affected. Constant observation of respiratory function is essential. Endotracheal intubation or tracheostomy with mechanical ventilation may be necessary if respiratory failure develops.

- Assess and document level of motor function every four hours and PRN.

- Observe for signs and symptoms of developing respiratory failure: Shallow respirations, tachypnea, flaring nares, restlessness, anxiety, panic, decreased tidal volume and vital capacity, increased blood pressure and pulse, diaphoresis, cyanosis, stridor, Cheyne-Stokes respirations.

- See Tracheostomy.

- If the patient is allowed to eat, observe for dysphagia. Keep suction equipment at the bedside. If dysphagia is present, keep NPO and notify physician.

- Minimize patient's exposure to infections. Restrict staff and visitors with infections and/or transmissable illnesses. Keep room temperature at a moderate level. Wash hands before patient care and maintain aseptic technique in all procedures.

- Prevent muscle deformities during paralysis by maintaining good body alignment.

- Provide full range of motion exercises *after* acute phase and only as ordered.
- Prevent skin breakdown and pressure sores (see The Immobilized Patient).
- Assess for signs and symptoms of urinary retention: Absent voiding, bladder distention, voiding 25–50 cc more than one time per hour.
- Assess and support the patient's psychosocial needs. Explain the nature of the disease and that most patients recover fully. Recovery may take several months. Keep a positive and hopeful attitude. Encourage the family and friends to visit frequently and interact with the patient as much as possible. If the patient has a tracheostomy, provide reassurance and reduce anxiety. Keep the call light or other call devices within reach, respond promptly, and provide communication aids as necessary.

PATIENT AND FAMILY TEACHING

- Explain the potential for a long recovery period (up to 6 months). Stress the importance of following the prescribed exercises.
- If the patient is to be transferred to a rehabilitation unit, explain the difference in the nature of patient care from an acute medical-surgical unit.

MULTIPLE SCLEROSIS

POTENTIAL PROBLEMS

Respiratory Insufficiency	Vomiting
Pneumonia	Emotional Instability
Coma	Euphoria
Muscle Spasticity	Depression
Incoordination	Bowel/Bladder Incontinence
Vertigo	Urinary Retention
Impaired Vision, Speech,	Bladder Infections
and Sensations	Contractures
Skin Breakdown	Psychosocial Problems

KEY NURSING INTERVENTIONS

- Assess patient for complications of ACTH and/or prednisone therapy: Hypokalemia, hypernatremia, peripheral edema, gastrointestinal bleeding, diabetes, and the activation of tuberculosis.

- Prevent exacerbation. Provide frequent rest periods. Avoid muscle fatigue and/or overexertion when doing daily exercises. Ensure a calm, quiet environment.

- Prevent pressure sores, skin breakdown and contractures (see The Immobilized Patient).

- Prevent accidental injury due to skin sensory loss. Avoid contact with extreme temperatures and sharp objects.

- Observe for signs and symptoms of urinary retention: Absent voiding, bladder distention, voiding 25–50 cc more than one time per hour, feeling of fullness or discomfort, restlessness.

- Help prevent urinary incontinence. Have the patient void on a regular schedule. Start at every hour and gradually lengthen intervals. Regulate fluid intake to specific times and keep the patient well hydrated.

- Observe for signs and symptoms of bladder infection: Frequency, dysuria, urgency, pyuria, bacteriuria, positive urine culture, urethral discharge.

- Establish a regular bowel program for incontinence or constipation. Enemas or suppositories may be needed every other day (see The Immobilized Patient).

- If the patient has visual disturbances (ophthalmoplegia, blindness, nystagmus, diplopia), keep call light within easy reach, orient patient to location of items on bedside stand, assist with meals and ambulation. For diplopia, alternate covering one eye with patch every other day.
- Assess and support patient's psychosocial needs. Encourage independent activities within limits to promote good self esteem. Include the patient in care plan. Assist the patient and family in coping with changes in lifestyle, physiological losses and mood alterations. Help the patient and family develop realistic goals and expectations. Refer the patient and family to the National Multiple Sclerosis Society.

PATIENT AND FAMILY TEACHING

- Advise the patient to avoid known factors precipitating exacerbation, especially fatigue and infections.
- Instruct the patient to take frequent rest periods each day.
- Stress that daily exercises are important to maintain muscle strength and prevent contractures.
- Encourage adherence to bowel and bladder programs.
- Instruct the patient to ambulate with feet wide apart to improve steadiness.
- Instruct the patient and family to inspect skin daily for evidence of trauma and pressure sores.
- Instruct the family and patient in the proper use of assistive devices, i.e., braces, walkers, crutches.
- If the bedridden patient is to be cared for at home, demonstrate how to prevent pressure sores, contractures and skin breakdown (see The Immobilized Patient).

SPINAL CORD INJURY

POTENTIAL PROBLEMS

Respiratory Arrest
Respiratory Insufficiency
Spinal Shock
Autonomic Hyperreflexia
Pulmonary Embolism
Vein Thrombosis
Cord Compression
Paralysis
Paralytic Ileus

Exacerbation of Injury
Pneumonia
Atelectasis
Bowel & Bladder Incontinence
Urinary Retention
Skin Breakdown
Contractures
Pain
Psychosocial Problems

FOR SKELETAL TONGS

Infection at Puncture Sites
Misalignment of Pulleys and
  Weights
Loosening of Screws on
  Halo Traction

FOR STRYKER FRAME AND CIRCOLECTRIC BED

Dislodgement of Tubes
Collapse of Frame

KEY NURSING INTERVENTIONS

- Assess neurological system by performing neurologic checks with vital signs and PRN. Neurologic checks should include the following: Level of consciousness, respiratory patterns, pupil size and reaction to light, and extremity movements (see Neurological Assessment).

- Observe for signs and symptoms of respiratory insufficiency: Weak cough, inability to clear secretions, paradoxical movements of diaphragm or intercostal spaces when coughing, decreased lung expansion and vital capacity, cyanosis, worsening blood gasses, and altered mental status.

- Assess patient for signs and symptoms of spinal shock: Decreasing blood pressure, loss of sensory and motor function below level of injury, bladder and bowel distention, loss of sweating below level of injury, hyperthermia. This occurs following the injury and may last up to six weeks.

- If SPINAL SHOCK occurs: Maintain patent airway and adequate ventilation, suction secretions, maintain circulatory volume by IV crystalloids and colloids, insert nasogastric tube as ordered to suction gastric contents and relieve distention, and monitor urinary output.

- Assess sensory and motor functions every 2–4 hrs. and document patient's response (see Neurological Assessment). Deterioration in sensory and motor functions is a sign of cord compression and should be reported immediately.

- Observe for signs and symptoms of autonomic hyperreflexia in patients with injury at or above T6: Severe headache, diaphoresis, bradycardia, severe hypertension, piloerection. This is a medical emergency.

- If AUTONOMIC HYPERREFLEXIA occurs, place patient in upright position, administer antihypertensives, remove sensory stimuli that may be causing it (distended bowel or bladder, pain, extreme temperatures and tactile skin stimuli, visceral contraction or distention).

- Assess patient for signs and symptoms of thrombophlebitis: Pain, redness and swelling of affected extremity. Check for positive Homans' sign, which is pain in calf upon dorsiflexion of the foot.

- Observe for signs and symptoms of pulmonary embolism: Chest pain, shortness of breath, dyspnea, tachypnea, tachycardia, cyanosis, cardiopulmonary arrest.

- Prevent contractures by the following: Use of foot boards, trochanter rolls and passive range of motion *only as ordered.*

- Prevent respiratory complications by encouraging coughing, deep breathing, and adequate fluid intake.

- Assess and support patient's psychosocial needs. Help the patient progress through the grieving process. Foster a hopeful atmosphere, especially when the prognosis is uncertain. Allow the patient as much control over activities of daily living and other functions within prescribed limitations. Provide sensory stimulation to prevent deprivation. Allow the patient to express anger, depression, and frustrations without becoming alienated. Help the patient set realistic goals for the future with the assistance from the health care team. For patients on Stryker frame and CircOlectric bed, explain turning procedure beforehand to allay anxiety and fear.

  - *For Skeletal Tongs:* Keep pulleys and cords unobstructed. Weights should hang freely. Observe for signs of infection at puncture sites. Observe back of head for pressure areas and massage potential pressure areas frequently. Keep patient in the center of the bed.

- *For Stryker Frame:* Use pillows and pressure protectors where needed. Tighten bolts and straps securely before turning the patient. Assure free tubing movement prior to turning. Provide skin care after each turning and turn patient every 2 hrs. as ordered. Keep call light within reach.

- *For Halo Traction:* Observe pin insertion site for signs of infection. Maintain torque screwdriver at bedside for screw tightening PRN. Headache and pain at pin sites is to be expected for several days after insertion.

- *For CircOlectric Bed:* Maintain brakes in ON position AT ALL TIMES. Unplug bed when not turning patient. Use pillows and pressure protectors where needed. Provide skin care after each turning and turn patient every 2 hrs. as ordered. Keep call light within reach.

PATIENT AND FAMILY TEACHING

- Involve family in patient care.
- Prepare patient and family for transfer to a rehabilitation center. Emphasize the difference in patient care from the acute facility and that independent behaviors will be encouraged.
- Explain to patient and family the purpose of the Stryker frame, skeletal traction and CircOlectric bed.

RUPTURED DISC

POTENTIAL PROBLEMS

Pain	Pressure Sores
Traction Malfunction	Recurrent Injury
Neurologic Deficit	Psychosocial Problems

KEY NURSING INTERVENTIONS

- Usually a ruptured disc is treated with strict bed rest and traction. (For surgical treatment, see Laminectomy and Spinal Fusion.)

- Assess the patient for signs and symptoms of neurologic deficit: Muscle weakness, loss of sensation, tingling sensations, motor deficits, unrelieved pain in extremities.

- If a cervical collar is being used, avoid hyperextension of the neck. A neutral or slight flexed position is desired.

- Maintain proper body alignment at all times.

- When moving the patient for washing, changing linens or placing on a bedpan, always logroll using at least three people.

- For low back pain, keep the head of bed elevated 20–30 degrees and the knees slightly flexed with pillows or semi-Fowler's bed position. Avoid the prone position as this puts the spine in a hyperextended position.

- For traction keep the head of bed elevated as ordered. For lumbar traction the legs should also be elevated. Keep pulleys and cords unobstructed. Weights should hang freely. Observe the skin around traction straps for irritation. Do not shave a beard on a male patient who is to have cervical traction. The beard acts as padding. If at any time traction increases pain, discontinue it and notify physician.

- When not in traction, encourage frequent change of position in bed.

- Assess and support the patient's psychosocial needs. A ruptured disc is painful and treatment may be slow. Administer pain medication as ordered but also discuss other methods of pain control such as relaxation techniques, diversional activities, imaging and adherence to strict bed rest. Allow the patient as much control over the daily routine as possible. Encourage the family to visit frequently and bring nonstrenuous activities to help relieve boredom.

PATIENT AND FAMILY TEACHING

- Instruct the patient to avoid hyperextension of the neck and back.
- Demonstrate proper lifting techniques and exercises to help strengthen muscles.
- Inform the patient and family of the purpose, function, and safe operation of traction equipment.

LAMINECTOMY, SPINAL FUSION

POTENTIAL PROBLEMS

Respiratory Arrest	Urinary Retention
Aspiration	Skin Breakdown
Shock	Paralytic Ileus
Hemorrhage	Infection
Paralysis	Pain
Pulmonary Embolus	Psychosocial Problems

KEY NURSING INTERVENTIONS

- See Preoperative and Postoperative Care.

- Prepare bed and equipment before the patient arrives (i.e., CircOlectric bed, Stryker frame, air mattress, traction equipment, suction devices).

- Maintain correct body alignment at all times (see Stryker frame and CircOlectric bed). When transferring patient to another bed, washing, changing linen, or placing on bedpan, always logroll using at least three people.

- Avoid flexion of the head, back, and knees. For comfort the legs may be elevated with flexion at the hips only.

- Observe for signs and symptoms of neurologic deficit: Muscle weakness, loss of sensation, tingling sensations, motor deficits, unrelieved pain in extremities.

- For cervical laminectomy, maintain a patent airway by frequent observation and oropharyngeal suctioning as needed.

- Observe dressings and incision site for bleeding and infection.

- Observe for signs and symptoms of urinary retention: Feelings of discomfort or fullness, distended bladder, absent voiding, frequent voiding of 20–50 ml of urine every hour or less.

- Assess and support the patient's psychosocial needs. Spinal surgery can be very anxiety-producing. If appropriate, inform the patient that full recovery is possible if a proper medical regime is following including proper bed rest, body alignment, and body mechanics. Help the patient deal with pain and prolonged rest periods by providing diversional activities. Encourage the family to visit frequently. Be sure to explain all procedures to the patient before performing them.

PATIENT AND FAMILY TEACHING

- Explain the purpose and stress the importance of body alignment and logrolling.
- Explain the procedure and function of special equipment.
- Demonstrate proper lifting techniques and exercises to help strengthen muscles.
- Instruct the patient to avoid straining, over-exercising, lifting heavy objects or sitting for long periods.

RESPIRATORY SYSTEM

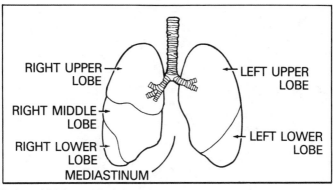

Lobes of Right and Left Lungs

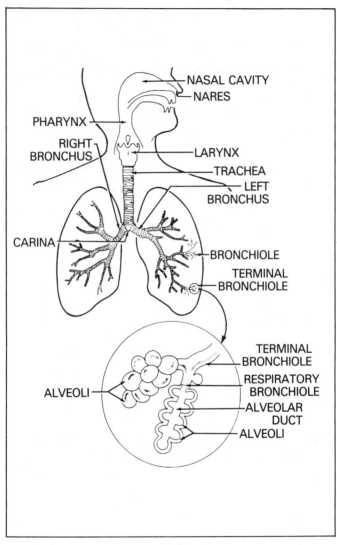

Anatomy of Respiratory System

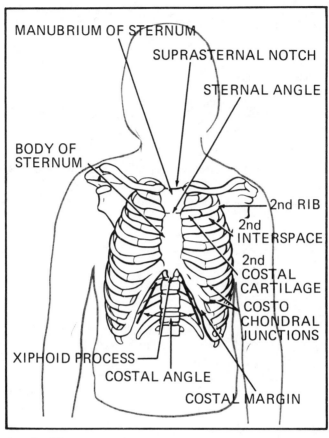

Anterior Thorax

RESPIRATORY SYSTEM—PHYSIOLOGY SUMMARY

I. RESPIRATION

A. External Respiration

1. Air Exchange
   —*Inspiration*

   a) The diaphragm and external intercostal muscles contract to increase thoracic space.

   b) Intrathoracic pressure becomes less than atmospheric pressure and air moves into the lungs.

   c) Oxygen pressure in the alveoli becomes greater than oxygen pressure in the pulmonary capillaries surrounding the alveoli.

   d) Oxygen flows into capillaries.

   —*Expiration*

   a) Carbon dioxide pressure in the capillaries becomes greater than in the alveoli and diffuses out into the alveoli.

   b) The diaphragm and external intercostal muscles relax to decrease thoracic space.

   c) Intrathoracic pressure becomes greater than atmospheric pressure, and air passively moves out of the lungs.

2. Factors Affecting Air Exchange

   a) Amount of air in alveoli.

   b) Amount of functional surface area of membranes.

   c) Pressure gradient between alveoli and venous blood.

   d) Respiratory rate and volume.

   e) Volume of air which reaches alveoli upon inspiration.

B. Internal Respiration

Gas exchange in the tissues occurs according to the pressure gradients as it does in the lungs. When intracellular pO_2 decreases, oxygen dissociates from the hemoglobin and diffuses out of the blood into the cells. When intracellular pCO_2

increases due to catabolism, it diffuses out of the cell into the blood.

II. RESPIRATORY CONTROLS

A. The Respiratory Center

Consists of neurons located in the pons and medulla oblongata. It is divided into (1) the medullary rhythmicity area, (2) the apneustic area, and (3) the pneumotaxic area. Involuntary respirations and rhythm are controlled by these areas.

B. Hering-Breuer Reflex

Depth and rhythm are controlled by stimulation of baroreceptors in the lungs following inspiration and expiration.

C. pCO_2

Increasing pCO_2 stimulates chemoreceptors located in the medulla, carotid tissues, and the aorta causing faster respirations. Decreasing pCO_2 inhibits chemoreceptors causing slower respirations.

D. pH

Central and peripheral centers are sensitive to a decreasing pH (acidosis), causing an increase in the depth and rate of respirations.

E. pO_2

Exremely low pO_2 levels, below a critical level, will cause decreased or absent respirations as hypoxic neurons are unable to conduct impulses to respiratory muscles. Slight decreases in pO_2, now below a critical level, will cause stimulation of chemoreceptors and increase respirations.

F. Cerebral cortex

Voluntary control of respirations occurs as impulses are transmitted from motor areas of the cerebrum to the respiratory centers in the medulla.

III. RESPIRATORY MECHANICS

A. Vital capacity

The volume of air that can be inspired after maximum expiration.

B. Total lung capacity

The total amount of air in the lungs after maximum inspiration (about 6.0 liters).

C. Tidal volume

The amount of air normally inspired (about 500 cc).

D. Residual volume

The amount of air that cannot be forcibly exhaled (about 1.0 liter).

E. Inspiratory reserve volume

The amount of air that can be inspired after regular inspiration (about 2.5 liters).

F. Expiratory reserve volume

The amount of air that can be forcibly expired after regular expiration (about 2.0 liters).

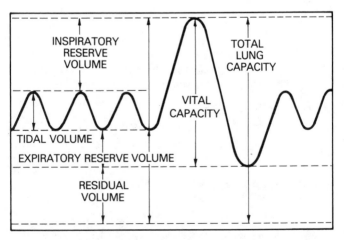

Respiratory Mechanisms

RESPIRATORY SYSTEM ASSESSMENT

I. HISTORY

A. Past history of respiratory problems

1. What type?
2. What therapy was utilized? Did it work?

B. Recent History

1. Shortness of breath?

   a) Episodes of difficulty breathing?

   b) When do they occur?

   c) How many pillows are used at night?

2. Presence of cough?

   a) Productive: Loose sounding, producing sputum.

   b) Hacking: A series of forceful expirations may be harsh or raspy.

   c) Paroxysmal: Spasmodic hacking.

   d) Brassy: Coughing with a harsh buzzing sound.

   e) Habitual: Continuous, usually due to an irritant.

   f) Habit cough: Usually related to nervousness.

3. Sputum?

   a) Mucoid: Clear, thin. Indicates early bronchitis.

   b) Mucopurulent: Thick, viscid, greenish color, frothy, nonoffensive. Indicates pneumonia, later bronchitis, or tuberculosis.

   c) Purulent: Thick, viscid, yellowish, offensive smelling. Indicates lung abscess, advanced tuberculosis, bronchiectasis, pneumonia.

   d) Nummular: Mucopurulent with small semi-solid masses that sink in water. Indicates advanced tuberculosis.

   e) Rusty: Mucopurulent. Very viscid, rust-tinged. Indicates pneumonia.

   f) Prune Juice: Dark brown and offensive smelling. Indicates late pneumonia or gangrene of lung.

g) Hemoptysis: Bright red and frothy. Indicates cancer, tuberculosis, pneumonia, pulmonary embolism, mitral stenosis, or aneurysm rupturing into bronchial tubes.

C. Level of Activity

1. Describe a typical day in terms of activity.
2. Is the patient on breathing exercises?

D. Pain

Use PQRST mnemonic.

P— Provokes.	What makes the pain worse or better? What was the patient doing prior to the onset of pain?
Q—Quality.	Subjective description of pain by the patient. Use the patient's own words, i.e., burning, stabbing, pressure.
R— Radiation.	Where is the pain located and does it radiate anywhere?
S— Severity.	Ask the patient to judge the pain on a scale of 1 to 10 with 10 being the worst pain ever felt.
T— Time.	How long has the patient had this pain? When did the pain begin and end?

G. Habits

1. Smoking. How long has the patient smoked? How many packs per day?
2. Alcohol. How long has the patient ingested alcohol? How much and what type per day?

H. Medications

1. List medications, including over-the-counter drugs.
2. Allergies.

I. Nutrition

Describe a typical:

1. Breakfast.
2. Lunch.
3. Dinner.
4. Snacks.

II. BACKGROUND INFORMATION

A. Lab Values

Check for abnormal values or worsening trends.

B. Arterial Blood Gases

Check the pH, pO_2, pCO_2, and HCO_3 for normal limits.

C. EKG

See Cardiovascular Assessment.

D. Diagnostic Studies

Identify abnormal reports of diagnostic studies, i.e., x-rays, biopsies, fluid aspirations, pulmonary function studies, lung scans, bronchoscopy, etc.

E. Chart

Check old chart for past relevant information.

III. INSPECTION

The patient should be sitting upright and uncovered to the waist. Provide support only if needed.

A. Trachea

Should be midline.

B. Chest Symmetry

Should have bilateral chest expansion upon inspiration. Check slope of ribs. Look for deformities.

C. Configuration

Anterior-posterior diameter should be shorter than bilateral diameter. Look for barrel, funnel, or pigeon-shaped chest and spinal deformities.

D. Intercostal Spaces

Look for bulging or retractions.

E. Skin

Odor, mottling, patterns, scars, irregularities.

F. Respiratory Pattern

Check the rate and rhythm. Look for nasal flaring, pursed-lip breathing, retractions, or splinting because of pain.

1. Normal: Inspiration and expiration times are equal and regular. Rate: 12 to 20 per minute.

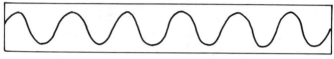

2. Tachypnea: Rapid and shallow.

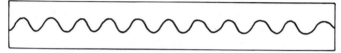

3. Hyperventilation or Kussmaul's: Increased rate and depth.

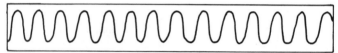

4. Bradypnea: Slowed but regular.

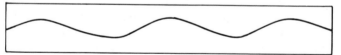

5. Apnea: Absence of respiration, usually periodic.

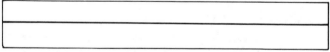

6. Cheyne-Stokes: Periods of increased deep breathing followed by apnea.

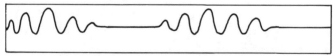

7. Obstructive breathing: With COPD the expiratory phase is longer.

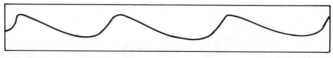

8. Biot's: Interrupted breathing associated with head injury.

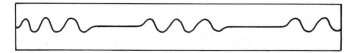

IV. PALPATION

A. Palpate

Palpate gently, then deeper all over thorax for areas of tenderness.

B. Chest expansion

Place both hands on either side of the chest at the bases and ask the patient to inhale deeply. Hands should move equally upward and slightly outward.

C. Tactile fremitus

Vibrations are felt on the chest by the examiner's palm when the patient says "ninety-nine," or "one, two, three." Normally, fremitus is felt strongest over the bronchi and diminishes as the hands approach the bases.

V. PERCUSSION

A. Percuss

Percuss along the same areas as for auscultation.

B. Listen

Listen for dullness, resonance, hyperresonance, and tympany. The lungs should have resonance throughout, except over the heart and scapulae. Consolidation, atelectasis, and effusion sound dull while pneumothorax and COPD sound hyperresonant.

VI. AUSCULTATION

A. Technique

The patient should first cough to clear the upper airway. Listen in each area for one full breath while the patient breathes in and out of his mouth.

1. Anteriorly: Auscultate the trachea, then down and across to each apex, proceeding in a zigzag pattern to the diaphragm, comparing side to side.
2. Posteriorly: Avoid the scapulae and move down and across, comparing from side to side.

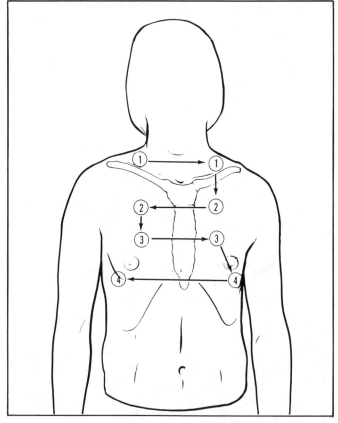

Anterior Respiratory Auscultation Pattern

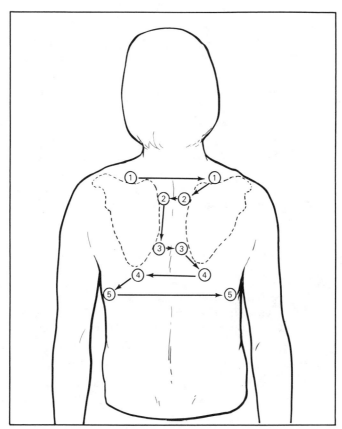

Posterior Respiratory Auscultation Pattern

B. Normal Breath Sounds

1. Tracheal or bronchial: Heard over the trachea down to the main bronchi. Expiration is greater than inspiration with a high-pitched sound.

2. Bronchovesicular: Heard over the main bronchi. Expiration equals inspiration and is lower in pitch and not as loud as tracheal sounds.

3. Vesicular: Heard throughout the rest of the lungs. Inspiration is greater than expiration and the sound is lower and softer.

C. Abnormal or Adventitious

1. Diminished: The lungs may be clear but the sounds are distant or not as loud. May be due to thick chest wall or low tidal volume.

2. Rales: Can be heard as crackling or fine, and gurgling or coarse. Usually heard in the bases or at the level of edema. They are usually inspiratory.

3. Rhonchi: Heard as low-pitched expiratory sounds caused by secretions or narrowing in the larger bronchioles.

4. Wheezes: Similar to rhonchi only higher pitched and are caused by constriction of more distal airway passages. May be expiratory, inspiratory, or both.

5. Friction rub: A continuous rubbing or grating sound coincident with respirations. May be similar to fine rales but is usually accompanied by pain upon inspiration.

D. Spoken and Whispered Sounds

Procedure: Have patient say "ninety-nine" or "eee" and auscultate chest in various areas. Normally, sounds are muffled. The following qualities indicate consolidation or effusion.

1. Bronchophony: A spoken syllable heard clearly.

2. Egophony: The sound "eee" changes to "aaa."

3. Whispered pectoriloquy: Clear transmission of the whispered voice.

EPISTAXIS

POTENTIAL PROBLEMS

Shock   Hypertension
Aspiration of Blood   Psychosocial Problems
Nausea and Vomiting

KEY NURSING INTERVENTIONS

- Instruct the patient to pinch the nose firmly for 10–20 minutes minimum until more aggressive measures can be taken by the physician. Maintain a high-Fowler's position. Take frequent blood pressures. Epistaxis may be due to a hypertensive crisis.

- Observe for signs and symptoms of shock: Increased pulse, decreased blood pressure, dizziness, diaphoresis, agitation, restlessness, inability to stop bleeding, frequent swallowing.

- Instruct the patient to expectorate the blood rather than swallow. Blood is very irritating to the stomach and may cause nausea and vomiting.

- Assist the physician with nasal packing or cauterization. Supplies that may be necessary are: Cocaine or epinephrine spray, head lamp, Vasoline gauze, nasal balloons or Foley catheters, nasal forceps, silver nitrate applicator sticks or other cautery equipment.

- Assess and support patient's psychosocial needs. Hemorrhage can cause the patient to be extremely fearful, apprehensive and feel powerless over control of the body. Be reassuring and confident when providing emergency care. Keep patient informed of progress. Avoid family encounters and other situations that may increase anxiety. Remain with patient until hemorrhage subsides, then check on patient frequently.

PATIENT AND FAMILY TEACHING

- Demonstrate how to pinch the nose in case of a repeat episode.
- Instruct the patient to avoid hot liquids, coughing, sneezing, bending over, and straining for a few days post bleeding.
- Stress the importance of antihypertensive medications if hypertension is present.

TONSILLECTOMY, ADENOIDECTOMY

POTENTIAL PROBLEMS

Respiratory Distress	Pain
Airway Obstruction	Shock
Aspiration	Infection
Hemorrhage	Psychosocial Problems
Dehydration	

KEY NURSING INTERVENTIONS

- See Preoperative and Postoperative Care.

- Position patient on side with face slightly prone following general anesthesia. Position patient with head elevated 45 degrees following local anesthesia. After patient is fully conscious following general anesthesia, change to semi-Fowler's position.

- Keep working suction, oral and nasal airways at bedside.

- Assess patient for signs and symptoms of airway obstruction: Stridor, crowing, decreased inspiratory and expiratory volumes, chest retractions, tachypnea, cyanosis.

- Observe for signs and symptoms of hemorrhage and shock: Frequent swallowing, red or dark brown emesis in large amounts; decreased blood pressure; increased pulse; cool, clammy, pale skin; restlessness; agitation. Carefully inspect the throat with a flashlight for bleeding.

- Maintain fresh ice collar to throat intermittently.

- Encourage bed rest, voice rest and quiet activities postoperatively.

- Take rectal temperatures immediately postoperatively.

- Do not allow patient to use straw for fluids (increases risk of bleeding).

- When able, start diet with ice chips and room temperature water. Advance to bland, soft diet per physician's order. Avoid hot, spicy, citrus, raw or hard foods.

- Assist patient with oral mouth rinses TID.

- Assess and support patient's psychosocial needs. Pain management will help the patient's coping mechanisms. Encourage family or significant other contact. Frequently check on patient postoperatively.

Inform patient of care plan activities. Provide a quiet, restful environment. Advise visitors to avoid prompting patient to talk following surgery.

PATIENT AND FAMILY TEACHING

- Instruct patient not to cough or clear throat.
- Tell patient to avoid hot, spicy, citrus, hard, raw and other irritating foods.
- Advise patient to brush teeth and rinse mouth TID. Gargling should be avoided.
- Instruct patient and family to observe for bleeding at home and to notify physician or go to an emergency room.

LARYNGECTOMY, RADICAL NECK DISSECTION

POTENTIAL PROBLEMS

Airway Obstruction   Infection
Hemorrhage   Pneumonia
Tracheoesophageal Fistula   Dehydration
Pain   Psychosocial Problems
Malnutrition

KEY NURSING INTERVENTIONS

- See Preoperative and Postoperative Care.

- See Tracheostomy.

- Observe for signs and symptoms of airway obstruction: Stridor, panic, agitation, decreased breath sounds unilaterally, cyanosis, tachypnea, tachycardia. It may be due to aspiration or a pressure dressing that is too tight. Keep working suction equipment at bedside.

- Observe for signs and symptoms of postoperative bleeding and hemorrhage: Red blood at laryngectomy tube, frequent swallowing, blood-soaked dressings, red blood in nasogastric drainage, agitation, cyanosis, diaphoresis, decreased blood pressure, increased pulse.

- Protect the suture lines. Suction nasal and oral secretions gently. Never suction past the mouth or insert a nasogastric tube without an order.

- Observe for signs and symptoms of tracheoesophageal fistula: Coughing or choking during feedings, bleeding, food particles in tracheal suctioning.

- Supervise initial oral fluid intake. Some coughing and choking may occur until the patient learns to swallow.

- To help compensate for neck muscle weakness, elevate the head of the bed 30–45 degrees. Support the head and neck when repositioning the patient.

- Assess and support patient's psychosocial needs by supporting the patient and family in the grieving process. Patients undergoing this type of surgery experience ''loss'' on many levels: Physiological, psychological and socioeconomic. Provide a means of communication to minimize patient's frustrations. Anticipating patient's needs will also reduce frustrations. Answer call light immediately. Understand that although the patient is unable to talk, the sense of hearing remains intact. Speaking loudly will only contribute to the patient's poor self-concept. A relaxed and calm manner will promote adaptation to new methods of communicating. Allow the patient to finish writing sentences. Explain all new procedures to the patient. Professional psychiatric help may be necessary for the severely depressed patient. Allow the patient to express anger. When appropriate, arrange for a laryngectomee to visit and refer patient to the International Association of Laryngectomees, American Cancer Society, The Lost Chord Club, and New Voice Club.

PATIENT AND FAMILY TEACHING

- If indicated, demonstrate how to remove and insert the laryngectomy tube. Reinsertion is easier with slight flexion of the neck. Usually the stoma is formed by eight weeks and a tube is only necessary at night.

- If home nasogastric tube feedings are indicated, demonstrate proper insertion technique.

- When the patient is ready, demonstrate tracheostomy suctioning. Use a table mirror so the patient can see. Stress the importance of aseptic technique.

- Instruct male patients to avoid lacerations and aspiration when shaving. Be cautious and use an electric shaver.

- Instruct the patient to notify the physician for signs and symptoms of infection of suture lines, pneumonia, and other complications.

- Encourage the patient to continue with speech therapy.

- Advise the patient to maintain good oral hygiene.

- Recommend chewy foods in the diet to help increase muscle tone.

- Advise the patient to wear a protective plastic cover when showering. Swimming should be avoided.

TRACHEOSTOMY

POTENTIAL PROBLEMS

Airway Obstruction	Infection
Respiratory Insufficiency	Tracheal Necrosis
Aspiration of Secretions	Aphasia
Accidental Extubation	Tracheoesophageal Fistula
Hemorrhage	Dehydration
Pneumothorax	Subcutaneous Emphysema
Atelectasis	Mediastinal Emphysema
Dry Mucous Membranes	Psychosocial Problems

KEY NURSING INTERVENTIONS

- See Preoperative and Postoperative Care.

- Maintain a patent airway by keeping head elevated 45 degrees and suctioning secretions every hour and PRN as needed. Encourage patient to cough up secretions when possible. Auscultate lungs for effectiveness of coughing and suctioning (see Respiratory Assessment).

- Observe for signs and symptoms of airway obstruction: Noisy respirations, decreased inspiratory and expiratory volumes, restlessness, use of accessory muscles of respiration.

- Adhere to aseptic suctioning and cleaning technique.

- Note color, character and amount of suctioned secretions. Report excess bleeding to physician.

- Clean inner cannula, if present, and provide stoma care every 2–4 hrs. × 24 hrs. postoperatively, then TID to BID.

- Assess patient for signs and symptoms of respiratory insufficiency: Decreased pO_2; increased pCO_2; anxiety; restlessness; increasing blood pressure and pulse; shallow, rapid respirations; use of accessory muscles with respiration; rales; wheezes; diminished breath sounds; asymmetrical chest movements.

- Prevent tracheal trauma by suctioning gently. Insert catheter with inspirations and with suction off. Apply intermittent suction while withdrawing catheter to prevent damage to the mucosa.

- Keep tracheostomy obturator at the head of bed at all times.
- Keep an extra tracheostomy tube of the same size and type in the room.
- Deflate cuffs that are NOT low pressure every 1 hr. for 5 mins. unless contraindicated. Do not overinflate.
- Assure inflation of cuff prior to PO fluids and for 30 mins. after feeding to prevent aspiration.
- Secure tracheostomy ties with a square knot. (Do not use bows.)
- Change tracheostomy ties PRN using two people—one to hold the tracheostomy tube and one to change the ties. *DO NOT* change ties for 24 hrs. after surgery to allow for stabilization.
- Do not attempt to *force* an accidentally dislodged tracheostomy tube back into the trachea. Obtain qualified help while assuring airway patency and effective ventilation.
- Observe for signs and symptoms of hemorrhage: Bloody secretions and stomach bleeding lasting longer than 8 hrs. postoperatively, increasing pulse, decreasing blood pressure, restlessness, and pallor.
- Assess patient for development of tracheoesophageal fistula: Choking or coughing when eating or drinking and PO intake aspirate from tracheostomy.
- Assist patient with frequent oral hygiene.
- Provide communication devices. Ask ''Yes'' or ''No'' questions. Keep call light within reach.
- Encourage fluids as ordered. Hold head downward to ease swallowing.
- Assess and support patient's psychosocial needs. Feelings of apprehension are common postoperatively. Provide nursing care in a calm and reassuring manner. Be patient when patient attempts to communicate. Help patient deal with feelings of loss and altered body image. Encourage family and significant other contact. Check on patient frequently, offering cheerful assistance.

PATIENT AND FAMILY TEACHING

- Instruct patient in deep breathing and coughing techniques.
- If tracheostomy is permanent for discharge (i.e., sleep apnea), demonstrate placement and care of tracheostomy tube. When the patient is ready, teach clean suctioning technique using a portable suction machine and a mirror.
- Instruct patient in leg and foot exercises while in bed.

THORACIC SURGERY

POTENTIAL PROBLEMS

Respiratory Arrest	Circulatory Insufficiency
Cardiac Arrest	Atelectasis
Airway Obstruction	Pneumonia
Tension Pneumothorax	Gastric Distention
Respiratory Insufficiency	Dehydration
Cardiac Arrhythmias	Infection
Myocardial Infarction	Chest Tube Malfunction
Pulmonary Embolus	Muscle Atrophy
Pulmonary Edema	(Operative Side)
Hemorrhage	Psychosocial Problems

KEY NURSING INTERVENTIONS

- See Preoperative and Postoperative Care.

- See Chest Tubes.

- Assess patient for signs and symptoms of respiratory insufficiency: Decreased pO_2, increased pCO_2, anxiety, restlessness, dyspnea, increasing blood pressure and pulse rate tachypnea, use of accessory muscles of respiration, wheezes, rales, diminished breath sounds, decreased tidal and minute volumes, and asymmetrical chest movements—except with pneumonectomy where asymmetry is normal.

- Observe for signs and symptoms of tension pneumothorax: Chest pain, tachypnea, dyspnea, neck vein distention, tracheal deviation, absent lung sounds, increased CVP, decreased blood pressure, cardiopulmonary arrest. This is a life-threatening situation. Notify physician immediately.

- Observe for signs and symptoms of circulatory insufficiency: Hypotension, high CVP (greater than 10 is indicative of cardiac failure or hypervolemia), low CVP (less than 5 is indicative of hypovolemia), pallor, cyanosis, increased pulse, increased respiratory rate, dyspnea, decreased urinary output (less than 30 cc/hr.). This may be due to hypovolemia or to myocardial pathology.

- Maintain patent airway by encouraging patient to cough and deep breathe every hour postoperatively. Suction mouth and throat if patient is unable to clear secretions effectively. Auscultate lungs to determine the need for suctioning and the effectiveness of patient coughing (see Respiratory System Assessment). Coughing and deep breathing are the most important interventions.

- Observe for signs and symptoms of airway obstruction: Noisy respirations, decreased inspiratory and expiratory volumes, restlessness.

- Monitor for cardiac arrhythmias.

- Prevent complications of thoracic surgery by effective pain management. Controlling pain permits increased ventilation, coughing and deep breathing exercises and position changes. (Usually small, frequent doses of meperidine are prescribed. Morophine is contraindicated.) Observe for respiratory depression following each dose of narcotic.

- When vital signs are stable, elevate head 30–40 degrees. Turning should be done according to physician's orders. (Generally, patients may lie on both sides post lobectomy, on *un*operated side following wedge resections, and turn partially to either side following pneumonectomy.)

- Inspect and percuss bowel for signs of gastric distention: Enlarged, tight abdominal girth and hyperresonance.

- Assess patient for signs and symptoms of pulmonary embolism: Chest pain, dyspnea, fever, hemoptysis, elevated CVP, distended neck veins, rapid respirations, hypoxia, tachycardia, hypotension, apprehension, diaphoresis, nausea, and wheezes. This is a medical emergency.

- Initiate passive range of motion (ROM) exercises to arm on affected side every four hours until patient can tolerate and perform active ROM.

- Assess and support patient's psychosocial needs. Patients having thoracic surgery may be extremely anxious regarding the chest tubes and prognosis. Additionally, pain intensifies existing apprehensions and may interfere with proper care. Nursing care should be reassuring and promote comfort. Help the patient and family deal with changes in body image and body functions. Help establish realistic goals and expectations. Pain control and psychological support will help to overcome such fears. Family contact is most important and should be encouraged but kept within patient tolerance.

PATIENT AND FAMILY TEACHING

- Coughing and deep breathing should be taught preoperatively and reinforced postoperatively. Using a pillow to splint the chest, place in

Fowler's position, instruct the patient to take a deep breath and cough forcefully, holding incision area and tightening abdominal muscles. Assist patient every hour in doing this.

- Inform patient of the purpose for chest tubes. Advise the patient to move carefully to avoid tube dislodgement.

- Explain the reason for ROM exercises to arm on affected side. When patient is ready, instruct in active ROM exercises.

- Teach patient leg and feet exercises while on bed rest. Whem ambulating, explain the benefits of ambulation towards preventing complications.

CHEST TUBE DRAINAGE

POTENTIAL PROBLEMS

Tension Pneumothorax
Abnormal Air Leaks
Crepitus
Reflux of Drainage into
    Chest
Chest Tube Obstruction
Psychosocial Problems

Infection
Malfunction of Equipment
Pain
Muscle Atrophy of Extremity
    On Affected Side

KEY NURSING INTERVENTIONS

- Assess patient for signs and symptoms of tension pneumothorax: Chest pain, tachypnea, dyspnea, neck vein distention, tracheal deviation, absent lung sounds, increased CVP, decreased blood pressure, cardiopulmonary arrest. This is a life-threatening situation. Notify physician immediately.

- Position patient in low- to semi-Fowler's position. Turn patient to *affected* side, keeping a folded bath blanket under the patient to protect the tubes from the patient's body weight and prevent obstruction. Change position frequently.

- Tape all tubing connection sites.

- Prevent dependent loops in tubing by fastening tubing to the bedding with rubber bands and safety pins. Excess tubing can be coiled on the bed. Allow for freedom of movement.

- Maintain patent tubing by "milking" towards drainage container every hour and PRN.

- Keep drainage container below chest at all times.

- Keep container or bottles secure in appropriate bracket to prevent accidental breakage.

- Observe for fluctuations of fluid in water seal chamber as a sign of proper functioning. Normally, fluctuations will stop when there is re-expansion of the lung (usually within 48–72 hours of chest tube insertion). Fluctuations may stop due to the following problems: Obstructed tubing from clot formation, kinking, patient's position or to suction malfunction.

- Never allow drainage section to overfill. If it is necessary to change the drainage section, set up necessary equipment and clamp chest tubes close to patient's chest during the change using two padded clamps. Remove clamps *immediately* after the change. Clamping chest tubes too long may cause tension pneumothorax.

- Keep two padded clamps at bedside at all times.

- Observe for abnormal air leaks in system by looking for *continuous* bubbling in water seal chamber. (Intermittent bubbling is normal and indicates that air is being removed from the pleural cavity. As the lungs re-expand, the bubbling will stop.) Identify source of air leak. Start at insertion site and work down the system. If the leak cannot be identified, notify physician.

- Check insertion site and surrounding area for crepitus and progressive subcutaneous emphysema.

- Notify physician immediately if rapid continuous bubbling occurs (indicative of pleural tear).

- Observe suction section for bubbling in the water as a sign of normal suction functioning. If bubbling in this section stops, the suction unit may be malfunctioning or the patient may have an air leak. (Identify air leak vs. suction malfunction.) Air leak into pleural cavity is indicated by the start of bubbling when the chest tube is clamped near insertion site. Air leak in the system should be ruled out by examining connecting sites, rubber stoppers and bottles. If a new suction machine is applied and there is still absence of bubbling, notify physician.

- Check system every shift for amount of suction ordered by physician. (In a two- or three-bottle system, the long tube is extended into the water at a depth ordered by the physician, usually 20–30 cm. Keep this tube open to air at all times. In a Pleur-Evac the suction chamber should be filled to the precribed level.)

- If suction is not ordered, maintain open air vent.

- Clamping chest tubes should be avoided or performed only momentarily to avoid tension pneumothorax.

- Encourage ROM to upper extremity of affected side every two hours as tolerated.

- Mark drainage level on drainage container with date and time every hour for the first 24 hrs., then a minimum of every shift. Notify physician of excessive drainage.

- Encourage patient to cough and deep breathe every 1–2 hrs.

- Assess and support patient's psychosocial needs. Provide reassurance regarding all procedures related to the chest tube. Medicate patient for pain when indicated to help decrease anxiety. Encourage family or significant other to be with patient and provide sensory stimulation. Keep patient informed of progress and all new orders. Provide care in a relaxed and calm manner.

PATIENT AND FAMILY TEACHING

- Instruct patient to cough and deep breath every 1–2 hrs. Provide a pillow and instruct patient in splinting.
- .Explain all procedures to the patient.
- Teach patient leg and feet exercises while in bed.
- Advise patient to avoid rapid position changes to avoid tube dislodgement.
- See Thoracic Surgery.

CHRONIC OBSTRUCTIVE PULMONARY DISEASE, EMPHYSEMA, CHRONIC BRONCHITIS, ASTHMA

POTENTIAL PROBLEMS

Respiratory Arrest
Arrhythmias
Respiratory Acidosis
Congestive Heart Failure
Pulmonary Edema
Spontaneous Pneumothorax
Respiratory Infection

Cor Pulmonale
Hypoxia
Shortness of Breath
Chest Pain
Malnutrition
Psychosocial Problems

KEY NURSING INTERVENTIONS

- Observe for signs and symptoms of worsening pulmonary obstruction: Shortness of breath, decreased level of consciousness, confusion, agitation, cyanosis, chest pain, increased use of accessory muscles, decreased breath sounds, increased wheezing, irregular pulse, arrhythmias, decreasing pH, increasing pCO_2, decreasing pO_2.

- Help the patient breathe easier during acute episodes. Place the patient in high-Fowler's position or dangle the legs over the side of the bed. Provide a padded overbed table for support. Encourage pursed-lip breathing. Stay with the patient. Administer low-flow oxygen and other respiratory treatments. Caution: Respiratory arrest may occur if a high concentration of oxygen is delivered to chronically hypoxic patients. Never administer nasal oxygen over 2 liters per minute unless otherwise ordered by physician.

- Prepare for tracheal intubation if patient is acute and not responding to therapy.

- Prevent further complications and/or exacerbations by providing an irritant-free environment; eliminate smoke, dust, and flowers; keep the patient away from people with respiratory infections; encourage coughing, deep breathing, and expectoration of sputum; administer postural drainage; suction secretions, if necessary.

- Provide small, frequent meals so the patient does not tire during eating.

- Administer bronchodilators with caution. Observe for nervousness, irregular pulse, tachycardia, ventricular and other arrhythmias, and hypertension.

- Assess and support the patient's psychosocial needs by informing the patient that although this is a chronic condition, it may be controlled by carefully following a plan of care. Observe for depression, anger, and anxiety. Understand that this is common due to being chronically short of breath. Attempt to incorporate patient's idiosyncrasies, especially regarding treatment modalities, into the care plan. This will increase cooperation which will benefit both the patient and the nurse. Help the patient adapt to changes in lifestyle due to being chronically ill.

PATIENT AND FAMILY TEACHING

- Attempt to involve the spouse or significant other in patient care and discharge planning.

- The best time for patient teaching is when the patient is least short of breath.

- Demonstrate diaphragmatic and pursed-lip breathing. Tell the patient to do this during periods of shortness of breath.

- Instruct the patient to avoid situations or environments that may trigger an attack or increase the chance of infection: Smoke, dust, fumes, extreme temperatures, people with upper respiratory tract infections, and crowded areas with poor ventilation. Have the patient stay indoors when air pollution levels are high.

- If the patient is to go home with IPPB, aerosols, oxygen or other equipment, demonstrate their use. Make sure the patient knows how to use them safely.

- Demonstrate postural drainage and chest percussion to the family.

- Instruct the patient to report signs and symptoms of respiratory tract infections so that early therapy may be initiated.

- Stress the importance of medications. Make sure the patient knows the name, dose, schedule, and side effects. Demonstrate how to use an inhaler and advise the patient not to overuse it.

PNEUMONIA

POTENTIAL PROBLEMS

Airway Obstruction	Endocarditis
Respiratory Failure	Myocarditis
Atelectasis	Pericarditis
Empyema	Meningitis
Dehydration	Congestive Heart Failure
Delayed Resolution	Pleural Effusion
Delirium	Pain
Septic Shock	Psychosocial Problems
Superinfections	

KEY NURSING INTERVENTIONS

- Identify patients who have increased susceptibility to pneumonia: Postsurgical patients, immunotherapy, COPD, congestive heart failure, cancer of the lung, prolonged bed rest, fractured ribs, elderly patients, tracheostomy, mechanical ventilation, pain under the diaphragm or any situation that may cause shallow respirations.

- Maintain a patent airway by: Suctioning secretions, elevating head of bed, coughing and deep breathing, postural drainage, chest percussion, and encouraging the patient to expectorate sputum.

- Observe for signs and symptoms of hypoxia: Confusion, restlessness, hallucinations, decreased pO_2, cyanosis of tongue, lips, and nail beds.

- Observe for signs and symptoms of other complications: Septic shock, atelectasis, pneumothorax, empyema, congestive heart failure, delirium, meningitis, respiratory failure, endocarditis, myocarditis, pericarditis.

- Provide an adequate supply of tissues and disposal containers. Change disposal containers frequently.

- Maintain appropriate isolation (see Infection Control).

- Collect sputum specimen as ordered. Avoid collecting saliva (see Specimen Collection).

- Keep the patient well hydrated by the following: Maintain I.V. fluids as ordered, encourage PO fluid intake to at least 2000 cc per day, and maintain accurate intake and output.

PATIENT AND FAMILY TEACHING

- Inform the patient that recovery may be slow. Increase activity gradually. Instruct the patient to avoid overexertion and to get plenty of rest.
- Demonstrate and explain the importance of coughing and deep breathing, chest percussion, and postural drainage.
- Discourage smoking and excessive alcohol intake.
- Stress the importance of good nutrition and staying well hydrated. Drink at least 2000 cc per day if not restricted.
- Inform the patient that one episode of pneumonia increases the chances of recurrent infections. Avoid extreme temperatures and persons with upper respiratory tract infections.

PULMONARY EMBOLUS

POTENTIAL PROBLEMS

Chest Pain   Shortness of Breath
Congestive Heart Failure   Dyspnea
Arrhythmias   Psychosocial Problems
Cardiopulmonary Arrest

KEY NURSING INTERVENTIONS

- Identify the patient who is at high risk for developing pulmonary emboli: Postsurgical patients, pelvic trauma, lower extremity trauma, obesity, oral contraceptive therapy, pregnancy, prolonged bed rest, thrombophlebitis, congestive heart failure, myocardial infarction, cancer, sickle cell anemia.

- Observe for signs and symptoms of pulmonary embolus: Sudden or gradual onset of severe chest pain, dyspnea, shortness of breath, cyanosis, neck vein distention, tachycardia, hypotension, arrhythmias, decreased lung sounds unilaterally, shock, decreased pO_2, increased pCO_2, cardiopulmonary arrest.

- If signs and symptoms continue to worsen, prepare for possible endotracheal intubation, cardiopulmonary arrest, and/or surgery. If the patient remains stable, prepare patient for possible diagnostic studies which may include a chest x-ray, arterial blood gases, EKG, ventilation-perfusion lung scan, and pulmonary angiography.
  NOTE: The clinical manifestations of pulmonary embolism may be vague and may mimic other serious conditions, i.e., myocardial infarction, pneumothorax, tension pneumothorax, cardiac tamponade, congestive heart failure and COPD.

- See Thrombophlebitis for prevention and more key nursing interventions.

- See Anticoagulant Therapy if the patient is placed on Coumadin or heparin.

- Assess and support the patient's psychosocial needs by providing reassurance and staying with the patient during the acute stage.

PATIENT AND FAMILY TEACHING

- See Thrombophlebitis and Anticoagulant Therapy.

CARDIOVASCULAR SYSTEM

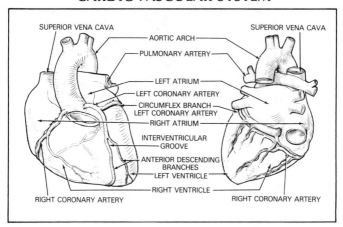

Anterior View

Posterior View

The Coronary Arteries

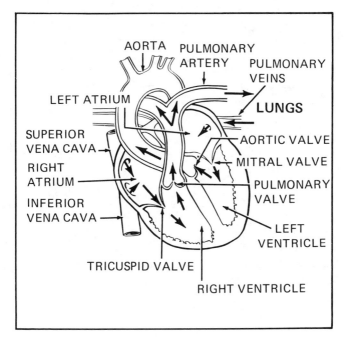

Internal Anatomy of the Heart

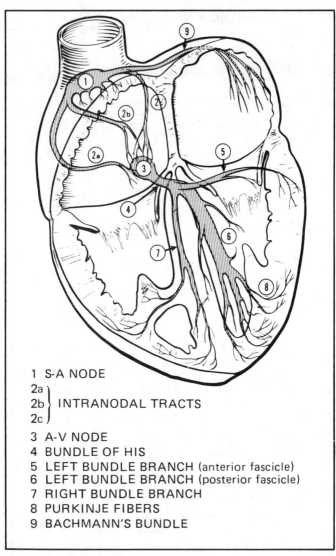

1 S-A NODE
2a ⎫
2b ⎬ INTRANODAL TRACTS
2c ⎭

3 A-V NODE
4 BUNDLE OF HIS
5 LEFT BUNDLE BRANCH (anterior fascicle)
6 LEFT BUNDLE BRANCH (posterior fascicle)
7 RIGHT BUNDLE BRANCH
8 PURKINJE FIBERS
9 BACHMANN'S BUNDLE

The Heart's Conduction System

CARDIOVASCULAR SYSTEM— PHYSIOLOGY SUMMARY

I. MYOCARDIAL CHAMBERS

A. The Right Atrium

1. Posteriorly located.
2. Thin walled.
3. Has a low pressure of 2 to 7 mm Hg.
4. Receives blood from the superior vena cava, the inferior vena cava, the coronary sinus, and thesbian veins.
5. Separated from the right ventricle by the tricuspid valve.

B. The Right Ventricle

1. Anteriorly located.
2. Thin walled.
3. Has a pressure of 20/0–5 mm Hg.
4. Empties into the pulmonary artery through the pulmonic valve.

C. The Left Atrium

1. Thicker walled than the right atrium.
2. Has a pressure of 5 to 10 mm Hg.
3. Receives oxygenated blood through the pulmonary veins.
4. Separated from the left ventricle by the mitral valve.

D. The Left Ventricle

1. Muscular wall is three times as thick as the right ventricle.
2. Has a pressure of 120/0–10 mm Hg.
3. Empties blood into the aorta through the aortic valve.

II. MYOCARDIAL BLOOD FLOW

A. The Right Coronary Artery

1. Extends from the aorta to the right side of the heart into the groove between the right atrium and the right ventricle.

2. Supplies 60% to 70% of blood to the sinoatrial node through its small branches.

3. Supplies the anterior surface of the heart through its large branches.

4. Supplies the posterior surface of the right ventricle through a large branch.

5. Supplies 85% to 95% of blood to the atrioventricular node through small branches.

6. Occlusion causes an inferior wall myocardial infarction.

B. The Left Coronary Artery

Extends from the aorta and divides into two branches, the left anterior descending, and the circumflex arteries.

C. The Left Anterior Descending Artery

1. Supplies the anterior surface of the right heart, the anterior portion of the left ventricle, and interventricular septum.

2. Occlusion causes an anterior or anterior septal myocardial infarction.

D. The Circumflex Artery

1. Supplies the free wall of the left ventricle.

2. Supplies 25% to 40% of the sinoatrial node and 10% to 15% of the atrioventricular node.

3. Occlusion causes a posterior myocardial infarction.

III. CARDIAC CONDUCTION

A. The S-A Node (the pacemaker)

Located on the rear wall of the right atrium, sends out nervous impulses through anterior, middle, and posterior internodal pathways at a rate of 70 to 80 times per minute.

B. Wave of Impulse

Crosses the atria, causing them to contract; it extends to the A-V node, located at the junction of the atria and ventricles.

C. The A-V Node

Transmits the impulses to the ventricles through the bundle of His, located in the septum.

D. The Bundle of His

Divides into the right and left bundle branches and then into a network of fibers called Purkinje fibers.

E. The Purkinje Fibers

Carry the impulses to the ventricles and cause them to contract.

IV. REGULATION

A. Neurohormonal Controls

1. The autonomic nervous system supplies the heart through the medulla, sympathetic, and parasympathetic (right and left vagus) nerves.

2. Sympathetic nerves innervate both the atria and the ventricles. Norepinephrine is the neurotransmitter released by sympathetic nerves which increases the heart rate, increases conduction from the S-A node, and shortens the refractory period.

3. Parasympathetic nerves (vagus) innervate primarily the S-A node, A-V node, and atrial muscle fibers. Acetylcholine is the neurotransmitter released by parasympapthetic nerves which slows conduction from the S-A node to the A-V node, and decreases the strength of atrial contraction.

4. Under stress, the adrenal medulla secretes epinephrine and norepinephrine (catecholamines), which increase the heart rate and contraction.

5. Arterial pressoreceptors, located in the carotid sinuses and the aortic arch, communicate with the medulla oblongata. When arterial pressure becomes too high, the heart rate slows and blood pressure decreases. The reverse also occurs.

6. Venous pressoreceptors, located in the proximal vena cava and right atrium, communicate with the medulla oblongata. When venous pressure increases, the heart rate also increases along with the strength of contraction. The reverse also occurs.

7. The cerebral cortex and hypothalamus communicate with the medulla, causing vasoconstriction and increased heart

rate in response to fear and anger, and vasodilation and increased heart rate in response to embarrassment.

B. Chemoreceptors

Chemoreceptors, located in the carotid bodies and aortic arch, respond to the following:

1. Decreased oxygen.
2. Increased carbon dioxide.
3. Increased hydrogen ion concentration (acidosis) all of which cause vasoconstriction and increased blood pressure.

C. Temperature

1. An increase in temperature causes an increase in heart rate.
2. A decrease in temperature causes a decrease in heart rate.

V. PHARMACOLOGIC RECEPTORS

A. Alpha Receptors

Norepinephrine activates alpha receptors, which causes vasoconstriction.

B. Beta Receptors

Beta receptors are activated by both epinephrine and norepinephrine, which causes the following:

1. Increased heart rate.
2. Vasodilation.
3. Increased myocardial contractility.

CARDIOVASCULAR ASSESSMENT

I. HISTORY

A. Past History of Cardiovascular Problems

1. What type?
2. What therapy was utilized? Did it work?

B. Recent History

1. Progressive weakness?

    a) Increasing fatigue after activity?
    b) Need for more sleep?

2. Shortness of breath?

    a) Episodes of difficulty breathing?
    b) When do they occur?
    c) How many pillows are used at night?

3. Syncope?

    a) Episodes of dizziness, fainting, blackouts?
    b) How often do they occur?

4. Presence of diaphoresis, nausea, vomiting?

    a) What are the circumstances of occurrence?
    b) Does it occur with chest pain?

C. Pain

Verbally assess the patient with chest pain, especially post myocardial infarction. Use the PQRST mnemonic to evaluate pain.

P—Provokes.   What makes the pain worse or better? What was the patient doing prior to the onset of pain?

Q—Quality.   Subjective description of pain by the patient. Use the patient's own words, i.e., burning, stabbing, pressure.

R—Radiation.   Where is the pain located and does it radiate anywhere?

S—Severity. Ask the patient to judge the pain on a scale of 1 to 10 with 10 being the worst pain ever felt.

T—Time. How long has the patient had this pain? When did the pain begin and end?

D. Lifestyle

1. Occupation.
2. Level of emotional stress.
3. Family situation.
4. Presence of Type A personality traits.

E. Activity Level

1. Describe a typical day in terms of activity.
2. Is the patient involved in cardiac rehabilitation or an exercise program?

F. Nutrition

1. Describe a typical breakfast, lunch, dinner, and snacks.
2. Does the patient use salt with meals?

G. Habits

1. Smoking. How long has the patient smoked? How many packs per day?
2. Alcohol. How long has the patient ingested alcohol? How much and what type per day?

H. Medications

1. List medications, including over-the-counter drugs.
2. Allergies.

II. BACKGROUND INFORMATION

A. Lab Values

Check laboratory studies for abnormal values or worsening trends

1. CBC:
   Note especially white blood count, hemoglobin and hematocrit for infectious or anemic trends.

2. Electrolytes:
   Check potassium level, especially if the patient is on diuretics or potassium supplements.

3. Cardiac enzymes:
   Look for trends in elevation of CPK, LDH, SGOT; check isoenzyme studies.

4. Coagulation studies:
   Check PT for oral anticoagulants and PTT for heparin therapy.

5. BUN:
   Evaluate kidney function.

6. Urinalysis:
   Especially note the specific gravity and the presence of protein.

7. Blood gases:
   Check the pH, pO_2, pCO_2, and HCO_3 for normal limits.

8. Serum drug levels:
   Digitalis, Quinidine, Pronestyl, Lidocaine.

B. EKG

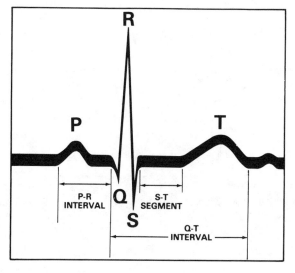

Normal Waveform

Identify possible acute changes or life-threatening arrhythmias. Systematically evaluate EKG

1. Rate:
   Should be between 60 and 100.

2. Normal Sinus Rhythm:
   Look for presence of P waves. There should be one for each QRS complex. P-to-P and R-to-R intervals should be the same.

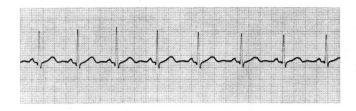

3. Irregular Rhythms:

   a) Atrial Fibrillation:
      No obvious P waves. Most common cause of an irregular pulse.

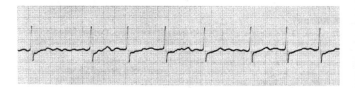

   b) Sinus Arrhythmia:
      Identical P waves. Varies with respirations.

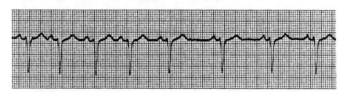

c) Wandering Pacemaker:
   P waves change shape.

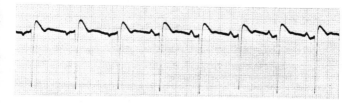

4. Premature Beats:

a) PAC:
   Early P wave followed by normal QRS.

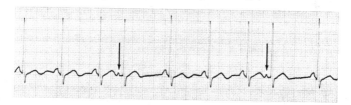

b) PJC:
   Same as above only with an inverted P wave or absent P wave.

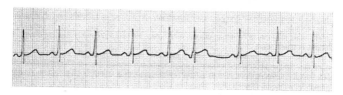

c) PVC:
   Wide, early QRS followed by compensatory pause with no P wave present.

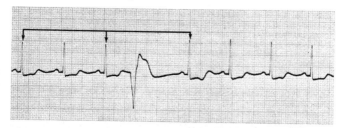

5. Pauses:

   a) Nonconducted PAC:
      Look for different T wave before pause caused by premature P wave. Most common cause of a pause.

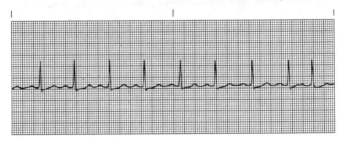

   b) Escape Beats:
      May be atrial, nodal, or ventricular. Always late and occurs after a pause of one complete cycle.

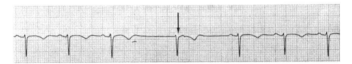

   c) Sinus Arrest:
      Pause in the normal rhythm that does not return to expected next beat.

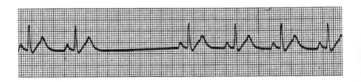

6. Rapid Rhythms:

   a) Sinus Tachycardia:
      Sinus rhythm with rate 100 to 150.

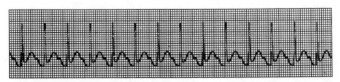

b) Atrial Tachycardia:
   Rate of 150 to 250. Narrow QRS and may or may not see
   P waves.

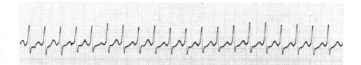

c) Atrial Flutter:
   Rate of 150 or greater. Presence of sawtooth P waves.

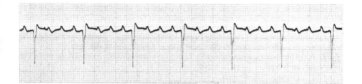

d) Junctional Tachycardia:
   Rapid and regular with absent or no P waves.

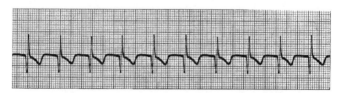

e) Ventricular Tachycardia:
   Rapid, wide complexes in succession.

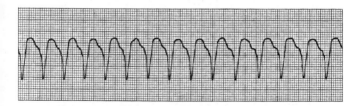

f) Ventricular Fibrillation:
   Very erratic. May be fine or coarse.

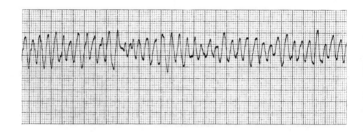

7. Heart Block:

a) SA Block:
Pause in normal rhythm that returns at expected next beat.

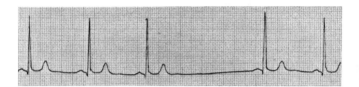

b) First-Degree AV Block:
Normal sinus rhythm, with PR interval greater than .20 seconds.

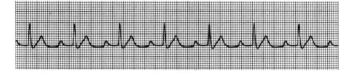

c) Second-Degree AV Block:
More P waves than QRS complexes. May be 1:2, 1:3, 1:4.

d) Mobitz Type I or Wenckebach:
Progressive prolongation of PR interval until there is no QRS. R-to-R interval shortens until there is no QRS.

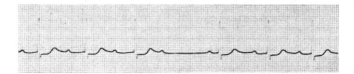

e) Mobitz Type II:
Usually wide QRS complexes and PR interval is constant. P waves produce a QRS until a beat is dropped.

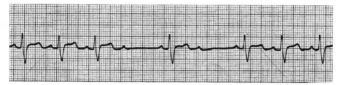

f) Third-Degree AB Block or Complete Heart Block:
P-to-P and R-to-R intervals are regular but at different rates. Ventricular rate is usually slow.

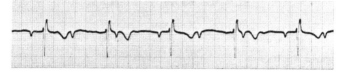

C. Diagnostic Studies

Identify abnormal results of diagnostic studies.

D. Chart

Check old chart for past relevant information.

III. INSPECTION

A. Sensorium

Should be alert and oriented.

B. Cardiac Area

Inspect for pulsations and other abnormalities.

C. Neck Veins

There should be no distention while sitting. Veins should fill and distend as the head of the bed is lowered to the supine position. Check for the presence of waves.

IV. PERCUSSION

Percuss the outline of the heart. Cardiomegaly is present if the apex is percussed past the midclavicular line. Only the left border of the heart may be percussed due to the sternum.

V. PALPATION

A. Apical Impulse

Palpate for the apical impulse or the point of maximal impulse. This is normally at the fifth intercostal space and 7–9 cm from the midsternum.

B. Thrills and Murmurs

Palpate for thrills or murmurs over each of the four heart valve areas. (See VI, B.) Determine when the thrill occurs in the cardiac cycle by palpating the carotid pulse. These findings should correlate with auscultation.

C. Peripheral Pulses

Palpate peripheral pulses for symmetry, quality, and regularity. Peripheral pulses: Carotid, brachial, radial, ulnar, femoral, popliteal, dorsalis pedis, and posterior tibialis.

D. Pulse Deficit

Check for pulse deficit by simultaneously palpating the radial while auscultating the apical pulse. The difference between the two is the pulse deficit.

VI. AUSCULTATION

A. Technique

The room must be quiet. Use both the bell and the diaphragm of the stethoscope over each valve area. The bell is for low-pitched sounds, while the diaphragm is for higher-pitched sounds.

B. Location of Valve Areas

1. Aortic area—Second right intercostal space close to sternum.

2. Pulmonic area—Second left intercostal space close to sternum.

3. Tricuspid area—Fifth left intercostal space close to sternum.

4. Mitral area—Over apex or fifth left intercostal space, about midclavicular line.

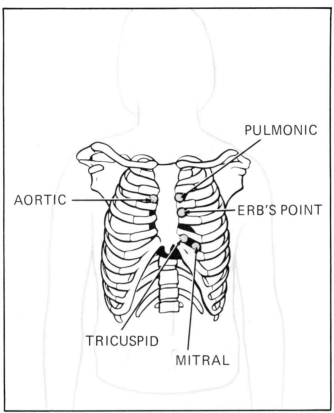

Areas for Cardiac Auscultation

C. Normal Heart Sounds

Normal heart sounds are probably caused by closure of valves. The normal heart is silent during diastole and systole.

1. S_1, the first heart sound, is caused by the closure of both the mitral and tricuspid valves. It is usually heard throughout the whole heart area but best heard over the apex or mitral area. This is the recognized beginning of the cardiac cycle and should be used as a reference point.

2. S_2, the second heart sound, is caused by the valve closure of the aortic and pulmonic valves. This sound is best heard over the respective valve areas. A splitting of these sounds is normal during inspiration.

D. Abnormal Heart Sounds

Extremely abnormal heart sounds should be identified. Classification and diagnosis is difficult and only necessary for specialized nursing.

1. Quiet or muffled heart sounds. May be caused by a thick chest wall, severe fluid overload, or cardiac tamponade.

2. Gallops are low in pitch and may sound similar to S_1 and S_2 heart sounds. It may sound as though the heart has an extra third sound, or a horse's gallop. If the extra sound occurs during ventricular filling, it is called an S_3; if it occurs during atrial contraction or right before S_1, it is called an S_4. Gallops are best heard over the apex and are a cardinal sign of congestive heart failure.

3. Snaps and clicks are caused by the rapid displacement of a valve from high pressure due to stenosis. They are high-pitched and are often associated with murmurs.

4. Murmurs are caused by turbulent flow through a valve due to congenital defects, narrowed valves, or from back flow through an unclosed valve. They may be high- or low-pitched. Murmurs are described by their place in the cardiac cycle, location, intensity, pitch, and radiation.

5. Friction rub may sound like two pieces of leather rubbing together. It is heard throughout the heart area and is associated with pericarditis.

ANGINA PECTORIS

POTENTIAL PROBLEMS

Unstable Angina   Hypoxemia
Myocardial Infarction   Nitrite Side Effects
Congestive Heart Failure   Beta-Adrenergic Side Effects
Arrhythmias   Psychosocial Problems

KEY NURSING INTERVENTIONS

- When anginal attack occurs, stop patient's activity and assist to sitting or lying position, have patient remain quiet until pain subsides, administer nitroglycerin as ordered (usually one tablet under tongue, which may be repeated every 5–10 minutes up to three tablets), and take blood pressure and pulse every 3–4 minutes.

- Assess nature of anginal attacks and document the following: When attack occurred in relation to patient's activity or other events, location of pain, duration, accompanying symptoms (nausea, diaphoresis, pallor, shortness of breath, etc.), elapsed time before pain was relieved.

- Monitor duration of pain and assess patient for reports of deviations from usual attacks. Pain lasting longer than 15 minutes or deviations may be indicative of myocardial infarction and must be reported immediately.

- Assess patient for developing congestive heart failure:
  Left-sided—Pulmonary congestion, dyspnea, orthopnea, paroxysmal nocturnal dyspnea, cough, fatigability, tachycardia, S_3 ventricular gallop, insomnia, restlessness.
  Right sided—Ankle edema, weight gain, pitting edema, upper abdominal pain due to liver enlargement, distended neck veins, anorexia, nausea, nocturia, weakness.

- Monitor pulse carefully for undocumented arrhythmias.

- Observe for side effects of nitroglycerin and report to physician: Headaches, dizziness, syncope, vomiting, visual disturbances, flushing.

- Observe for side effects of beta-adrenergic drugs (Inderal): Nausea, vomiting, mental depression, diarrhea, bradycardia, bronchospasm. **NOTE:** Inderal may precipitate congestive heart failure.
- Assess and support patient's psychosocial needs. Recognize that if the patient who has chronic angina is not allowed to keep nitroglycerin at the bedside for self-administration, the patient may become extremely anxious. Try to obtain permission from the physician in these instances. Severe attacks and side effects from medications may cause irritability and personality changes. Include family or significant other in care plan and discuss mood changes with family and physician. Knowledge of physiological reasons for angina will help reduce anxieties and fears.

PATIENT AND FAMILY TEACHING

- Teach patient and significant other correct nitroglycerin administration.
- Instruct patient to sit or lie down before taking nitroglycerin to reduce incidence of dizziness and faintness.
- Inform patient of the side effects of nitroglycerin and that they will lessen as tolerance to the drug increases.
- Advise patient not to take alcohol with nitroglycerin which may induce shock-like symptoms.
- Instruct patient to keep nitroglycerin fresh and to throw out expired bottles.
- Stress the importance of keeping nitroglycerin with the patient at all times and to protect it from light by keeping it in its brown bottle.
- Tell patient that pain which differs from the usual anginal attack or lasts longer than 15–20 minutes unrelieved by nitroglycerin should be reported to the physician immediately, and the patient should seek emergency treatment.
- Recommend that the patient avoid activities which precipitate anginal attacks. After meals the patient should rest.
- Inform patient of side effects of other prescribed medications and proper administration.
- Discuss precipitation conditions and high risk factors such as anxiety, being overweight, smoking, stressful lifestyle.

CONGESTIVE HEART FAILURE, PULMONARY EDEMA

POTENTIAL PROBLEMS

Refractory Heart Failure	Pulmonary Edema
Myocardial Infarction	Peripheral Edema
Pulmonary Infarction	Dyspnea
Digitalis Toxicity	Chest Pain
Thrombophlebitis	Pneumonia
Arrhythmias	Fatigue
Hypokalemia	Hyponatremia
Shock	Psychosocial Problems

KEY NURSING INTERVENTIONS

- Observe for signs and symptoms of acute pulmonary edema: Severe dyspnea; orthopnea; pallor, tachycardia; frothy, blood-tinged sputum; anxiety; diaphoresis; coarse rales; wheezes; cyanosis.

- *FOR PULMONARY EDEMA:*

  - This is a medical emergency. Notify physician immediately.

  - Maintain high-Fowler's position.

  - Administer high-flow oxygen per face mask as ordered.

  - Usual intravenous medications include vasodilators, diuretics, and aminophylline.

  - When using rotating tourniquets manually, assure that venous flow is obstructed but arterial flow remains intact and that tourniquets are rotated every 15 minutes.

  - Prepare to assist physician with intubation if dyspnea does not improve.

- Assess patient for signs and symptoms of cardiogenic shock: Pulmonary congestion, marked dyspnea, decreased tissue perfusion (cyanosis, pallor), hypotension.

- Assess patient for signs and symptoms of digitalis toxicity: Anorexia, nausea, vomiting, diarrhea, headache, fatigue, lethargy, depression, irritability, drowsiness, convulsions, arrhythmias. tachycardia or bradycardia, visual disturbances.

- See Digitalis Therapy.

- Promote bed rest as ordered. Keep necessary patient articles including call light within reach. Maintain a quiet, nonstressful environment. Use bedside commode as ordered. Provide comfort measures frequently (i.e., back rubs, dry pillow covers, position changes, etc.). Administer mild sedatives PRN as ordered for insomnia. Schedule daily activity to allow for uninterrupted rest periods.

- Prevent complications of bed rest (see The Immobilized Patient).

- Maintain prescribed diet (usually low-sodium, low-residue, bland diet in small, frequent feedings).

- Monitor laboratory studies (electrolytes, pH, blood urea nitrogen) for disturbances of diuretic therapy (see Fluid and Electrolyte Imbalances).

- Maintain fluid restriction as ordered. Use microdrip tubing on all intravenous solutions. Maintain accurate intake and output.

- Monitor blood pressure closely when vasodilators (i.e., nitrates, nitroprusside, hydralazine, prazosin) are used. Report sudden hypotension.

- Assist patient with nonlabored breathing. Place in high-Fowler's position. Assist patient to lean on padded overbed table.

- Monitor accurate daily weights. Use same scale and weigh patient at same time every day wearing the same type of patient gown.

- Assess and support patient's psychosocial needs. Advise patient and family to avoid situations which create anxiety and emotional upset. Explain all procedures and answer patient's questions as much as possible. Convey a reassuring attitude which will reduce fears and promote mental rest. Include significant other in care plan.

PATIENT AND FAMILY TEACHING

- Instruct patient and significant other to observe for signs and symptoms of recurrence after discharge: Weight gain, peripheral edema, orthopnea, dyspnea, lethargy, cough, nocturia, anorexia.

- Explain the signs and symptoms of digitalis toxicity. Stress the importance of correct digitalis administration and of reporting symptoms of toxicity immediately (see Digitalis Therapy).

- Inform patient of prescribed activity limitations.

- Advise patient to avoid obesity and excessive eating and drinking.
- Extreme climate temperatures are to be avoided to reduce cardiac workload.
- Explain the importance of following the medical regime outlined by physician and other health team members.

DIGITALIS THERAPY

POTENTIAL PROBLEMS

Digitalis Toxicity	Congestive Heart Failure
Hypokalemia	Arrhythmias

KEY NURSING INTERVENTIONS

- Assess patient for signs and symptoms of digitalis toxicity: Anorexia, nausea, vomiting, diarrhea, headache, fatigue, lethargy, depression, irritability, drowsiness, convulsions, arrhythmias, tachycardia or bradycardia, visual disturbances.

- Withhold digitalis and notify physician if pulse is less than 60 or greater than 100 per minute, signs of toxicity are present, or blood levels indicate higher than therapeutic levels.

- Check radial and apical pulse for rate and rhythm for one full minute before each digitalis administration.

- Check dosage and name of drug before administration.

- Monitor patient for developing congestive heart failure indicative of ineffective digitalis therapy:
  Left sided—Pulmonary congestion, dyspnea, orthopnea, paroxysmal noctural dyspnea, cough, fatigability, tachycardia, S_3 ventricular gallop, insomnia, restlessness.
  Right-sided—Ankle edema, weight gain, pitting edema, upper abdominal pain due to liver enlargement, distended neck veins, anorexia, nausea, nocturia, weakness.

- Observe for signs of hypokalemia (see Fluid and Electrolytes Imbalances).

- Identify and closely monitor patients with conditions producing increased sensitivity to digitalis: Diuretic therapy, hypokalemia, liver or kidney disease, vomiting, diarrhea, increased age of patient, acute myocardial infarction, chronic obstructive pulmonary disease, alkalosis, acidosis.

PATIENT AND FAMILY TEACHING

- Instruct the patient and family in the importance of monitoring patient's pulse for one full minute every day prior to digitalis administration. Demonstrate pulse locations and pulse-taking technique.

- Stress the importance of maintaining the prescribed schedule and not to take extra doses if one is missed.

- Review signs and symptoms of digitalis toxicity and advise contacting the physician if observed.

- Instruct patient in the proper administration of potassium supplements if prescribed. Emphasize the importance of potassium in effective digitalis therapy.

CARDIOGENIC SHOCK

POTENTIAL PROBLEMS

Cardiac Arrest	Shock Lung
Acidosis	Renal Failure
Cardiac Arrhythmias	Coma
Pulmonary Edema	Psychosocial Problems

KEY NURSING INTERVENTIONS

- Assess patient for signs and symptoms of cardiogenic shock: Poor tissue and organ perfusion, low systolic pressure (usually 90 mm Hg or less), tachycardia, arrhythmias, chest pain, cool and clammy skin, absent or diminished peripheral pulses, agitation, restlessness, confusion, somnolence, oliguria, S_3 or S_4 heart sounds. Notify physician and supervisor immediately.

- Observe for signs and symptoms of acute pulmonary edema: Severe dyspnea; orthopnea; pallor; tachycardia; frothy, blood-tinged sputum; anxiety; diaphoresis; coarse rales; wheezes; cyanosis.

- Check blood pressure, respirations, apical and peripheral pulses every 5–15 minutes until patient is transferred to CCU or condition stabilizes.

- Use microdrip tubing on intravenous line. Administer intravenous solution cautiously using mechanical controller if possible.

- Monitor cardiac rhythm. Observe for life-threatening arrhythmias (ventricular tachycardia, ventricular fibrillation, asystole, etc.).

- Prepare to do CPR if necessary. Have crash cart available.

- Attach urometer to urethral catheter bag and monitor urinary output frequently. Report urine output less than 30 cc/hour.

- Administer oxygen at prescribed flow rate.

- Position patient to minimize labored breathing. (Do *NOT* use Trendelenburg position).

- Usual medications include the following: Dopamine, norepinephrine, digitalis, nitroprusside, Lasix, and Levophed.

- Reassure patient by explaining procedures and maintaining a calm, confident manner. Answer patient's questions.

PATIENT AND FAMILY TEACHING

- Notify family of patient's transfer to CCU. Arrange for physician to speak to family.

BACTERIAL ENDOCARDITIS

POTENTIAL PROBLEMS

Congestive Heart Failure   Anemia
Aortic Valve Damage   Metastatic Abscess
Embolism/Infarction   Psychosocial Problems
  (Pulmonary, Peripheral,
  Bowel, Kidney, Spleen)

KEY NURSING INTERVENTIONS

- Assess patient for signs and symptoms of congestive heart failure:
  Left-sided—Pulmonary congestion, dyspnea, orthopnea, paroxysmal noctural dyspnea, cough, fatigability, tachycardia, S_3 ventricular gallop, insomnia, restlessness.
  Right-sided—Ankle edema, weight gain, pitting edema, upper abdominal pain, distended neck veins, anorexia, nausea, nocturia, weakness.

- Monitor patient for signs and symptoms of embolic phenomena:
  Splenic infarction—Enlarged and tender spleen, pain in upper abdomen.
  Renal infarction—Flank pain, hematuria.
  Cerebral infarction—Hemiparesis, visual disturbance, dysphasia.
  Peripheral infarction—Discoloration of extremity, coolness, diminished pulses, gangrene of toes or fingertips.
  Pulmonary infarction—Dyspnea, hemoptysis, coughing, chest pain.
  Myocardial infarction—Steady, severe chest pain unrelieved by rest or nitrates, diaphoresis, pallor, hypotension, dyspnea, nausea, vomiting, tachycardia or bradycardia, anxiety.

- Encourage adequate fluid and nutritional intake.

- Provide uninterrupted rest periods each day.

- While patient is on bed rest, prevent complications of inactivity. Encourage turning, coughing, and deep breathing. Encourage leg and foot exercises (see The Immobilized Patient).

- Prevent complications of long-term intravenous therapy. Use large veins when possible to minimize vessel trauma from potent antibiotics. Use iodine preparations to cleanse skin prior to venipuncture. Keep antimicrobial ointment on insertion site. Rotate intravenous site every three days.

- Administer antibiotics at exact times to prevent decline in blood levels.
- Assess and support patient's psychosocial needs. High fevers and prolonged, intensive antibiotic therapy may exhaust and frustrate the patient and family. Maintain a hopeful and optimistic attitude at all times. Spend time with patient to promote verbalization of feelings. Encourage social time with family and friends but do not allow patient to become too tired. Include significant others in care plan. Encourage self-care activities but prevent patient from becoming fatigued.

PATIENT AND FAMILY TEACHING

- Instruct patient prior to discharge in the importance of preventing relapse. Emphasize early treatment of illness such as sore throats, injuries, boils, etc.
- Stress adherence to medication regime as prescribed.
- Discuss the importance of rest and avoiding overexertion.
- Advise patient to discuss possible dental work involving gum bleeding with the physician beforehand.
- Emphasize a preventive approach in discharge planning.

PERICARDITIS

POTENTIAL PROBLEMS

Congestive Heart Failure   Pericardial Effusion
Cardiac Tamponade   Psychosocial Problems
Arrhythmias

KEY NURSING INTERVENTIONS

- Assess patient for signs and symptoms of pericardial effusion: Increased area of cardiac dullness, muffled heart sounds, distended neck veins.

- Observe for signs and symptoms of cardiac tamponade: Decreased systolic pressure, narrow pulse pressure, tachycardia, pulses paradoxus, distant heart sounds, dyspnea, orthopnea, cyanosis, restlessness, diaphoresis, distended neck veins.
  NOTE: Cardiac tamponade is a medical emergency. Report signs and symptoms to physician immediately.

- Assist dyspneic patients to breathe easier by maintaining semi-Fowler's position and providing a padded over-bed table to lean on.

- Prevent complications of immobility. Encourage coughing, turning, and deep breathing. Since these activities may aggravate pericardial pain, medicate patient for pain before encouraging patient. Encourage foot and leg exercises (see The Immobilized Patient).

- Notify physician if pericardial pain increases in intensity, frequency, or duration. This may be indicative of impending myocardial infarction.

- Assess patient for signs and symptoms of congestive heart failure: Pulmonary congestion, dyspnea, tachycardia, S_3 ventricular gallop, ankle edema, pitting edema, distended neck veins, abdominal pain, nausea, weakness.

- Provide uninterrupted rest periods in patient's daily schedule.

- Assess and support patient's psychosocial needs. Pericardial pain and dyspnea can cause extreme anxiety and fear which may be difficult for the patient to cope with. Keep patient well informed of medical and nursing plan of care. Approach patient with confidence. Encourage family support and socializing. Do not allow patient to become too tired.

PATIENT AND FAMILY TEACHING

- Instruct patient to stop activities which increase chest pain and dyspnea.
- Advise patient to rest at frequent intervals and especially after meals to minimize oxygen demands on the heart.
- If the patient is to take digitalis upon discharge, see Patient and Family Teaching for Digitalis Therapy.
- Include significant other in care plan and discharge planning.

MYOCARDIAL INFARCTION

POTENTIAL PROBLEMS

Cardiac Arrest   Pulmonary Embolism
Congestive Heart Failure   Shoulder-Hand Syndrome
Cardiogenic Shock   Psychosocial Problems
Arrhythmias

KEY NURSING INTERVENTIONS

Acute Stage on the Medical/Surgical Unit

- Notify physician and supervisor immediately upon recognition of clinical symptoms: Chest pain (constant, unrelieved by nitrates, and unrelated to respirations or exertion); cold, clammy skin with pallor; complaints of indigestion, hypotension, tachycardia or bradycardia, dyspnea, faintness, nausea, vomiting.
- Maintain strict bedrest.
- Record vital signs every 15 minutes until transferred to the CCU.
- Administer oxygen per nasal cannula as ordered (usually 4–6 liters/minute).
- Apply EKG monitor.
- Obtain 12-lead EKG as ordered.
- Keep crash cart outside room until transferred to the CCU.
- Initiate CPR if no pulse or respirations.
- See Cardiogenic Shock.
- Use microdrip tubing on intravenous fluids.
- Prepare to transfer to CCU.
- Assess and support patient's psychosocial needs. Denial is a common attitude in the initial stages of a myocardial infarction, which the nurse must not allow to interfere with good nursing judgment. Intense and prolonged chest pain may also evoke fear and apprehension in the patient. Proceed with necessary nursing interventions calmly and reassuringly.

Post-Acute Stage on the Medical/Surgical Unit

- Take apical pulse with vital signs. Assess rhythm for arrhythmias if no monitor is available on the unit.

- Assess patient for signs and symptoms of congestive heart failure:
  Left-sided—Pulmonary congestion, dyspnea, orthopnea, paroxysmal nocturnal dyspnea, cough, fatigability, tachycardia, S_3 ventricular gallop, insomnia, restlessness.
  Right-sided—Ankle edema, weight gain, pitting edema, upper abdominal pain, distended neck veins, anorexia, nausea, nocturia, weakness.

- Observe for signs and symptoms of pulmonary embolism: Chest pain, dyspnea, fever, hemoptysis, elevated CVP, distended neck veins, rapid respirations, hypoxia, tachycardia, hypotension, apprehension, diaphoresis, nausea, wheezes.

- Observe for signs and symptoms of shoulder-hand syndrome: Pain and tenderness in affected shoulder; weak, painful, and swollen affected hand.

- Encourage range of motion exercises to upper extremities to prevent shoulder-hand syndrome.

- Allow patient to participate in self-care hygiene activities. Activity limitations ordered by physician should be strictly adhered to.

- Provide uninterrupted rest periods.

- Prevent complications of bedrest (see The Immobilized Patient).

- Diet restrictions usually include no caffeine, cola, nicotine, high cholesterol, restricted sodium and avoidance of iced drinks.

- Meeting the psychosocial needs of the patient may include the following: Listening to expressed fears and anxieties, offering reassurance, providing information about after care and medication regime. Include significant other and family in care plan. Encourage nonfatiguing socializing. Include social worker and mental health nurse in care plan when necessary. Explore lifestyle changes and role changes necessary to adapt to post-myocardial infarction status. Refer patient and family to a cardiac rehabilitation program.

PATIENT AND FAMILY TEACHING

- Consult with physician regarding any limitations on patient teaching.

- Effective patient teaching should be done only when the patient is ready to learn without pain.

- Inform patient that depression is a normal and common feeling after a myocardial infarction if the patient is depressed.
- Instruct patient to avoid isometric-type activities which may strain the heart.
- Emphasize that activities causing chest pain, dyspnea or fatigue should be stopped immediately.
- Large meals should be avoided.
- All meals should be taken slowly. Advise patient to rest for approximately two hours after every meal to prevent strain on the heart.
- Reinforce dietary limitations. Consult with dietitian for patient teaching.
- Sexual intercourse should be resumed per physician's order. Usual instructions include stopping intercourse if dyspnea, chest pain, palpitations, fatigue or insomnia occur on the day following intercourse.
- Instruct patient to report to physician immediately if the following occurs: Chest pain is not relieved by nitroglycerin; dyspnea, ankle edema, dizziness, fatigue, tachycardia or bradycardia are experienced.
- Instruct patient in nitroglycerin administration guidelines (see Angina Pectoris).

CIRCULATORY SYSTEM

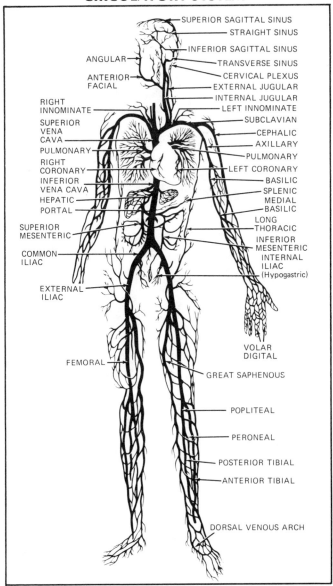

Veins

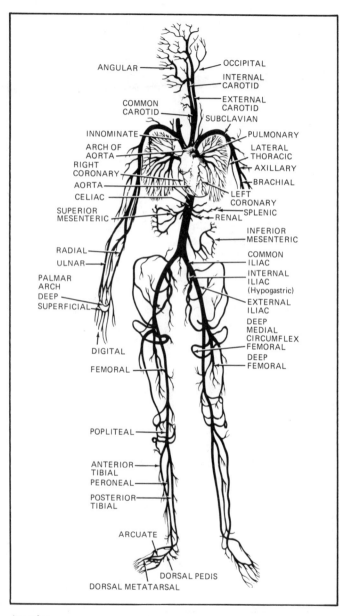

Arteries

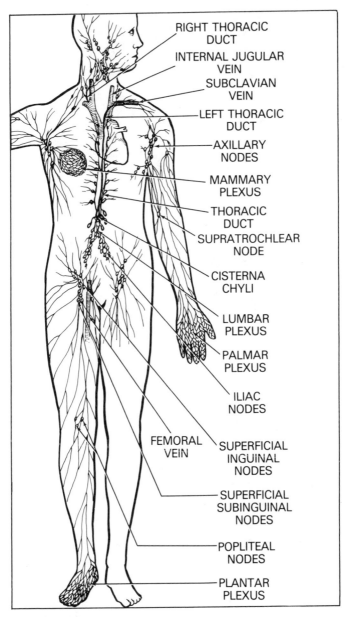

Lymphatic System

CIRCULATORY SYSTEM— PHYSIOLOGY SUMMARY

I. BLOOD

A. Components

Blood consists of plasma and cells. There are three types of cells.

1. Erythrocytes (RBC).
2. Leukocytes (WBC).
3. Thrombocytes (platelets).

B. Erythrocytes (RBC)

1. Transport O_2 and CO_2 via hemoglobin.
2. Formed in red bone marrow (in adults) in the following areas:

   a) Cranium.
   b) Ribs.
   c) Sternum.
   d) Vertebrae bodies.
   e) Proximal epiphyses of humeri and femurs.

3. Stages of cell development are:

   a) Stage I—Erythroblasts.
   b) Stage II—Reticulocytes.
   c) Stage III—Normoblasts.
   d) Stage IV—Erythrocytes.

4. Life span = approximately 120 days.
5. Erythropoisis (RBC formation) is stimulated by the following:

   a) A decreased number of RBC.
   b) Tissue hypoxia.

   This stimulates release of erythropoitin from kidneys, which stimulates red bone marrow activity.

6. Iron, amino acid, copper, vitamin B compounds, and gastric intrinsic factor are necessary for RBC production.

C. Leukocytes (WBC)

1. There are two types of leukocytes.

	Normal Concentration
a) Granular	
(1) Juvenile neutrophils (bands)	4%
(2) Segmented neutrophils (segs)	62%
(3) Eosinophils	2.3%
(4) Basophils	0.4%
b) Nongranular	
(1) Monocytes	5.3%
(2) Lymphocytes	30%

2. WBC function as a defense mechanism through phagocytosis and the formation of antibodies.

3. They are formed in bone marrow and lymphatic tissue.

D. Platelets

1. Function to initiate blood coagulation.

2. Are formed in red bone marrow.

E. Plasma

1. The liquid in blood without the cells.

2. Contains water and solutes (proteins, glucose, amino acids, lipids, lactic acid, urea, uric acid, creatinine, O_2, CO_2, hormones, and enzymes).

3. Plasma proteins = Albumin, globulins, fibrinogen.

4. Plasma proteins are made in the liver.

F. Major Antigens and Antibodies

1. There are four major blood groups.

   a) Type A—A antigen on RBC; this contains anti-B antibodies.

   b) Type B—B antigen on RBC; this contains anti-A antibodies.

    c) Type AB—A and B antigens on RBC; neither A or B antibodies are present.

    d) Type O—Neither A or B antigens present; this contains anti-A and anti-B antibodies.

2. Rh-positive blood—Rh factor present on RBC.

3. Rh-negative blood—Rh factor not present on RBC.

4. Anti-Rh antibodies are produced slowly after an Rh-negative person is exposed to Rh-positive blood.

II. COAGULATION

A. Mechanisms

1. Blood coagulation is initiated through two types of mechanisms.

    a) Intrinsic = starts in the blood itself.

    b) Extrinsic = starts after trauma to tissues.

2. Both mechanisms produce prothrombin activator.

B. Clot Formation

1. Both prothrombin and fibrinogen are made in the liver along with other clotting factors. These are necessary for clot formation.

2. Once prothrombin activator is made, coagulation follows this pathway:

$$
\begin{array}{l}
\text{PROTHROMBIN ACTIVATOR} + Ca^{++} + \text{PLATELET FACTORS} \\
\qquad\qquad\downarrow \\
\text{PROTHROMBIN} \longrightarrow \text{THROMBIN} \\
\qquad\qquad\qquad\qquad\downarrow \\
\qquad\qquad\text{FIBRINOGEN} \longrightarrow \text{FIBRIN THREADS (clot)}
\end{array}
$$

III. CIRCULATION

A. Blood

1. Transported to all parts of the body from the heart through arteries.

2. Arteries become thinner and smaller in diameter as they become arterioles.

B. Capillaries

1. The median microscopic vessels between arterioles and venules.
2. They are one cell in thickness and surrounded by a semi-permeable membrane.
3. The arteriole side of the capillary unit allows oxygen and nutrients to be transported out into the tissues.
4. The venule side allows carbon dioxide and other waste byproducts to be transported into the vessels.

C. Venules

Become veins as they increase in size and thickness.

D. Systemic Circulation

Arises from the aorta and extends to all parts of the body except the lungs.

E. Pulmonary Circulation

1. The flow of blood from the right ventricle through the right and left pulmonary arteries and into the lungs.
2. This blood carries CO_2 which is released into the alveoli where oxygen is then picked up.
3. Pulmonary veins return oxygen-rich blood to the left atrium.

IV. BLOOD PRESSURE

A. Systolic Pressure

The pressure exerted by blood against the vessel walls during contraction of the ventricles.

B. Diastolic Pressure

The pressure exerted by blood against the vessel walls during relaxation of the ventricles.

C. Influencing Factors

Blood pressure is determined by:

1. Volume of blood in vessels.
2. Cardiac minute output.
3. Peripheral resistance.
4. Blood viscosity.
5. Arteriole diameter.

V. NEUROHUMERAL REGULATION

A. Blood Vessels

1. All are innervated by the sympathetic branch of the autonomic nervous system.
2. Only the heart involves both sympathetic and parasympathetic innervation.

B. Vasodilation

1. Occurs when pressoreceptors (baroreceptors), located in the aortic arch, carotid sinuses, and nearly every large artery in the thoracic and neck area, are stimulated.
2. Stimulation of pressoreceptors occurs with an increase in blood pressure.
3. These impulses travel to the medulla where the vasomotor center is inhibited and the vagus center is stimulated.
4. Vagus stimulation causes vasodilation.

C. Vasoconstriction

1. Occurs when the blood pressure decreases.
2. Pressoreceptor impulses decrease with low blood pressure which stimulates the vasomotor center, causing vasoconstriction.
3. Norepenephrine is the neurotransmitter which causes vasoconstriction.

D. Circulation

A low pO_2, pH, and a high pCO_2 stimulate chemoreceptors in the aortic arch and carotid arteries which stimulate the vasomotor center. The result is increased circulation.

VI. LYMPH CAPILLARIES AND VESSELS

A. Lymphatic Capillaries

1. Originate as microscopic blind-ended vessels and are located in the intercellular spaces throughout the entire body.

2. Carry lymph from the intercellular spaces to lymphatic vessels.

3. Those capillaries in the intestine are called lacteals and absorb digested fat called chyle.

B. Lymphatic Vessels

1. Larger, thicker-walled, and contain valves which allow lymphatic fluid to flow in one direction only.

2. Direct lymph to the thorax where the vessels merge into two main lymphatic ducts, the right lymphatic duct and the thoracic duct.

VII. LYMPHATIC DUCTS

A. The Right Lymphatic Duct

Receives lymph from the right upper quadrant of the body (the upper right lobe of the liver, the right lung, the right side of the heart, the right arm, the right side of the head and neck), drains into the right lymphatic duct which then empties into the right subclavian vein.

B. The Thoracic Duct

Receives lymph from the entire body (except the right upper quadrant) and empties into the left subclavian vein.

VIII. LYMPHATIC FUNCTION

A. Lymph Vessels

1. Return water and proteins from interstitial fluid to the blood. This is only a means for proteins to return to the bloodstream.

2. Drain into lymph nodes where lymph fluid is filtered and receives lymphocytes, monocytes, antibodies, and globulins.

B. Lacteals

Participate in digestion by absorbing digested fats.

IX. LYMPH NODES

A. Lymph Nodes

Small, oval-shaped bodies of lymphatic tissue located mainly in groups throughout the body.

B. Function

1. Slow the rate of lymphatic flow and allow the reticuloendothelial cells lining the vessels to filter the fluid and phagocytize noxious materials (cancer cells, inflammatory particles).

2. Form lymphocytes and monocytes which are carried to the blood by the lymph fluid along with antibodies and globulins.

X. SPLEEN

A. The Spleen

An oval-shaped organ located in the upper left abdominal quadrant beneath the diaphragm.

B. Function

1. Blood and platelet destruction. Reticuloendothelial cells destroy old red blood cells and abnormal platelets by phagocytosis. Iron and globin are saved and returned to the bloodstream.

2. Hemopoiesis. The spleen produces red blood cells in the fetus and afterbirth only in some diseases (hemolytic anemia).

3. Blood reservoir. The spleen is capable of storing several hundred milliliters of blood in the splenic pulp. In stressful situations, the sympathetic stimulation causes the smooth

muscle in the capsule to constrict and express most of the stored blood into the circulation.

4. Phagocytosis. Macrophages line the venous sinuses and the splenic pulp. Microorganisms and debris are phagocytized by these cells and removed from circulation.

XI. THE THYMUS GLAND

A. The Thymus Gland

A flat two-lobed organ located in the chest anterior to the aorta and posterior to the sternum.

B. Function

The thymus gland is involved in the production of antibodies and also manufactures lymphocytes.

CIRCULATORY SYSTEM ASSESSMENT

I. HISTORY

A. Past history of peripheral vascular or lymphatic conditions

1. What type?
2. What therapy was utilized? Did it work?

B. Recent History

1. Pain in extremities (hands and feet)?
2. Pain in joints?
3. Redness in area where lymph nodes are located?
4. Intolerance to heat or cold?
5. Blue hands or feet?
6. Swelling of the extremities?
7. Decreased sensation?
8. Skin changes (see Integumentary Assessment)?

C. Pain

Use PQRST mnemonic.

P—Provokes.   What makes the pain worse or better? What was the patient doing prior to the onset of pain?

Q—Quality.   Subjective description of pain by the patient. Use the patient's own words, i.e., burning, stabbing, pressure.

R—Radiation.   Where is the pain located and does it radiate anywhere?

S—Severity.   Ask the patient to judge the pain on a scale of 1 to 10 with 10 being the worst pain ever felt.

T—Time.   How long has the patient had this pain? When did the pain begin and end?

D. Habits

1. Smoking. How long has the patient smoked? How many packs per day?

2. Alcohol. How long has the patient ingested alcohol? How much and what type per day?

E. Medications

1. List medications, including over-the-counter drugs.
2. Allergies.

F. Nutrition

1. Describe a typical breakfast, lunch, dinner, and snacks.
2. Does the patient use salt with meals?

II. BACKGROUND INFORMATION

A. Lab Values

Check laboratory studies for abnormal values or worsening trends.

B. Diagnostic Studies

Check reports of diagnostic studies for positive findings.

C. Chart

Check old chart for past relevant information.

III. INSPECTION

See Integumentary System Assessment.

IV. PALPATION

A. Peripheral Pulses

Palpate peripheral pulses for symmetry, quality, and regularity. Peripheral pulses: Carotid, brachial, radial, ulnar, femoral, popliteal, dorsalis pedis, posterior tibialis.

B. Skin Temperature

Palpate the hands and feet for skin temperature, tenderness, and/or pitting edema.

C. Capillary Refill

Palpate fingernails for capillary refill. Normal refill is less than 2 seconds.

D. Pain

1. Deeply but carefully palpate the calf muscles for tenderness.

2. Check for Homans' sign by dorsiflexing the foot with the leg extended. If pain is elicited, thrombophlebitis may be present.

E. Lymph Nodes

Palpate for enlarged lymph nodes: Head, neck, axilla, brachial, breast, inguinal, and popliteal areas. Normally, lymph nodes are not palpable. Note the location, size, firmness, symmetry, temperature, and tenderness.

PERIPHERAL VASCULAR DISEASE

POTENTIAL PROBLEMS

Ischemic Pain	Amputation
Infection	Thrombophlebitis
Ulcers	Pulmonary Emboli
Gangrene	Psychosocial Problems

KEY NURSING INTERVENTIONS

- Place the patient in a position that will enhance circulation to the affected area. In general, elevate the head of the bed for arterial disease and elevate the foot of the bed for vascular disease. Avoid positions that will interfere with blood flow such as gatching the knees, poor body alignment, and prolonged periods in the same position.

- Inspect the extremities frequently for cuts, bruises, ulcers, gangrene, and infection.

- Provide a safe environment that will reduce the chance of injury. To protect the feet, make sure slippers are worn whenever the patient is out of bed.

- Encourage exercise and ambulation with frequent rest periods. Often the physician will have a set of prescribed exercises. Exercise is contraindicated in patients who have gangrene, ulcers, or infection of the extremities.

- Promote vasodilation by keeping the environment warm. Make use of thermal underwear, gloves, socks, and extra blankets, if needed. Avoid the use of heating pads and hot water soaks unless ordered by the physician.

- Avoid vasoconstriction. Help the patient to avoid stressful situations. Prevent exposure to cold.

- Prevent the formation of thrombophlebitis and pulmonary embolism (see Thrombophlebitis).

- Administer foot care BID. Use mild soap and moderate temperatures.

- Keep the skin moist. Apply topical skin lotions every day. Encourage a liberal fluid intake to 2000 cc/day unless contraindicated.

- Never attempt to cut the toenails. Notify the physician if the toenails become a problem.
- Apply and remove antiembolism stockings BID.
- Assess and support the patient's psychosocial needs. Peripheral vascular disease is usually a chronic situation that may cause frequent painful episodes. Often the patient's lifestyle has to be altered in order to help enhance circulation. The threat of vascular surgery and amputation is always present. Help the patient and family deal with these changes. Allow for ventilation of feelings and provide as much teaching as possible.

PATIENT AND FAMILY TEACHING

- Explain the purpose and stress the importance of exercise, rest, keeping warm, avoiding injury, and quitting smoking. Demonstrate prescribed exercises.
- Stress the importance of skin and foot care. Demonstrate how to take care of the feet.
- Inform the patient of signs and symptoms of trauma, ulcers, gangrene, and infection.
- Instruct the patient to avoid crossing the legs, restrictive clothing, and sitting or standing for long periods.
- If there is an underlying disease such as diabetes, be sure that the patient is well informed and knows how to manage it.
- Explain the reasons for not smoking if patient smokes.

HYPERTENSION, HYPERTENSIVE CRISIS

POTENTIAL PROBLEMS

Heart Failure	Hemiparesis
Myocardial Infarction	Nausea
Stroke	Vomiting
Renal Failure	Dizziness
Seizures	Headache
Epistaxis	Pulmonary Edema
Altered Level of	Psychological Problems
Consciousness	

KEY NURSING INTERVENTIONS

- Observe for signs and symptoms of hypertensive crisis: Systolic pressure greater than 190 mm Hg, diastolic pressure greater than 110 mm Hg, headache, pupillary changes, altered level of consciousness, blurred vision, vertigo, dizziness, hemiparesis, weakness, shortness of breath, pulmonary edema, bradycardia, nausea, vomiting, seizures.

- Take frequent blood pressures when patient is symptomatic with hypertension. Notify the physician.

- Keep head of bed elevated.

- Observe urinary output. Report oliguria or output less than 30 cc per hour.

- Administer antihypertensive medications as ordered. Take frequent blood pressures and observe for hypotension.

- Observe for hypokalemia if medications increase potassium excretion.

- Maintain a low-salt diet as ordered. Restrict fluid intake as ordered.

- Provide a calm, nonstressful environment.

- Assess and support the patient's psychosocial needs. Help the patient to recognize and avoid situations that may be stressful and thus increase the blood pressure. Point out that hypertension is never really cured, but adherence to a medical program, strict diet, and lower stress levels usually has a successful outcome.

PATIENT AND FAMILY TEACHING

- Explain the purpose and stress the importance of medications, diet, exercise, rest, stress reduction, and possible fluid restriction.

- Inform the patient of signs and symptoms of high blood pressure.

- Explain that complications such as heart failure, myocardial infarction, stroke, and renal disease may be prevented if hypertension is controlled.

- Demonstrate how to take a blood pressure at home. Encourage frequent blood pressure checks. Emphasize that blood pressure may be dangerously high even though there are no symptoms.

- Stress the importance of avoiding smoking, obesity, excessive alcohol, and emotional stress.

- Warn the patient of possible side effects of antihypertensive medications. Check the *Physician's Desk Reference*.

THROMBOPHLEBITIS

POTENTIAL PROBLEMS

Pulmonary Embolism   Complications of
Edema   Anticoagulant Therapy
Pain   Psychosocial Problems
Formation of Other Thrombi

KEY NURSING INTERVENTIONS

- Maintain strict bed rest for 4 to 7 days. This will allow the thrombus to attach to the vessel wall and decrease the chance of embolism.

- Elevate the legs 6 to 10 inches. This will allow blood to drain by gravity which helps prevent venous stasis and new thrombi from forming. The knees should not be gatched.

- Apply and remove antiembolism stockings as ordered.

- Encourage exercise and ambulation as soon as the chances of embolism are eliminated, usually within 4 to 7 days. Do not allow the patient to sit or stand for long periods.

- Apply warm, moist compresses as ordered to affected leg to enhance circulation and hasten recovery.

- Avoid massaging the legs. This could cause a thrombus to dislodge and become an embolism. Do not allow patient to sit or stand until risk of embolism is past and patient is allowed to walk. Foot and leg exercises are then to be encouraged.

- Prevent and observe for signs and symptoms of complications of anticoagulant therapy (see Anticoagulant Therapy).

- Observe for signs and symptoms of pulmonary embolism: Chest pain, shortness of breath, dyspnea, tachypnea, decreased pO_2, increased pCO_2, cyanosis, tachycardia, hypotension, cardiopulmonary arrest.

- Assess and support the patient's psychosocial needs. Help the patient and family deal with problems of prolonged bed rest and anticoagulant therapy. Discuss ways of preventing boredom with patient and family.

PATIENT AND FAMILY TEACHING

- See Anticoagulant Therapy.

- Explain the purpose and stress the importance of strict bed rest, anticoagulant therapy, warm compresses, elevation of extremity, anti-embolism stockings, and avoidance of massaging the legs.
- Encourage the patient to maintain an exercise program that includes walking when allowed.
- Inform the patient of signs and symptoms of recurrent thrombo-phlebitis and pulmonary embolism.
- Instruct the patient to avoid crossing the legs, restrictive clothing, and sitting or standing for extended periods.

HYPOVOLEMIC SHOCK

POTENTIAL PROBLEMS

Cardiac Failure	Acidosis
Adult Respiratory Distress Syndrome	Coma
	Cardiopulmonary Arrest
Cardiac Arrhythmias	Pulmonary Edema
Renal Failure	Psychosocial Problems

KEY NURSING INTERVENTIONS

- Identify patients who would be most susceptible to hypovolemic shock: Post surgery, post trauma, burns, ulcers, bleeding disorders, anticoagulant therapy, anemia, alcoholism, diabetes or any patient with an altered fluid intake.

- Observe for signs and symptoms of shock: Cool, clammy skin; altered level of consciousness; thirst; decreased urinary output; postural vital sign changes; weak, rapid, thready pulse; decreased blood pressure; decreased central venous pressure; tachypnea; metabolic acidosis; cyanosis; restlessness; agitation.
  NOTE: The skin may be warm and dry in patients who are in shock due to severe dehydration as in the hyperglycemic state of diabetes.

- Therapy will depend on the type and severity of fluid loss.

- Place the patient in Trendelenburg position, elevate the legs, or place the patient in the M.A.S.T. suit.

- Administer high-flow oxygen and/or assist ventilations as necessary.

- Initiate intravenous therapy as ordered. Use the largest needle or catheter possible. Hang an isotonic solution such as lactated Ringers or normal saline as ordered. (Use normal saline when administering blood.)

- Administer blood and other colloids as ordered (see Intravenous Therapy: Blood Administration Procedure).

- Assist the physician with central line insertion. Attach a central venous pressure manometer. This intravenous line can be used to administer fluids rapidly and measure central venous pressure. Avoid giving blood through central line if possible, especially if blood is not being warmed.

- Place the patient on a cardiac monitor and observe for arrhythmias.
- Insert indwelling urinary catheter and record hourly urinary output.
- Frequently assess the patient in the following areas in order to evaluate fluid replacement: Level of consciousness; skin color, temperature, moisture; urinary output; pulse; blood pressure; central venous pressure; arterial blood gases; hemoglobin; hematocrit; and other blood chemistries.
- Prevent fluid overload especially in children and elderly patients. Frequently check intravenous flow rates and document intravenous fluid intake. Observe for hypertension, bradycardia, distended neck veins, elevated central venous pressure, bounding pulse, and pulmonary edema.
- Keep patient NPO as ordered.
- Prepare for transfer to Surgery or Intensive Care.
- Assess and support the patient's psychosocial needs. Being in severe shock is an anxiety-producing experience for all involved, including the patient. The patient may be suddenly exposed to many hospital personnel performing a variety of procedures. As the patient's nurse, attempt to provide reassurance by remaining calm and briefly explaining procedures before they happen. Keep the family informed of the patient's status.

PATIENT AND FAMILY TEACHING

- Shock is usually secondary to some other condition. Refer to the appropriate condition for information on patient teaching.

VEIN LIGATION AND STRIPPING

POTENTIAL PROBLEMS

Hemorrhage	Pain
Infection	Pulmonary Emboli
Nerve Damage	Psychosocial Problems
Thrombosis	

KEY NURSING INTERVENTIONS

- Observe for and prevent postoperative complications (see Postoperative Care).

- Maintain elastic bandages from foot to groin as ordered. This helps prevent bleeding and promotes circulation to deep veins. The leg is kept wrapped for up to 7 days. Check circulation, sensation, and movement of the foot to be sure the bandages are not too tight.

- Keep the legs elevated 6 to 10 inches. Use pillows, shock blocks or electric beds. Avoid gatching of the knees.

- Encourage passive then active range of motion exercises. The patient should be encouraged to ambulate for short periods. This is usually begun 24 to 48 hours postoperatively.

- Observe incision sites, especially the groin, for signs and symptoms of bleeding: Blood-soaked dressings, hematomas, increased pulse, decreased blood pressure, diaphoresis, cyanosis, restlessness, agitation, decreased dorsalis pedis and posterior tibialis pulse.

- Observe incision sites when dressings are removed for signs and symptoms of infection: Redness, swelling, red streaks, pain, discharge from wound, fever, malaise.

- Observe for signs and symptoms of saphenous nerve damage: Pain, hypersensitivity, tingling, numbness. Nerve damage may be permanent or temporary, which may last up to three weeks.

- Observe for signs and symptoms of pulmonary embolism: Chest pain, shortness of breath, dyspnea, cyanosis, cardiopulmonary arrest, tachycardia, hypotension, neck vein distention, decreased pO_2, increased pCO_2.

- Assess and support the patient's psychosocial needs. Help the patient realize that circulation will be enhanced and the legs will probably look much better than before surgery.

PATIENT AND FAMILY TEACHING

- Stress the importance of wearing elastic bandages or support stockings for up to three weeks or more, depending upon the advice of the physician.
- Encourage the patient to maintain a prescribed exercise program which usually includes walking intermittantly for at least one month.
- Tell the patient to avoid crossing the legs and sitting or standing for extended periods of time.
- Inform the patient that 5 to 8 days postoperatively, the leg will become "black and blue." Provide assurance that this is normal as long as there are no signs or symptoms of bleeding or infection.

CAROTID ENDARECTOMY

POTENTIAL PROBLEMS

Neurologic Deficit	Hemorrhage
Cerebrovascular Accident	Infection
Respiratory Problems	Myocardial Infection
Hypo/Hypertension	Psychosocial Problems
Hematoma	

KEY NURSING INTERVENTIONS

- Observe for and prevent postoperative complications (see Post-operative Care).

- Observe for signs and symptoms of neurologic deficit. Compare to preoperative condition. Perform frequent neurologic checks, which should include the following: Level of consciousness, respiratory patterns, pupil size and reaction to light, equality of extremity strength and movement.

- Observe for signs and symptoms of respiratory problems due to swelling, bleeding, or constricting dressings: Pain in neck or throat, inability to talk or swallow, stridor, dyspnea, tachypnea or accessory muscle use.

- Observe for signs and symptoms of postoperative bleeding: Blood-soaked dressings, hematoma to neck, altered level of consciousness, decreased blood pressure, increased pulse, diaphoresis, agitation, restlessness.

- Maintain a stable blood pressure. Keep the head elevated and maintain an adequate fluid volume. Hypotension can cause decreased perfusion, emboli formation, and stroke. Hypertension can cause bleeding at operative site or the brain.

- Prevent infection. Use strict aseptic technique when changing dressings. Keep dressings clean and dry. Wash hands thoroughly before handling dressings.

- Assess and support the patient's psychosocial needs. Help the patient and family deal with changes in body image and lifestyle. Usually the patient will experience a decrease in disabling symptoms.

PATIENT AND FAMILY TEACHING

- Explain the purpose of elevation of the head.
- Stress the importance of diet, rest, exercise, and medications as prescribed.
- Advise patient to report complications after discharge to the physician immediately: Fever, extremity weakness, dizziness, fainting, slurred speech, headaches, chest pain, redness, or drainage from incision area.

FEMOROPOPLITEAL BYPASS GRAFT

POTENTIAL PROBLEMS

Thrombus Formation	Hemorrhage
Pulmonary Emboli	Infection
Distal Vascular Insufficiency	Decubitus Ulcers
Myocardial Infarction	Psychosocial Problems

KEY NURSING INTERVENTIONS

- Observe for and prevent postoperative complications (see Post-operative Care).

- Observe for signs and symptoms of postoperative hemorrhage: Blood-soaked dressings, hematoma to groin, leg or groin pain, diaphoresis, decreased blood pressure, increased pulse, decreased central venous pressure, oliguria, decreased hemoglobin and hematocrit, rest-lessness, agitation.

- Observe for signs and symptoms of infection: Purulent wound drainage, bleeding at incision site, pain, redness, swelling, red streaks, elevated temperature.

- Prevent infection. Use strict aseptic technique when changing dress-ings. Keep dressings clean and dry. Wash hands thoroughly with anti-microbial soap prior to patient contact.

- Frequently assess distal vascular and nervous function. Check for sensation, movement, capillary refill and distal pulses. Compare to preoperative condition. Report signs of vascular and nervous insuffi-ciency.

- Prevent thrombus formation. Keep legs elevated. Avoid gatching the knees. Apply antiembolism stockings, if ordered.

- Prevent complications of anticoagulant therapy, if utilized (see Anti-coagulant Therapy).

- Prevent decubitus ulcer formation (see Decubitus Ulcers).

- Observe for signs and symptoms of thrombophlebitis: Calf or leg pain, Homans' sign (dorsiflexion of the foot causes calf pain), redness, swelling, warmness of affected leg, fever.

- Observe for signs and symptoms of pulmonary embolism: Chest pain, shortness of breath, dyspnea, tachypnea, decreased pO_2, cyanosis, cardiopulmonary arrest.

- Assess and support the patient's psychosocial needs. Depending upon the age and physical condition of the patient, convalescence may be short or prolonged. Help the patient and family deal with temporary alterations in lifestyle. Make sure arrangements have been made if the patient is going to need help at home.

PATIENT AND FAMILY TEACHING

- Stress the importance of diet, proper fluid intake, exercise and rest.
- Inform the patient and family of signs and symptoms of infection, thrombophlebitis, and pulmonary embolism.
- Instruct patient in the prevention of thrombophlebitis: Not crossing legs, avoid sitting for long periods, avoid constricting socks or stockings which are not prescribed, doing foot and leg exercises while lying down (see Postoperative Care).

ANTICOAGULANT THERAPY

POTENTIAL PROBLEMS

Hemorrhage   Psychosocial Problems
Drug Interactions

KEY NURSING INTERVENTIONS

- Observe for signs and symptoms of bleeding and hemorrhage: Dark and tarry stools, red stools, hematemesis, hemoptysis, hematuria, epistaxis, bleeding gums, hematomas, ecchymosis, severe vaginal bleeding, surgical wound bleeding, puncture wound bleeding, neurological changes, abdominal pain, diaphoresis, increased pulse, decreased blood pressure, decreased hemoglobin and hematocrit, dizziness, change in level of consciousness, restlessness, agitation.

- Keep specific antidotes on hand: Protamine sulfate for heparin and Vitamin K for Coumadin.

- Observe coagulation studies for therapeutic drug values:
  Prothrombin time (PT) (used for Coumadin therapy) should be 2 to 2.5 times the normal (12–14 secs.) and 20% to 30% of the normal activity (80%–100%).
  Partial thromboplastin time (PTT) (used for heparin therapy) should be 2 to 2.5 times the normal (60–70 secs. or 25–37 secs. for APTT).
  Lee-White clotting time (used for heparin therapy) should be 15 mins. (normal is 7 mins.).

- Identify medications that may potentiate or inhibit anticoagulants: Salicylates, anabolic steroids, anti-inflammatory agents, barbiturates, and hypnotics. Check each medication with the *Physician's Desk Reference*.

- Identify patients for whom anticoagulant therapy may be contraindicated: Liver and kidney disease, hypertension, ulcers, clotting problems, post surgery, diabetes, post trauma and patients with aneurysms.

- Avoid multiple skin punctures. Apply pressure for 2 to 4 minutes following venous punctures. Avoid arterial punctures.

- Administer heparin per hospital protocol which usually includes: Cleaning the skin gently, checking dosage with another nurse, injecting heparin into subcutaneous fatty area in the abdomen at a 45-degree angle, not pulling back on the plunger, not rubbing the area, applying pressure if bleeding occurs, keeping a chart of injection sites and times.

- Administer IV heparin solutions with an infusion pump or controller. Frequently check rate and bottle fluid level. Leave heparin locks in place for at least two hours after last dose.

- Protect the patient from hazardous situations that could cause injury.

- Assess and support the patient's psychosocial needs: Help the patient and family deal with possible lifestyle changes from anticoagulant therapy.

PATIENT AND FAMILY TEACHING

- Instruct the patient to report signs and symptoms of bleeding to the physician: Blood in urine, black or red stools, nose bleeds, excessive bruising, bleeding gums, abdominal pain.

- Instruct the patient to avoid situations that could cause minor trauma, i.e., use of razors, excessive nose blowing, vigorous tooth brushing, contact sports, etc.

- Instruct the patient to inform the dentist and all other physicians of anticoagulant therapy.

- Have dietician discuss foods which counteract the effect of Coumadin (foods high in Vitamin K).

ANEMIA

POTENTIAL PROBLEMS

Congestive Heart Failure   Secondary Infections
Angina Pectoris   Dyspnea
Orthopnea   Dizziness
Headache   Anorexia
Skin Breakdown   Sore Mouth and Tongue
Blood Transfusion Reactions   Paresthesias

KEY NURSING INTERVENTIONS

- Arrange patient's daily schedule to provide uninterrupted rest periods. Assist patient in limiting excessive visitors, phone calls and anything that prevents rest periods.

- Prevent skin breakdown by encouraging patient to turn and change position frequently. Assist patient as needed. Observe pressure points (back of head, bony prominences, sacrum, etc.) for redness and signs of breakdown. Massage pressure areas gently with lotion. Use mild soap with bath (see The Immobilized Patient).

- Encourage nutritional intake. Arrange to have 6 small meals per day. Assist patients who are too weak to feed themselves.

- Assure good mouth care daily, especially when mouth and tongue are sore. Spicy and hot foods should be avoided. Arrange for family to bring a soft-bristle toothbrush and have patient brush teeth after each meal. Keep lips moistened with petroleum products. Keep mouthwash within reach for frequent rinsing.

- Keep chilled patients warm but avoid heating pads which may burn the skin. Paresthesias cause insensitivity to heat and burns can result from such devices.

- Protect patient from infections. Restrict hospital personnel and visitors with respiratory infections. Do not place patient in room with potentially infective patients.

- *FOR ANEMIA DUE TO BLOOD LOSS:*

  - Observe for reliable laboratory reflection of blood loss 1 to 2 days after hemorrhage. Erythrocytes, hemoglobin and hematocrit results are usually high the first 24 to 48 hours of blood loss and are unreliable.

- Usual treatment consists of stopping hemorrhage, replacing blood volume with IV blood products, iron supplements, nutritious dietary intake.

- *FOR IRON DEFICIENCY ANEMIA:*

  - Usual treatment consists of identifying the cause (blood loss or poor dietary iron intake), administration of iron, and increasing iron dietary intake.
  - Use Z-tract injection technique for parenteral iron administration.
  - Give PO iron with food to avoid gastric irritation. Foods high in ascorbic acid should be given with iron since ascorbic acid enhances iron absorption.

- *FOR PERNICIOUS ANEMIA:*

  - Usual treatment consists of Vitamin B-12 injection, diet high in iron, protein and vitamins, and rest.
  - Protect patient from burns and skin trauma since sensitivity to heat and pain is decreased.

- *FOR FOLIC ACID DEFICIENCY ANEMIA:*

  - Usual treatment consists of folic acid administration and Vitamin C administration.

- *FOR APLASTIC ANEMIA:*

  - Usual treatment consists of removal of myelotoxic agent, blood transfusions, steroid therapy to stimulate bone marrow activity, splenectomy.
  - Prevent infection. Restrict hospital personnel and visitors with *any* infections. Do not place patient in room with infective patients.
  - Observe for signs and symptoms of infection: Sore throat, sniffles, elevated temperature, mouth and skin sores, dysuria.
  - Prevent and control bleeding. Advise patient to do gentle oral care and use electric shaver; avoid injections, if possible.
  - Check stools for occult blood.

- *FOR SICKLE CELL ANEMIA:*

  - Usual treatment consists of IV fluid administration, oxygen, rest, analgesics.

- Encourage PO fluid intake.
- Monitor temperature for elevation.
- Protect patient from infection. Restrict hospital personnel and visitors with upper respiratory infections.

- Assess and support patient's psychosocial needs. Recognize that weakness and fatigue can cause irritability and inadequate coping abilities. Approach patient with understanding patience and avoid rushing activities. Allow for uninterrupted rest periods.

PATIENT AND FAMILY TEACHING

- Instruct patients with iron deficiency in foods high in iron (meat, fish, poultry, eggs, green leafy vegetables, potatoes, dried fruits, whole grains, enriched breads and cereals and dried beans). Have dietician provide written instructions.
- Instruct patients with folic acid deficiency in foods high in folic acid (green and yellow fresh leafy vegetables, citrus and berry fruits, organ meats, dried yeast and legumes). Have dietician provide written instructions.
- Instruct family and visitors in the importance of protecting patient from infections.
- Reinforce explanation of particular type of anemia.
- Instruct patient in proper administration of prescribed medications.

GASTROINTESTINAL SYSTEM

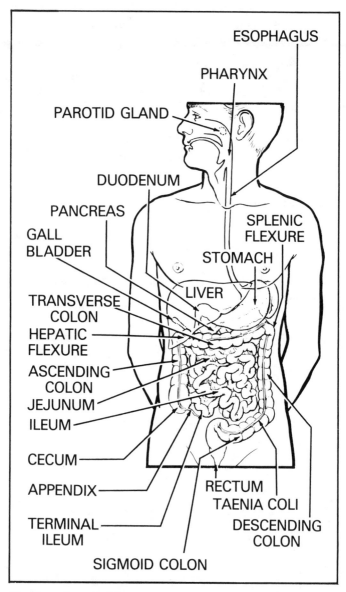

The Gastrointestinal System

GASTROINTESTINAL SYSTEM— PHYSIOLOGY SUMMARY

I. MOUTH

A. The Mouth

1. Chews food.
2. Mixes food with salivary enzymes.
3. Empties by swallowing.

B. Digestion

1. The salivary glands are innervated by the parasympathetic and the sympathetic nervous systems.
2. Stimulation by the parasympathetic system initiates watery secretions.
3. Stimulation by the sympathetic system initiates viscous secretions.
4. The salivary glands secrete the enzyme ptyalin, which hydrolyzes starch and glycogen in the mouth.
5. Salivary secretion increases with irritation of the esophagus, stomach, and duodenum and decreases with dehydration and emotional stress.
6. The brain stem controls secretions and responds to taste and sensory impulses.

II. STOMACH

A. The Stomach

1. Stores food.
2. Secretes gastric juice, mucus, and intrinsic factor.
3. Mixes food with gastric enzymes.
4. Absorbs digested foodstuffs.
5. Regulates emptying into small intestine.

B. Motility

1. Mixing movements are initiated in the middle area of the stomach about every 20 seconds.

2. Food is emptied into the duodenum by peristaltic waves from the antrum portion of the stomach.

3. Both mixing and peristaltic movements occur through parasympathetic innervation (vagus and sacral nerves).

4. Stomach emptying is regulated by:

   a) The degree of peristaltic activity of the pyloric pump.

   b) Distention of the stomach by food.

   c) The secretion of gastrin hormone by the stomach, which stimulates the pyloric pump.

   d) The enterogastric reflex (inhibits emptying when the duodenum is full; when the chyme entering the duodenum is too acidic, hyper- or hypotonic; and in the presence of excessive digested protein products.

   e) The secretion of enterogastrone hormone by the small intestine in the presence of fatty acids, which inhibits gastric motility and emptying.

   f) Increased fluidity of foods, which increases gastric emptying.

C. Secretions

1. The stomach secretes:

   a) Mucus, which protects stomach wall from digestive enzymes and contains intrinsic factor necessary for vitamin B–12 absorption.

   b) Pepsinogen, which becomes pepsin and digests proteins.

   c) Hydrochloric acid to provide an acid medium is necessary for pepsin activity.

   d) Small quantities of gastric lipase and amylase.

   e) The hormone gastrin from the antrum of the stomach.

   f) 2 to 3 liters of gastric juices every 24 hours.

2. Gastric secretions are controlled by two mechanisms, nervous and hormonal.

   a) The vagus nerve stimulates gastric glands to secrete pepsin, acid, mucus and the hormone gastrin.

   Cephalic: The vagus nerve is stimulated by taste, sight, smell of food or eating, and when the blood sugar level is below 50 mgm.

Gastric: The hormone gastrin is secreted from the antrum in the presence of partially digested proteins, alcohol, caffeine and by gastric distention. Gastrin enters the bloodstream and is carried back to the gastric glands to stimulate the release of acid and enzymes.

Intestinal: The presence of food in the bowel initiates reflex which cause gastric secretion.

b) Gastric secretions are inhibited by:

- The enterogastric reflex (see #B4).
- The release of enterogastrone hormone by the duodenum in the presence of fat, hypertonic or hypotonic solutions, and acid.

D. Digestion

1. *Proteins.* Pepsin begins the digestion of proteins by hydrolyzing them into proteoses, peptones and large polypeptides.

2. *Carbohydrates.* Carbohydrate digestion begun in the mouth by ptyalin continues in the stomach until ptyalin is inactivated by acid.

3. *Fat.* The amount of fat digestion in the stomach is extremely small.

E. Absorption

1. The stomach absorbs minimal amounts of water, glucose, alcohol and some drugs.

2. Calcium is absorbed in the stomach in an acid medium and in the presence of protein and vitamin D.

III. THE SMALL INTESTINE

A. The Small Intestine

1. Secretes digestive juices.
2. Completes digestion.
3. Absorbs nutrients.
4. Propels waste products into the large intestine.

B. Motility

1. Distention of the small intestine stimulates mixing contractions (segmentation) which mixes the chyme, facilitating increased digestion and absorption.

2. Parasympathetic stimulation increases mixing contractions and sympathetic stimulation inhibits contractions.

3. Peristaltic contractions propel the chyme through the small intestine at about 1 cm per minute. The small intestine is completely emptied in 3–10 hrs.

4. Distention initiates the gastroenteric reflex which causes peristalsis.

5. Irritation or over-distention causes a peristaltic rush (a powerful peristaltic wave travelling the full length of the small intestine) to occur in a few minutes.

C. Secretions

1. Brunner's glands, on the intestinal mucosa, secrete mucus to protect the intestinal wall from digestive juices.

2. The crypts of Lieberkuhn, throughout the intestine, secrete a neutral pH extracellular fluid to facilitate absorption.

3. Enterokinase and amylase enzymes are secreted by intestinal glands.

4. Epithelial cells secrete the following enzymes:

   a) Peptidases (break polypeptides into amino acids).

   b) Sucrase, maltase, lactase, isomaltase (split disaccharides into monosaccharides).

   c) Lipase (splits fat into glycerol and fatty acids).

5. Intestinal secretions are stimulated by:

   a) Distention of small intestine by chyme.

   b) Irritating stimuli.

   c) Parasympathetic (vagal) stimulation.

   d) Intestinal hormones.

D. Digestion

1. The liver, gallbladder and pancreas secrete enzymes into the small intestine which contribute to digestion.

2. *Proteins*. Partially digested proteins entering the small intestine are broken into amino acids by:

   a) Pancreatic enzymes (trypsin, chymotrypsin and carbooxypolypeptidase).

   b) Intestinal enzymes (amino polypeptidase and dipeptidases).

3. *Carbohydrates*. Partially digested carbohydrates entering the small intestine are broken into monosaccharides by:

   a) Intestinal enzymes.

   b) Pancreatic amylase acts on carbohydrates not partially digested in the mouth and splits them into disaccharides.

4. *Fats*.

   a) The liver secretes bile salts which act on fat globules to make them easily digested by lipase.

   b) Fat globules (triglycerides) are hydrolyzed by pancreatic and enteric lipases and changed into monoglycerides, free fatty acids and glycerol.

   c) Cholesterol is hydrolyzed by pancreatic cholesterol esterase.

E. Absorption

1. Water and electrolytes are absorbed by active transport and diffusion.

2. Carbohydrates are absorbed as monosaccharides by active transport.

3. Proteins are absorbed as amino acids by active transport.

4. Fats are absorbed:

   a) As monoglycerides and fatty acids by combining with bile salts, diffusing across the epithelium and then into the lymphatic system where they are then transported to the neck and emptied into the blood vessels.

   b) As fatty acids directly into the portal circulation.

5. Iron is converted to a ferrous state in the stomach and absorbed in the small intestine.

6. The duodenum absorbs calcium in an acid medium and in the presence of protein and vitamin D.

7. The small intestine is the main site of electrolyte absorption.

IV. THE LARGE INTESTINE

A. The Large Intestine

1. Absorbs water and electrolytes from chyme.

2. Stores feces until defecation.

B. Motility

1. Mixing movements called haustral contractions facilitate absorption while moving the feces towards the rectum.

2. Peristaltic contractions occur as mass movements several times a day and most prominently after breakfast.

3. Mass movements are caused by reflexes (gastrocolic and duodenocolic) as a result of: Distention of the stomach and duodenum, irritation of the colon, parasympathetic stimulation and overdistention of the colon.

4. When feces reach the rectum, the defection reflex is stimulated through the medulla and spinal cord.

C. Secretion

1. Mucus is secreted by goblet cells in response to tactile stimulation and by parasympathetic stimulation.

2. Mucus facilitates the formation of stools.

3. Mucus protects the intestinal wall from excoriation and bacteria, and its alkalinity protects it from the acid in feces.

4. The large intestine secretes water and electrolytes in response to irritation such as bacterial infection.

D. Digestion

1. Bacteria in the proximal large intestine digest small quantities of cellulose.

2. Bacteria assist in synthesizing Vitamin K, B-12, thiamine, riboflavin, and form gas in the colon.

3. Feces is the waste product of digestion and is composed of dead bacteria (30%), fat (10–20%), inorganic material (10–20%), protein (2–3%) and roughage (30%).

E. Absorption

1. The large intestine absorbs 80–90% of the water contents of chyme.

2. The proximal colon is where most of the absorption occurs.

3. Water absorption is facilitated by the absorption of sodium and chloride ions.

V. PANCREAS

A. The Pancreas

1. The pancreas is an endocrine gland secreting the hormones, insulin and glucagon into the bloodstream.

2. The pancreas is an exocrine gland secreting digestive juices containing the enzymes, trypsin, chymotrypsin, carboxypolypeptidase, amylase and lipase into a major duct emptying into the duodenum.

B. Secretion

Pancreatic secretion is stimulated by parasympathetic stimulation but mainly by the release of the hormones secretin and cholecystokinin in the duodenum in the presence of chyme.

VI. LIVER

A. The Liver

Is divided into the right and left main lobes by the falciform ligament.

B. Circulation

1. The liver receives oxygenated blood from the hepatic artery.

2. It receives venous blood carrying metabolic materials, toxins and nutrients from the digestive tract, spleen and pancreas, and from the mesenteric and splenic veins which join to form the portal vein.

3. Blood leaves the liver through the hepatic vein, which becomes the inferior vena cava at the right atrium.

C. Lobules

The functional units of the liver are called lobules.

D. Bile Ducts and Lymph Vessels

1. Supply the liver.
2. The bile ducts in the liver join, forming the right and left hepatic ducts.
3. These unite with the cystic duct from the gallbladder, forming the common bile duct which opens into the duodenum.

E. Liver functions

1. Synthesis

   a) The liver synthesizes cholesterol, a precursor to bile formation.

   b) The liver synthesizes 500–1000 ml of bile salts each day.

   c) The liver synthesizes the coagulation factors fibrinogen and prothrombin and other clotting factors in the presence of Vitamin K.

   d) In the fetus and in abnormal conditions of the adult, the liver produces erythrocytes.

2. Storage

   a) The liver stores Vitamins A, D, E, K, B-12, and other vitamins.

   b) The liver stores iron.

   c) In the presence of insulin, glucose is transported to liver cells where it is converted into glycogen and stored until glucose is needed.

   d) The liver is capable of storing up to 400 ml of blood.

3. Phagocytosis

   Kupffer cells in the liver carry out phagocytosis of bacteria, foreign bodies and old erythrocytes.

4. Detoxification

   The liver converts harmful toxins into less harmful materials through conjugation, methylation, oxidation and reduction.

5. Metabolism

   a) Carbohydrates
     The liver regulates blood glucose concentration by storing glycogen and gluconeogenesis. The liver converts galactose into glucose.

   b) Fats
     The liver converts excess carbohydrates into fat, forms cholesterol and phospholipids and lipoproteins, and oxidizes fatty acids to form acetoacetic acid.

   c) Protein
     The liver forms urea to remove ammonia from the body, deaminates amino acids, forms plasma proteins, and different amino acids through transamination.

VII. GALLBLADDER

A. The Gallbladder

Is a depository for bile.

B. Bile

1. Bile is composed of water, cholesterol, bilirubin, fatty acids, lecithin, bile salts and electrolytes.

2. Bile is concentrated in the gallbladder by chloride and bicarbonates.

3. Bile is released by the action of cholecystokinin, a hormone released in the duodenum that causes the gallbladder to contract.

4. After bile is released into the intestine, the bile salts are absorbed into the portal vein and reabsorbed into the liver to be reused.

VIII. METABOLISM

A. Carbohydrate

1. Two-thirds of ingested glucose is converted to glycogen in the liver (glycogenesis).

2. Glycogen is broken down when glucose is needed by the body (glycogenolysis).

3. Glycogen is made in the liver from non-carbohydrate materials by glucocorticoids from the adrenal cortex and thyroxine (glyconeogenesis).

4. Circulating glucose is used by the cells for energy (glycolysis), converted to lactose in mammary glands, converted to fat (lipogenesis), and used to make other substances.

B. Protein

1. Amino acids are absorbed into the bloodstream and transported into body cells.

2. Amino acids are used to synthesize proteins (protein anabolism).

3. Amino acids can be stored in tissues for a short time, especially in the liver and muscles.

4. Amino acids can be converted into glucose for energy or into fat through deamination in the liver.

5. Amino acids can be altered and new amino acids and ketoacids formed through transamination in the liver.

6. Ammonia formed through deamination is converted in the liver to urea and excreted in the urine.

C. Fat

1. Fat metabolism begins with hydrolysis, producing fatty acids and glycerol.

2. After hydrolysis, fatty acids are oxidized to form coenzyme A, which is then converted to a ketone, acetoacetic acid.

3. Acetoacetic acid is changed to form two more ketone bodies, acetone and beta-hydroxybutyric acid.

4. Fat metabolism is carried out in the liver.

5. Ketone bodies are finally transported in the blood to body tissues where they are oxidized the same as glucose.

6. Glycerol enters tissue cells and is used for energy, the same as glucose.

7. Fat can be stored in the liver or in fat depots.

8. Stored fat remains dynamic, changing positions and depositions. Fat becomes stationary in states of starvation and increased energy demands.

9. Cholesterol is absorbed through the intestine through the action of bile salts and is manufactured in the liver. Cholesterol participates in the synthesis of cortisol and progesterone.

GASTROINTESTINAL SYSTEM ASSESSMENT

I. HISTORY

A. Past History of Gastrointestinal Problems

1. What type?
2. What therapy was utilized? Did it work?

B. Recent History

1. Nausea, vomiting, and diarrhea?

   a) Before or after meals?

   b) Precipitating factors, ie: after emotional stress, medications, treatments, procedures, or specific foods?

   c) Describe frequency, color, amount, consistency, and odor.

2. Gas?

   a) Belching and/or flatulence?

   b) Frequency?

3. Constipation?

   a) When was the last bowel movement?

   b) Formed or loose?

   c) Does the patient use laxatives and/or enemas?

4. Bleeding?

   a) Vomitus may be bright red, brown, blood-tinged, "coffee grounds," or positive for occult blood.

   b) Stool may be bright red, blood-tinged, dark and tarry, or positive for occult blood.

5. Abdominal Masses?
   (See Palpation)

C. Pain

Use PQRST mnemonic.

P— Provokes.   What makes the pain worse or better? What was the patient doing prior to the onset of pain?

Q—Quality.   Subjective description of pain by the patient. Use the patient's own words, i.e., burning, stabbing, pressure.

R—Radiation.   Where is the pain located and does it radiate anywhere?

S—Severity.   Ask the patient to judge the pain on a scale of 1 to 10 with 10 being the worst pain ever felt.

T—Time.   How long has the patient had this pain? When did the pain begin and end?

D. Menstrual Cycle

1. When was the last menstrual period?
2. Was it normal?
3. Are the periods regular?
4. How long do they last?
5. Use of oral or other contraceptives?

E. Habits

1. Smoking. How long has the patient smoked? How many packs per day?
2. Alcohol. How long has the patient ingested alcohol? How much and what type per day?

F. Medications

1. List medications including over-the-counter drugs.
2. Allergies?

G. Nutrition

Ask the patient to describe a typical breakfast, lunch, dinner and snacks in order to assess nutritional status.

II. BACKGROUND INFORMATION

A. Lab Values

Check lab values for abnormal results or worsening trends.

B. Diagnostic Studies

Identify abnormal reports of diagnostic studies, i.e., x-rays, scans, endoscopies, sigmoidoscopies, etc.

C. Chart

Check old chart for past relevant information.

III. INSPECTION

A. Preparation

1. Patient must be supine.

2. The urinary bladder should be empty.

3. Relax the patient by explaining the procedure. Provide as much privacy as possible. For comfort, place a pillow behind the head and knees. Use warm hands and stethoscope.

B. Technique

1. Expose the entire abdomen. Cover the breasts and pubic area with a gown and bed sheet.

2. Inspect the skin for color, jaundice, pigmentations, hair distribution, scars, rashes, striae, lesions, and surgical wounds.

3. Describe the contour or shape of the abdomen, i.e., cachexic, obese, flat, round, distended, or concave.

4. Observe for symmetry, masses, herniations, visible peristalsis or pulsations.

IV. AUSCULTATION

A. Technique

1. Auscultate before percussion or palpation to prevent stimulating peristalsis.

2. Auscultate systematically in all four quadrants or nine regions. Use the diaphragm because bowel sounds are high pitched.

B. Normal Sounds

1. Bowel sounds heard every 5 to 20 seconds.

2. Bowel sounds should be heard in all four quadrants.

3. Borborygmi (occasional stomach growling).

C. Abnormal Sounds

1. Hypoactive bowel sounds are heard less than one sound per minute. This may indicate a paralytic ileus, peritonitis, hemorrhage, obstruction, mesenteric infarct, post abdominal surgery, or no food in the bowel. To determine absence of bowel sounds, auscultate for a full three minutes.

2. Hyperactive bowel sounds are heard as almost continuous. This may be heard with vomiting, diarrhea, above a bowel obstruction, or just after eating.

3. Vascular sounds. Arterial bruit may indicate vascular disease, heart murmurs, or an aneurysm. A venous hum may be heard in the presence of liver disease.

V. PERCUSSION

A. Technique

Percuss the same areas for auscultation. Listen for areas of dullness and tympany.

B. Normal

The stomach, large and small bowel should be tympanic. The liver, spleen, bladder, and a gravid uterus are dull.

1. Stomach. A tympanic gas bubble may be percussed in the left lower anterior rib cage.

2. Spleen. Splenic dullness may be percussed on the left side at the 10th rib just posterior to the mid-axillary line. The spleen is difficult to percuss. Dullness in this area may indicate an enlarged spleen.

3. Liver. Begin percusion over tympanic bowel along the mid-clavicular line and proceed upwards until a dull sound is percussed. Continue upwards until the dullness diminishes and the tympany of the lung fields is percussed. Next percuss along the mid-sternal line and the mid-axillary line in the same manner. Normal values for length are:
   6 to 12 cm for mid-clavicular line,
   4 to 8 cm for mid-sternal line.

C. Abnormal

1. Liver. A liver span at the mid-clavicular line greater than 12 cm may indicate hepatomegaly. Incorrect liver spans

may be due to gas in the colon, air under the diaphragm, or a pleural effusion.

2. Spleen. Splenic dullness heard below the costal margin may indicate an enlarged spleen.

VI. PALPATION

A. Light Palpation

Palpate no deeper than one centimeter. Feel for areas of tenderness, masses, and involuntary guarding.

B. Deep Palpation

Palpate for normal anatomy, enlarged anatomy, masses, and pain.

C. Normal

1. Liver. In most normal adults, the liver is not palpable. Standing on the right side of the patient, place the left hand behind the patient at the posterior costal margin. Place the right hand just below the anterior costal margin. Ask the patient to inhale deeply. The diaphragm will contract and push the liver downward. The lower edge of the liver may be palpable and extend to the left upper quadrant. Another technique is to stand on the right side of the patient near the shoulder area. Place the fingertips of both hands so that they may hook around the costal margin. Ask the patient to inhale.

2. The spleen and pancreas are not normally palpable.

3. Kidney. Place the left hand behind the patient below the costal margin and the right hand at the right mid-abdominal region. Ask the patient to inhale. The lower pole of the right kidney may be palpated. The left kidney is not normally palpable.

4. The urinary bladder is not normally palpable.

5. Aorta. In the thin adult, the abdominal aorta may be palpated slightly left of the midline as a long, thin pulsatile mass. It should be thin and consistent. A large pulsatile mass may indicate an aortic aneurysm.

D. Abnormal

1. Tenderness. Abdominal structures that are tender may indicate inflammation, infection, or pathology.

2. Rebound tenderness is slow, deep palpation with a quick release of the hand. If pain is more severe upon release, rebound tenderness is present.

3. Enlargement. If the liver, gallbladder, spleen, pancreas, left kidney, or urinary bladder are palpable, it may indicate pathology.

4. Large pulsatile masses may indicate an abdominal aortic aneurysm.

5. Abdominal Masses. Palpate systematically. Describe the masses in terms of location, size, mobility, firmness, and movement with respirations. To distinguish an abdominal mass from one in the abdominal wall, ask the patient to flex his stomach muscles. A mass in the abdominal wall will still be palpable, while a deeper mass will not be palpable.

6. Normal structures may be mistaken for masses, ie: gravid uterus, aorta, muscles, feces-filled colon, distended bladder, and the sacral promontory.

7. Presence of a fluid wave indicates ascites.

VII. RETROSIGMOID EXAMINATION

A. Inspection

Place the patient in the left lateral Sims position. Observe the perianal area for fissures, hemorrhoids, scars, lesions, skin irritation, ulcers, and rectal prolapse.

B. Palpation

1. Palpate the perianal area for tenderness and masses.

2. Perform a digital exam by inserting a gloved, lubricated index finger.

   a) Feel for areas of tenderness, tumors, polyps, and abscesses.

   b) Palpate the prostate gland in males and the cervix in females just anterior to the rectum. Describe the size, shape, firmness, and note any tenderness.

c) Palpate for fecal impactions and remove them carefully.

d) If bleeding is suspected, test stool for occult blood.

ESOPHAGEAL CONDITIONS: STRICTURES, ACHALASIA, HIATUS HERNIA, NEOPLASM, VARICES, DIVERTICULUM, INFLAMMATION

POTENTIAL PROBLEMS

Airway Obstruction	Aspiration
Fluid and Electrolyte Imbalances	Malnutrition
	Hemorrhage
Dysphagia	Pain
Aphagia	Psychosocial Problems
Regurgitation	

KEY NURSING INTERVENTIONS

- Observe for signs and symptoms of respiratory distress: Inability to speak, stridor, gurgling respirations, decreased lung sounds, tachypnea, apnea, cyanosis, cardiopulmonary arrest.

- Prevent respiratory problems by keeping suction equipment at bedside, elevating head of bed, and encouraging coughing and deep breathing.

- Observe for signs and symptoms of fluid and electrolyte imbalances (see Fluid and Electrolytes).

- Observe for signs and symptoms of esophageal bleeding: Hematemesis, blood in stool, decreasing hemoglobin and hematocrit, diaphoresis, restlessness, agitation, increased pulse, decreased blood pressure.

- Assist the physician in inserting special nasogastric tube (see Nasogastric Tubes).

- Document color and amount of nasogastric tube aspirate. Check for occult blood.

- When the patient is allowed to eat, offer small, frequent meals. Avoid high fiber, spicy, hot, cold, or irritating foods. Encourage patient to thoroughly chew foods and to take fluids with meals. Do not offer foods at least two hours before sleeping. Document which foods are tolerated best.

- Administer frequent oral hygiene, especially if the patient has dysphagia. Provide a container so that the patient may expel saliva and secretions. Change container frequently.

- Prepare the patient for possible diagnostic studies or surgery as ordered. (See Diagnostic Procedures, Pre- and Postoperative Care.)

- Assess and support the patient's psychosocial needs by helping the patient and family deal with body changes inherent in the patient's condition, i.e., halitosis, difficulty swallowing, regurgitation, and eating habits. Eating may become a frightening experience. Provide a calm environment during meals and stay with the patient if necessary.

PATIENT AND FAMILY TEACHING

- Encourage small, frequent meals. Instruct the patient to avoid irritating foods, smoking, alcohol and aspirin. Explain the importance of relaxing during meals.

- Instruct the patient to report unresolving symptoms or bleeding to the physician.

- Develop a plan to help the patient learn how to swallow.

NASOGASTRIC TUBES: LEVINE, SALEM SUMP, MILLER-ABBOTT, LINTON, SENGSTAKEN-BLAKEMORE

POTENTIAL PROBLEMS

LEVINE/SALEM SUMP/ MILLER-ABBOTT

Pneumonia
Electrolyte Imbalance
Dislodgement
Esophagitis
Abdominal Distention
Nasal Inflammation
Throat Irritation
Dry Mucous Membranes
Psychosocial Problems

LINTON/SENGSTAKEN- BLAKEMORE

Respiratory Distress
Pulmonary Aspiration
Esophageal Rupture or Injury
   (SENGSTAKEN-
   BLAKEMORE)
Abdominal Distention
Pressure Sores
Restlessness
Dry Mucous Membranes
Psychosocial Problems

KEY NURSING INTERVENTIONS

LEVINE/SALEM SUMP/MILLER-ABBOTT

- Assess patient and laboratory reports for signs and symptoms of electrolyte imbalance (see Fluids and Electrolytes).
- Check suction machine for proper functioning and pressure setting. Assess abdomen for distention.
- Maintain secure anchored tube (taped to nose and pinned to gown).
- Keep suction bottles below patient's midline at all times.
- Moisten lips and nostril with cream or ointment. Assist patient in rinsing mouth and brushing teeth frequently. Keep tubing around nostril clean.
- Maintain semi-Fowler's position unless contraindicated.
- If patient complains of sore throat, discuss the possibility of anesthetic throat lozenges or gargles with the physician.

- Observe and document the color, odor, and quantity of gastric secretions and notify physician of changes. Include irrigant in intake and output record.

- Prevent complications of bed rest (see The Immobilized Patient).

- *FOR SALEM SUMP:*

  - Maintain suction on intermittent high pressure (120 mm Hg) or continuous low pressure.

  - Following irrigation with saline, reconnect suction and irrigate air vent with 30 cc of air while suction is on.

  - Keep air vent pigtail of tube above patient's midline at all times.

- *FOR MILLER-ABBOTT:*

  - Usual advancement is 2–4 inches at prescribed intervals.

  - Tape tube *only* as ordered.

LINTON/SENGSTAKEN-BLAKEMORE

- Observe for signs and symptoms of respiratory distress: Dyspnea, use of accessory respiratory muscles, cyanosis, pallor, decreased inspiratory and expiratory volumes, decreasing pO_2 and increasing pCO_2.

- If acute respiratory distress occurs, deflate balloon and notify physician. If necessary, remove tube as ordered.

- Monitor balloon pressures to maintain at ordered level. Doubly clamp balloon channels with rubber-shod clamps.

- Deflate balloons not under traction for 5 mins. every 8–12 hrs. as ordered. Do not deflate balloons under traction.

- Observe patient and laboratory results for signs and symptoms of electrolyte imbalance (see Fluids and Electrolytes).

- Keep head of bed elevated slightly unless contraindicated by condition.

- Encourage deep breathing exercises but *NOT* coughing.

- Document quality and quantity of drainage. Include irrigant in intake and output record.

- Check suction machine for proper functioning. Maintain collection bottles below patient's midline at all times.

- Assist patient with oral hygiene. Keep lips moistened with ointment or lip balm.

- Assess and support patient's psychosocial needs. Explain all procedures to patient and family. Encourage family to visit patient and lend support. Maintain an atmosphere of hope and optimism.

- *FOR SENGSTAKEN-BLAKEMORE:*

  - Observe for chest pain as a sign of esophageal injury or rupture. Notify physician immediately and deflate tube as ordered.

  - Check each balloon for accurate amount of pressure every 30 mins. if sphygomomanometer is used; otherwise, clamp tube with two hemostats. (Pressure is usually 20–40 mm Hg.)

  - Check for secure traction.

  - Irrigate through gastric lumen only. Use iced normal saline for gastric lavage. Document quality of return.

- *FOR LINTON:*

  - Maintain prescribed amount of air in gastric balloon (usually 400 cc). Doubly clamp balloon channel with rubber-shod clamps.

  - Irrigate gastric lumen only. Used iced normal saline for gastric lavage.

  - Maintain secure traction with either helmet or sponge rubber.

PATIENT AND FAMILY TEACHING

- Explain all procedures to patient and family.

- If soft restraints are used, stress the reasons for their use to the family and patient.

- Instruct patient not to cough while the tube is in place.

ABDOMINAL SURGERY: CHOLECYSTECTOMY, SPLENECTOMY, ENTEROSTOMY, APPENDECTOMY, GASTRIC RESECTION, EXPLORATORY LAPAROTOMY

POTENTIAL PROBLEMS

Pulmonary Embolism	Thrombophlebitis
Hemorrhage	Evisceration
Shock	Dumping syndrome
Pneumonia	Paralytic Ileus
Atelectasis	Abscess Formation
Fluid and Electrolyte	Pain
Imbalance	Psychosocial Problems
Infection	
Peritonitis	

KEY NURSING INTERVENTIONS

- See Preoperative and Postoperative Care.

- Observe for signs and symptoms of hemorrhage and shock: Abdominal pain, hematemesis, shoulder pain, abdominal rigidity, blood-soaked dressings, diaphoresis, altered mental status, restlessness, agitation, increased pulse, decreased blood pressure.

- Observe for signs and symptoms of pulmonary embolism: Chest pain, shortness of breath, dyspnea, tachypnea, tachycardia, cyanosis, cardiopulmonary arrest.

- Observe for signs and symptoms of thrombophlebitis: Pain, redness, and swelling of affected extremity. Check for positive Homans' sign, which is pain in the calf upon dorsiflexion of the foot.

- Observe for signs and symptoms of peritonitis: Worsening abdominal pain, rebound tenderness, nausea, vomiting, fever, decreased bowel sounds.

- Prevent respiratory complications by encouraging frequent changes of position, coughing, deep breathing, assuring adequate fluid intake, and ambulation as soon as possible. Attempt these exercises 30–60 minutes after pain medication. Have the patient splint the abdomen with a pillow to help reduce pain when coughing and deep breathing.

- Minimize the risk of pulmonary embolism and thrombophlebitis. Maintain low-Fowler's position and avoid gatching the knees. Never massage the legs. Use anti-embolism stockings and avoid crossing the legs.

- Assess for urinary retention and/or renal failure. Keep the patient well hydrated by checking IV flow rates and encouraging PO fluid intake when allowed. Report output less than 30–50 cc per hour.

- When the patient is allowed to eat, provide a progressive bland diet. Be sure to assess for bowel sounds and/or passage of flatus. Small frequent meals are best.

- Assess and support the patient's psychosocial needs by being aware that a common fear of patients who have had abdominal surgery is that their "insides" will fall out upon coughing or standing. Be supportive and inform the patient that this will not happen. Help the patient and family deal with changes in body image and loss of function.

FOR CHOLECYSTECTOMY:

- Maintain a patent drainage or T-tube by avoiding the supine position. Place the patient in low or semi-Fowler's position. Attach tube to drainage bag or bottle. Avoid kinking or twisting of tube, and allow enough tube length to allow free movement in bed.

- Document quality and amount of bile drainage.

- After 5–7 days, the physician may order the tube clamped before and after meals. Document how the patient tolerates this. Observe for abdominal pain, nausea, and vomiting.

- Observe for signs and symptoms of biliary obstruction: Jaundice of skin and sclera, and changes in color and consistency of stools.

- Observe skin around tube insertion and prevent skin breakdown by checking and changing the dressings frequently.

FOR SPLENECTOMY:

- These patients are especially prone to thrombus formation and sepsis due to high platelet counts and alterations in white blood cell formation. Observe closely for pulmonary emboli, mesenteric emboli, and sepsis.

FOR GASTRIC RESECTION:

- Observe for signs and symptoms of dumping syndrome caused by rapid emptying of gastric contents: Nausea, vomiting, diarrhea, diaphoresis, palpitations, tachycardia, bradycardia, and syncope.

FOR ENTEROSTOMY:

- See Ileostomy/Colostomy.

PATIENT AND FAMILY TEACHING

- If the patient is to go home with dressings, tubes, or drainage bags, demonstrate their use and proper care.
- Instruct the patient to eat small, frequent meals and to chew food well. If the patient is to have a special diet, provide a list of acceptable foods or arrange for a visit from the hospital dietician.
- Encourage fluid intake to at least 2000 cc per day unless restricted.
- Instruct the patient to report signs and symptoms of complications to physician: Abdominal pain, chest pain, shortness of breath, dizziness, fainting, sweating, pain or swelling in lower extremities, fever, chills, prolonged vomiting or diarrhea, changes in bowel movements, yellowing of skin or eyes, and pain, redness or swelling of incision.
- Encourage the patient to be as active as possible but to avoid strenuous exercise, over-exercising, and heavy lifting until allowed by physician.

ULCERS: GASTRIC, PYLORIC, AND DUODENAL

POTENTIAL PROBLEMS

Pain

Fluid and Electrolyte
   Imbalance

Malnutrition

Hemorrhage

Obstruction

Alcoholism

Nausea

Vomiting

Perforation

Psychosocial Problems

KEY NURSING INTERVENTIONS

- Observe for signs and symptoms of fluid and electrolyte imbalances (see Fluid and Electrolytes).

- Observe for signs and symptoms of hemorrhage or perforation: Sudden severe abdominal pain, abdominal rigidity, shoulder pain, hematemesis, diaphoresis, increased pulse, decreased blood pressure.

- Promote bed rest by providing a quiet, tranquil environment with long periods of rest.

- Insert nasogastric tube as ordered for nausea and vomiting or for saline lavage in the case of gastric bleeding.
  NOTE: Do not insert if esophageal varices or diverticula are suspected.

- Document color, amount, and frequency of nasogastric secretions, emesis and stool. Check for occult blood.

- Administer antacids as ordered and with caution. Use low-sodium antacids. Observe for constipation with aluminum preparations and diarrhea with magnesium preparations.

- Assess and support the patient's psychosocial needs by promoting positive lifestyle changes to help reduce stress. Have the patient arrange for someone else to take care of the household or business while in the hospital. Attempt to make the patient realize that unless stress is reduced, the chance of a recurring ulcer is high. Some ulcers are caused by alcoholism. If this is the case, refer the patient to a local rehabilitation program.

PATIENT AND FAMILY TEACHING

- Stress the importance of eating six small meals per day. Advise the patient to avoid stressful situations, alcohol, smoking, caffeine, and aspirin.
- Inform the patient and family of signs and symptoms of gastric bleeding or hemorrhage. Instruct patient to seek medical care immediately if signs and symptoms occur.

SMALL AND LARGE BOWEL INFLAMMATION: GASTROENTERITIS, REGIONAL ENTERITIS, ULCERATIVE COLITIS, CROHN'S DISEASE, DIVERTICULITIS, IRRITABLE COLON

POTENTIAL PROBLEMS

Fluid and Electrolyte
   Imbalances
Nausea
Vomiting
Diarrhea
Fever
Hemorrhage
Toxic Megacolon

Malnutrition
Fistulas
Abscesses
Anorexia
Pain
Peritonitis
Psychosocial Problems

KEY NURSING INTERVENTIONS

- Observe for fluid and electrolyte imbalances (see Fluid and Electrolytes).

- Observe for signs and symptoms of complications (peritonitis, perforation, toxic megacolon, hemorrhage, abscesses, and fistula formation): Severe abdominal pain, fever, abdominal distention, rigidity, diaphoresis, increased pulse, decreasing blood pressure, shoulder pain, bowel contents in urine, open draining wounds.

- Promote rest of the bowel. Keep patient NPO as ordered. Promote bed rest by keeping emesis basin, bedpan, or bedside commode at bedside. Administer hyperalimentation as ordered (see Total Parenteral Nutrition).

- Provide good skin care, especially in states of malnutrition. Observe for excoriation in perianal area due to severe diarrhea.

- Document color, amount, frequency and presence of blood in emesis and/or stools.

- When the patient is allowed to resume oral intake, initiate a progressive diet. Offer foods in small frequent amounts. Avoid cold fluids, irritating foods, smoking, and alcohol. Give foods low in residue.

- Assess and support the patient's psychosocial needs by helping the patient realize that these diseases are characterized by periods of exacerbation and remissions (except for gastroenteritis) and that there is no cure. Help the patient adapt to new eating habits and possibly a change in lifestyle to help reduce stressors. To help avoid the embarrassment of frequent vomiting and diarrhea, provide a private room if possible, be supportive, and remove emesis and/or stool promptly. If the patient has an ileostomy, refer to an enterostomal therapist.

PATIENT AND FAMILY TEACHING

- Attempt to involve the family or significant other in patient care and discharge planning.
- Teach the patient to become more aware of early signs and symptoms of exacerbations so that treatment may be initiated sooner.
- Instruct the patient to eat low-residue foods and eat six small meals per day. Avoid irritating foods, cold liquids, alcohol and smoking. Arrange for a visit by the hospital dietician.

INTESTINAL OBSTRUCTION, PARALYTIC ILEUS

POTENTIAL PROBLEMS

Fluid and Electrolyte
   Imbalance
Dehydration
Peritonitis
Perforation

Intestinal Gangrene
Shock
Pain
Psychosocial Problems

KEY NURSING INTERVENTIONS

- Observe for signs and symptoms of fluid and electrolyte imbalance (see Fluid and Electrolytes).

- Observe for signs and symptoms of perforation, strangulation, and shock: Sudden, severe, and prolonged abdominal pain, abdominal rigidity, fever, diaphoresis, altered mental status, increasing pulse, decreasing blood pressure.

- Keep the patient NPO and insert nasogastric tube as ordered or assist the physician in passing an intestinal tube (see Nasogastric Tubes).

- Assist the patient in turning from side to side to help aid passage of fluid and gas past the obstruction.

- Document color, amount and frequency of nasogastric secretions, emesis, and stool. Check for presence of occult blood.

- If the patient is allowed to eat, give food in small amounts. Check for bowel sounds in all four quadrants after every meal.

- If necessary, prepare the patient for surgery (see Abdominal Surgery and/or Ileostomy-Colostomy).

- Assess and support the patient's psychosocial needs by explaining the purpose and procedure of nasogastric tube insertion. If an enterostomy is to be performed, help the patient deal with changes in body image and lifestyle (see Ileostomy-Colostomy).

PATIENT AND FAMILY TEACHING

- If an enterostomy is present, stress the importance of eating small, frequent amounts and thoroughly chewing all foods.

- When allowed, encourage fluids for good hydration.
- Instruct the patient to avoid constipation by staying as active as possible.

COLOSTOMY, ILEOSTOMY

POTENTIAL PROBLEMS

Hemorrhage
Fluid and Electrolyte
   Imbalance
Obstruction
Infection/Peritonitis
Retraction
Prolapse
Stricture
Skin Breakdown

Wound Dehiscence
Stomal Ischemia
Malnutrition
Drug Malabsorption
Diarrhea
Renal Calculi
Pain
Psychosocial Problems

KEY NURSING INTERVENTIONS

- See Preoperative and Postoperative Care.

- See Abdominal Surgery.

- Observe stoma for color and size. Stoma should be pink to bright red. Dark blue-black or purple-red must be reported immediately. Stoma should remain above the surface level of the skin. Prolapse and major hemorrhage must be reported immediately.

- Observe incision for signs and symptoms of infection: Redness, purulent drainage, fever, tenderness.

- Assess patient for signs and symptoms of obstruction: Distention, abdominal pain, vomiting, absence of stool, malodor.

- Prevent skin irritation and wound infection. Evaluate appliance for proper fit. (Stomal opening of bag should be ⅛-1⁄16 inch larger than stoma.) Assure a good seal using effective skin barriers (Stomahesive, Karya ring, etc.). When leakage occurs, change bag immediately. Try different types of appliances as needed. (Use transparent, drainable appliances.)

- Assess patient for signs and symptoms of fluid and electrolyte imbalance (see Fluids and Electrolytes).

- If nasogastric tube is present, monitor aspirate for color, consistency, amount and odor.

- Auscultate bowel for return of peristalsis.

- Palpate bowel for resistance, rigidity, rebound tenderness and involuntary guarding (indicative of peritoneal irritation).

- Assess patient tolerance to PO intake when nasogastric tube is removed.

- Encourage adequate fluid intake, especially with ileostomy patients.

- Assess the quality and quantity of stools. Report diarrhea to surgeon. (For *ILEOSTOMY*, stools will be watery at first and later become semisolid or paste-like at about 500 cc/day. For *COLOSTOMY*, stools will be watery in the ascending colon, pasty in the transverse colon and increasingly solid down the descending colon.)

- Control odors. Use air fresheners when changing ostomy bag. Avoid odorous foods such as cabbage, onions, eggs, and fish. Odor-proof bags can be used along with oral deodorizing agents (chlorophyll, bismuth subcarbonate, bismuth subgallate, parsley and spinach).

- Observe wound for signs of dehiscence (sudden, profuse serosanguinous drainage from incision around 5th to 8th day postoperatively).

- Properly apply and secure appliance. Measure stoma prior to application. Wash and thoroughly dry skin around stoma. Skin barrier should be used if bag does not have one. Apply open-ended bag at a 45-degree angle while on bedrest and 90 degrees when ambulatory. Prevent wrinkles in adhesive part of bag and in patient's skin when applying bag. Remove all air from bag before sealing.

- Assess and support patient's psychosocial needs. Alteration in body image and loss of normal body functioning are the two greatest psychological hurdles for patient adaptation. Nursing care should be individualized since each patient's coping mechanisms, previous experiences and ability to adjust are different. Interventions should focus on helping the patient cope. Create an open atmosphere that encourages discussion of feelings. Help the patient explore fears, anxieties, and frustrations. Reassure patient that sex, work, exercise, and most other activities may be resumed as soon as strength increases and other medical conditions permit. Refer patient to United Ostomy Association. Arrange for a visit by a patient with a similar ostomy when patient is ready. Do not force the patient into learning situations until the patient is ready. Include family or significant others in care plan.

- *FOR INTERNAL ILEAL RESERVOIR:*

  - A catheter is left in the stoma for approximately 2 weeks postoperatively and connected to low suction to keep the reservoir empty and prevent pressure on suture lines.

  - Irrigate catheter q 4–6 hrs. with normal saline as ordered.

  - Report cessation of drainage along with reports of cramping and distention.

- *FOR ILEOSTOMY:*

  - Encourage thorough mastication of food to prevent food blockage.

  - Observe stools for undissolved medications and for effectiveness of medications. Notify physician of signs of malabsorption.

- *FOR COLOSTOMY:*

  - Irrigate *only* as ordered.

  - Insert irrigating catheter tip no more than 3 inches.

  - Never force catheter into stoma.

  - Allow fluid to enter *slowly*.

  - Allow 20 mins. for initial return. Close irrigating sleeve and allow 45 mins. for completion of return. (Drinking warm water and abdominal massage will help stimulate peristalsis).

PATIENT AND FAMILY TEACHING

- Attempt to involve significant other in patient teaching.

- Demonstrate proper stoma care, skin care, and application of bags. Tell patient to carry extra bags, skin barrier and cement at all times.

- Inform patient of local ostomy supply distributors.

- Stress the importance of adequate fluid intake (3000 cc/day).

- Advise patient to avoid spicy foods, carbonated beverages, beer, beans, cabbage, onions, radishes, cucumbers, and chewing gum which cause gas.

- Recommend deodorizing foods such as cranberry juice, yoghurt, buttermilk, and parsley.

- Advise trying new foods one at a time so that if a problem develops, it can be easily identified.

- Instruct patient to report signs of infection: Fever, swelling, redness, tenderness, drainage.

- Signs and symptoms of obstruction should be reported (abdominal distention, absence of bowel elimination, abdominal pain, vomiting).

- *FOR ILEOSTOMY:*

  - Instruct patient to chew food thoroughly to prevent food blockage.
  - Changing the ileostomy appliance is easiest before meals or before going to bed.

- *FOR COLOSTOMY:*

  - Instruct patient in irrigating technique as ordered.

RECTAL SURGERY: HEMORRHOIDS, PILONIDAL CYST, FISTULAS, ABSCESSES, TUMORS

POTENTIAL PROBLEMS

Hemorrhage	Constipation
Pain	Urinary Retention
Infection	Psychological Problems

KEY NURSING INTERVENTIONS

- See Preoperative and Postoperative Care.

- Observe for signs and symptoms of postoperative bleeding or hemorrhage: Blood-soaked dressings, frank rectal bleeding or blood in stools, severe rectal pain, diaphoresis, increasing pulse, decreasing blood pressure.

- Prevent infection of surgical wounds by using aseptic technique during dressing changes and keeping perianal area clean.

- Help decrease postoperative pain and promote healing. Provide sitz baths with a comfortable water temperature. Avoid the same position for long periods. Apply cool or warm compresses as ordered. Avoid constipation by providing a high fiber diet and increasing fluids to at least 2000 cc per day. Avoid cathartics and enemas.

- Help avoid urinary retention by good fluid intake and, if possible, allowing the patient to stand or sit on the toilet to void.

- Assess and support the patient's psychosocial needs by being aware that rectal problems may be embarrassing for the patient. Provide privacy when doing dressing changes or conversing about the patient's rectal problem. Since the first bowel movement may be a frightening experience, assure the patient that you will be available to provide needed moral support.

PATIENT AND FAMILY TEACHING

- Instruct the patient to avoid rubbing the perianal area after defecation. Instead make use of sitz baths and pat the area dry with soft tissue.

- Have the patient avoid constipation by a diet high in fiber, staying well hydrated, staying as active as possible, and using stool softeners only as ordered.
- Advise the patient to avoid cathartics, enemas, and sitting for long periods.

CHOLECYSTITIS, CHOLELITHIASIS, CHOLEDOCHOLITHIASIS

POTENTIAL PROBLEMS

Pain	Fever
Fluid and Electrolyte	Peritonitis
Imbalances	Perforation
Malnutrition	Infection
Nausea	Jaundice
Vomiting	

KEY NURSING INTERVENTIONS

- Observe for signs and symptoms of fluid and electrolyte imbalance (see Fluid and Electrolytes).

- Observe for signs and symptoms of perforation and peritonitis: Increased abdominal pain, rebound tenderness, nausea, vomiting, fever, decreased bowel sounds, tachycardia.

- Insert nasogastric tube to low suction as ordered to help relieve nausea and vomiting. This will eliminate gastric juices which stimulate bile secretion. Document color and amount of gastric secretions.

- Prevent respiratory complications (may be due to pain under the diaphragm) by encouraging frequent change of position, coughing, and deep breathing. Attempt these exercises 30–60 minutes after pain medication.
  NOTE: Avoid morphine since this may cause the pain to worsen.

- Prepare the patient for diagnostic studies and/or surgery if ordered (see Diagnostic Studies and/or Abdominal Surgery.)

- Assess and support the patient's psychosocial needs. The patient with abdominal pain may have to undergo many diagnostic studies in order to diagnose the problem. This can be very taxing on the patient. Attempt to schedule these tests to allow for periods of rest. Let the patient know how long the test will take and what will be required. Help the patient and family deal with changes in body image and function, especially if jaundice is present and pain is severe.

PATIENT AND FAMILY TEACHING

- Explain the purpose and procedure of the nasogastric tube prior to insertion.

- Provide a list of foods low in fat. Encourage meals in small, frequent amounts. Arrange for visit from hospital dietician if needed.

- Instruct the patient to report signs and symptoms of complications (see Abdominal Surgery).

HEPATITIS, CIRRHOSIS

POTENTIAL PROBLEMS

Jaundice	Pneumonia
Fluid and Electrolyte Imbalances	Ascites
	Altered Mental Status
Bleeding Tendencies	Coma
Anorexia	Anemia
Nausea	Skin Breakdown
Vomiting	Pruritus
Weakness	Alcoholism
Esophageal Varices	
Psychosocial Problems	

KEY NURSING INTERVENTIONS

- Observe for signs and symptoms of fluid and electrolyte imbalances related to NPO, nasogastric suctioning, and/or anorexia (see Fluid and Electrolytes).

- Observe for signs and symptoms of hemorrhage and shock related to bleeding tendencies: Blood in emesis or stool, abdominal pain, abdominal rigidity, shoulder pain, diaphoresis, altered mental status, restlessness, agitation, increased pulse, decreased blood pressure.

- Observe for signs and symptoms of impending hepatic failure or hepatic encephalopathy: Confusion, stupor, tremor of hands, hyper-reflexia, hallucinations, coma.

- Insert nasogastric tube and attach to low suction as ordered for nausea and vomiting.
  NOTE: Nasogastric tube insertion is contraindicated if esophageal varices are suspected, especially in the patient with cirrhosis.

- Document color, amount, frequency, and characteristics of nasogastric secretions, vomitus, and stool. Check for occult blood.

- Prevent respiratory complications which may be related to ascites or pain under the diaphragm by encouraging frequent change of position, coughing, deep breathing, and measuring abdominal girth to check for worsening ascites.

- Place the patient in appropriate isolation as indicated (see Infection Control).

- Promote bed rest by explaining its importance, providing a quiet environment and limiting visitors to specific hours during the day.

- When the patient is allowed to eat, offer meals in small, frequent amounts. Consult with hospital dietician if special diet is ordered (usually low fat and protein). Provide low salt diet for ascites or edema.

- Administer skin care BID and PRN. Check for and document presence of ecchymosis, breakdown, and pruritus.

- Assess and support the patient's psychosocial needs by attempting to involve the family or significant other in patient care and discharge planning. Help them plan for a long convalescence and possible change in lifestyle due to prolonged absence from school and/or work. Explain the purpose and procedure of isolation, if necessary. Help the patient and family deal with negative attitudes towards liver disease. Avoid labeling the patient as a drug addict, alcoholic, homosexual, or unclean. If an underlying problem is present such as alcoholism, refer the patient to a local rehabilitation program.

PATIENT AND FAMILY TEACHING

- Provide a list of allowed foods. Stress the importance of eating even though there is no appetite. Small frequent meals are best. Encourage fluid intake to 2000 cc per day if not restricted.

- Instruct the patient to report signs and symptoms of complications to physician: Blood in emesis or stool, abdominal pain, anorexia, increased malaise or weakness, shortness of breath, prolonged vomiting or diarrhea, sweating, dizziness, altered mental status, and hallucinations.

- Stress the importance of good personal hygiene and prevention of infection to others. Demonstrate good hand washing, proper handling and disposal of food and patient excretions. Explain mode of transmission for hepatitis.

- Instruct the patient never to donate blood.

- Tell the patient to avoid alcohol completely. Always check with the physician before taking over-the-counter medications, especially acetaminophen.

- Encourage slow, progressive activity. Stress the importance of rest. Emphasize that a relapse may occur if activity is increased too rapidly.

- Arrange for family to receive gammaglobulin injections or hepatitis B vaccines if indicated. Consult with the nurse epidemiologist or physician.

PANCREATITIS

POTENTIAL PROBLEMS

Shock   Hyperglycemia
Internal Hemorrhage   Pain
Abscess Formation   Respiratory Problems
Electrolyte Imbalances   Psychosocial Problems

KEY NURSING INTERVENTIONS

- Pancreatitis usually causes severe abdominal pain. Strong narcotics may be required. Avoid the use of opiates (morphine) which can cause biliary-pancreatic duct spasm, making the pain worse.

- Observe for signs and symptoms of complications:

  Hemorrhage and shock from internal bleeding due to leakage from pancreas: Abdominal pain; cool, moist skin; increasing pulse; decreasing blood pressure; pallor; dizziness upon sitting or standing; agitation; restlessness.

  Fluid and electrolyte imbalances. Observe for changes in laboratory values, especially potassium, sodium, glucose, amylase, calcium, and magnesium (see Fluid and Electrolytes).

  Acid-base imbalance from hyperglycemia: Polydipsia; polyuria; glycosuria; hot, dry skin; altered mental status; acetone breath (see Diabetes Mellitus).

  Respiratory problems from pain and edema under diaphragm: Shallow respirations, tachypnea, shortness of breath, decreased pO_2.

- Check nasogastric tube aspirate. Document odor and amount of drainage.

- Observe and document stools for presence of steatorrhea: Frequent, frothy, foul-smelling.

- When the patient is allowed to eat, provide a low-fat diet in small, frequent amounts.

- A large percentage of pancreatitis is caused by alcohol abuse. If this is the case, close observation for alcohol withdrawal (delirium tremens) is essential. This can be life-threatening (see Alcoholism).

- Assess and support the patient's psychosocial needs. Be careful not to label the patient with pancreatitis as an alcoholic or drug addict. Many patients with this disease do not have these problems. However, chronic pancreatitis causes chronic abdominal pain, and it is not uncommon for these patients to become dependent on narcotics for pain relief. Alcohol abuse will precipitate an attack or aggravate the situation. These are serious and difficult problems to deal with both in and out of the hospital. It usually takes a team effort of nurses, physicians, psychological experts, and significant others to effectively deal with these problems.

PATIENT AND FAMILY TEACHING

- Explain the importance of maintaining a low-fat diet in small, frequent amounts.
- Inform the patient and family of signs and symptoms of complications (abdominal pain, nausea, vomiting, fever, polydipsia, polyuria, altered mental status, jaundice).
- Stress the importance of avoiding alcohol. Continued use will cause recurrence of pancreatitis.
- Provide a list of local alcohol and/or drug rehabilitation programs if indicated.

ALCOHOLISM, DELIRIUM TREMENS

POTENTIAL PROBLEMS

Cardiac Failure

Malnutrition

Neuropathies

Fluid and Electrolyte
  Imbalances

COPD

Pancreatitis

Hepatitis

Psychosocial Problems

Cirrhosis

Esophageal Varices

Gastrointestinal Bleeding

Pneumonia

Skin Breakdown

Anemias

Bleeding Tendencies

KEY NURSING INTERVENTIONS

- Alcoholism is not a gastrointestinal disorder. However, since its abuse directly affects the gastrointestinal system, it is probably most appropriate to include it in this section. It should be stressed that any patient may have a problem with alcohol and may be found almost anywhere in the hospital setting with almost any type of accompanying condition.

- Since alcohol affects the whole body, a complete assessment of all systems is essential, including an in depth psychosocial assessment.

- Observe for problems from the effects of alcohol:

  Gastrointestinal: Nausea, vomiting, diarrhea, abdominal pain, malnutrition, esophageal varices, gastrointestinal bleeding, ulcers, pancreatitis, hepatitis, cirrhosis, ascites.

  Neurological: Polyneuropathies: Decreased sensation in hands and feet, burns to skin from poor sensation, muscle pain. Wernicke-Korsakoff syndrome: Noncortical nystagmus, diplopia, walking and motor disturbances, poor memory, confusion, confabulation, frank psychoses.

  Cardiovascular: Poor cardiac output, congestive heart failure, hypertension, hypotension, tachycardia, vascular collapse.

  Respiratory: Pneumonia, COPD, tuberculosis.

  Fluid and Electrolyte Imbalance: Fluid shifts, hypocalcemia, hypomagnesemia (see Fluid and Electrolyte Imbalances).

Integumentary: Poor hygiene, skin breakdown, rashes, dermatitis, petachiae, ecchymosis, jaundice.

Hematologic: Anemias, bleeding tendencies, difficulty in fighting infections.

- Encourage nutritional and fluid intake if the patient can tolerate oral intake.

- Assess and support the patient's psychosocial needs. Build a trusting relationship with the patient by being nonjudgmental about past behavior. An alcoholic patient may withdraw or be belligerent, angry, or manipulative. Setting limits on undesirable behavior is an important intervention. However, to be effective, these behavioral limits must be realistic and communicated to the patient, visitors, family and the rest of the staff. Realize that it is difficult to treat alcoholism in the acute care setting while still dealing with the organic component that originally brought the patient to the hospital. Stress to family and friends never to bring in alcoholic beverages for the patient as this only prolongs and aggravates the problem. Only through a long-term team effort of the nurse, physician, family, psychiatric help, and a rehabilitation program can the alcoholic be successfully treated.

- *FOR DELIRIUM TREMENS:*

  - Observe for signs and symptoms of delirium tremens: Onset is usually 24–72 hours after the last drink, acute anxiety, anger, irritability, agitation, restlessness, tremors, tachycardia, sweating, fever, visual and auditory hallucinations, seizure activity.
    NOTE: This is a medical emergency.

  - If the patient has delirium tremens: Check vital signs every 30–60 minutes and PRN; Administer sedatives and anticonvulsants as ordered to prevent injury, exhaustion, seizures, and further deterioration (Valium, Librium, chloral hydrate, dilantin, magnesium sulfate); place the patient in a low-stimulus environment; avoid bright lights and many shadows which may precipitate or aggravate hallucinations; Maintain seizure precautions (see Seizure Disorders).

  - Assess and support the patient's psychosocial needs. Stay with the patient during acute episodes. Provide reassurance that hallucinations are not real even though they seem to be. Tell the patient that this is not going to last forever. Arrange for a family member or sitter to stay with the patient at all times, especially if suicidal tendencies have been expressed. Restrain the patient only if necessary. Arrange for a visit from Social Service or other counseling, if necessary. It usually takes a team effort of health care professions to deal with acute alcoholism.

PATIENT AND FAMILY TEACHING

- Attempt to involve the family or significant other in patient care and discharge planning.

- Provide a list of local alcohol rehabilitation programs and the family-oriented counseling agencies.

- When the patient is ready, explain the harmful systemic effects and problems caused by alcohol. Stress the importance of a well-balanced diet with proper fluid intake.

ENDOCRINE SYSTEM

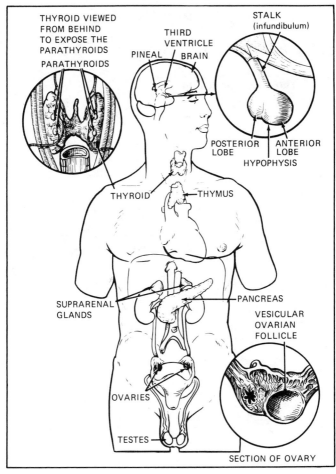

Endocrine System

ENDOCRINE SYSTEM—PHYSIOLOGY SUMMARY

I. PITUITARY GLAND

A. The Posterior Pituitary

1. The posterior pituitary is directly connected to the hypothalamus.

2. It does not secrete hormones but stores two hormones which are secreted by the hypothalamus, oxytocin and ADH.

3. The hypothalamus stimulates the posterior pituitary to release the hormones via nerve fibers.

4. Oxytocin (Pitocin) actions are as follows:

   a) Stimulates uterine contraction at childbirth and stimulates smooth muscles to maintain the labor process.

   b) Stimulates the glandular cells of the lactating breast to release milk into the ducts.

5. ADH (antidiuretic hormone or vasopressin) actions are as follows:

   a) Arterial constriction, thus increasing blood pressure.

   b) The reabsorption of water in the distal tubule of the kidney.

   c) Gastrointestinal smooth muscle stimulation.

B. The Anterior Pituitary

1. The anterior pituitary secretes the following:

   a) STH (somatotropin)—growth hormone.

   b) ACTH (adrenocorticotropin).

   c) TSH (thyrotropin).

   d) Prolactin (lactogenic).

   e) FSH (follicle stimulating hormone).

   f) LH (luteinizing hormone).

   g) ICSH (interstitial cell stimulating hormone).

   h) MSH (melanocyte stimulating hormone).

2. STH—somatotropin—growth hormone:

   a) Participates in protein, carbohydrate, fat, and calcium metabolism in the presence of adequate amounts of insulin.

   b) Controls bone growth prior to epiphyseal closure.

3. ACTH—adrenocorticotropin hormone:

   a) Regulates the adrenal cortex.

   b) Controls cortisol (hydrocortisone) production by the adrenal cortex.

4. TSH—thyrotropin hormone:

   a) Controls secretion of thyroxine by the thyroid gland.

   b) TSH secretion is regulated by thyroxine level (a feedback mechanism whereby increased TSH levels cause the release of thyroxine and an increased level of thyroxine causes inhibition of TSH release).

5. LTH—prolactin—luteotropic hormone:

   a) Stimulates breast growth.

   b) Maintains lactation.

   c) Preserves the corpus luteum which causes progesterone secretion.

   d) Secretion of LTH is stimulated by suckling.

6. FSH—follicle stimulating hormone (also called a gonado-tropic hormone):

   a) Controls development of ovaries and testes.

   b) Controls graafian follicles, causing development of ovarian cells and estrogen production.

   c) Participates in spermatozoa development.

7. LH—luteinizing hormone (also called a gonadotropic hormone; in males, also called ICSH—interstitial cell stimulating hormone)

   a) Controls production of testosterone by males.

   b) Controls production of progesterone by females.

8. MSH—melanocyte stimulating hormone
   Possibly participates in skin pigment regulation.

II. THYROID GLAND

A. The Thyroid Gland

Is composed of two lobes which become enlarged normally during stress, pregnancy, and puberty.

B. Two hormones are produced

1. Thyroxine (T_4)
2. Tri-iodothyronine (T_3)

C. Thyroid Hormone

1. Thyroxine and tri-iodothyronine perform the same functions and can be termed collectively as thyroid hormone.
2. Thyroid hormone is produced by the combination of sodium or potassium iodine and the amino acid tyrosine.
3. Release of thyroid hormone is regulated by TSH from the anterior pituitary.
4. Thyroid circulates in the blood as a protein-bound hormone.

D. Thyroid hormone actions

1. Participation in metabolic processes.
2. Regulation of metabolic rate.

III. PARATHYROID GLAND

A. Parathyroid Hormone

1. Is secreted by the parathyroid gland and regulates calcium ion concentration.
2. It therefore participates in the following:

   a) Bone formation
   b) Blood coagulation
   c) Maintaining cell permeability
   d) Maintaining neuromuscular irritability

B. Regulation

1. The release of parathyroid hormone is regulated by a negative feedback mechanism.

2. Decreased plasma calcium levels stimulate parathyroid release, which then removes calcium from the bones to raise the plasma level.

3. High levels of plasma calcium inhibit parathyroid release.

IV. PANCREAS (ISLETS)

A. Pancreatic islets

1. Produce two hormones, insulin and glucagon.

2. There are three types of islet cells

   a) Alpha

   b) Beta

   c) Delta

B. Beta cells

1. Produce the hormone insulin.

2. Insulin regulates blood glucose levels and participates in carbohydrate metabolism by enabling glucose to enter the cell, thus decreasing the blood level of glucose.

C. Alpha cells

1. Produce the hormone glucagon.

2. Glucagon regulates blood glucose levels by stimulating the liver to break down glycogen into glucose, thus increasing the blood glucose level.

D. Regulation

1. The release of both insulin and glucagon is controlled by the glucose level of the blood.

2. A high glucose level stimulates the release of insulin, and a low glucose level stimulates the release of glucagon.

V. ADRENAL GLANDS

A. The adrenal gland

Is composed of two parts

1. The cortex (outer part).

2. The medulla (inner part).

B. The adrenal cortex

Secretes:

1. Mineral corticoids (aldosterone).

2. Glucocorticoids (cortisol or hydrocortisone).

3. Androgens (testosterone).

C. Aldosterone

Regulates water and electrolyte metabolism by its actions on the kidney.

1. It causes increased reabsorption of sodium, which in turn increases the osmotic pressure of extracellular fluid.

2. Low sodium concentration stimulates the secretion of aldosterone, and high sodium concentration inhibits aldosterone secretion.

3. Decreased extracellular fluid concentration causes increased secretion of aldosterone and vice versa.

4. Aldosterone causes increased secretion of potassium, which can cause weakness and arrhythmias.

5. Aldosterone also causes potassium excretion and sodium retention in perspiration and saliva.

D. Cortisol

Participates in glucose, protein, and fat metabolism, but the exact mechanism is unknown. It is responsible for increasing the rate of gluconeogenesis and amino acid metabolism.

E. Androgens

Responsible for masculine characteristics. Testosterone is secreted by the testes.

F. The adrenal medulla

Secretes:

1. Epinephrine

2. Norepinephrine

G. Epinephrine

Causes an increase in blood sugar by converting stored liver glycogen to glucose and by converting muscle glycogen into lactic acid for further glucose production in the liver (see Gastrointestinal Physiology Summary).

H. Norepinephrine

Acts on the sympathetic nerves to stimulate various functions (see Nervous System Physiology Summary).

I. Innervation

Both epinephrine and norepinephrine are released in response to sympathetic innervation and stimulation.

VI. OVARIES

Secrete two hormones

1. Estrogen.

2. Progesterone.

(See Reproductive Physiology Summary).

VII. TESTES

The testes secrete the hormone testosterone (see Reproductive System Physiology Summary).

VIII. PINEAL GLAND

It is believed that the pineal gland participates in anterior pituitary function.

IX. PLACENTA

A. The placenta

Secretes the following:

1. Chorionic gonadotropin.

2. Estrogen.

3. Progesterone.

B. Chorionic gonadotropin hormone

Responsible for maintaining the corpus luteum which, in turn, secretes estrogen and progesterone.

C. Estrogen

Secretion increases throughout pregnancy and peaks prior to birth. Its functions in pregnancy are the following.

1. Increasing uterine musculature.

2. Increasing uterine vasculature.

3. Enlargement of vagina and external sex organs.

D. Progesterone

Levels reach a peak prior to birth and function as follows.

1. Increases nutritional supplies to the ovum.

2. Inhibits uterine muscular growth.

ENDOCRINE SYSTEM ASSESSMENT

The endocrine system is highly complex and difficult to assess. Since most of the glands are small and inaccessible, they do not lend themselves to traditional auscultation, percussion, and palpation. Each endocrine disorder has its own specific hormone imbalance and thus a specific set of signs, symptoms, and potential problems; there may be some common manifestations observed, however. A thorough history, physical inspection, observation of laboratory values, and familiarization with the involved gland are the best modes of assessing the endocrine system.

I. HISTORY

A. Past history of endocrine problems

1. What type?
2. What therapy was utilized? Did it work?

B. Recent History

Ask the patient and family for presence of the following:

1. Personality changes, i.e., feelings of nervousness, depression, anger, emotional outbursts.
2. Weakness, fatigue, exhaustion.
3. Headaches.
4. Anorexia.
5. Polyuria.
6. Menstrual problems.
7. Sexual problems.
8. Intolerance to temperatures.
9. Musculoskeletal problems.
10. Past surgeries.

C. Medications

1. List medications, including over-the-counter drugs.
2. Allergies.

D. Nutrition

Describe a typical:

1. Breakfast.

2. Lunch.

3. Dinner.

4. Snacks.

II. BACKGROUND INFORMATION

A. Lab Values

Check laboratory studies for abnormal values or worsening trends.

B. Diagnostic Studies

Identify abnormal results of diagnostic studies.

C. Chart

Check old chart for past relevant information.

III. INSPECTION

A. Appearance

Observe for the following:

1. Dwarfism, gigantism, acromegaly.

2. Abnormal hair growth.

3. Abnormal skin pigmentation.

4. Unusual changes in physical appearance, i.e., moon face, exophthalmos, obesity, buffalo hump.

5. Dehydration.

6. Edema.

B. Personality changes

Question the patient and significant others for:

1. Acute anxiety.

2. Mood swings.

3. Inappropriate affect.

4. Neuroses.

5. Psychoses.

HYPOTHYROIDISM (MYXEDEMA), MYXEDEMA COMA

POTENTIAL PROBLEMS

Myxedema Coma	Decubitus Ulcers
Bradycardia	Muscle Aches
Hypoventilation	Constipation
Hypotension	Weight Gain
Hypothermia	Menorrhagia
Convulsions	Lethargy
Heart Disease	Psychosocial Problems
Dry Skin	

KEY NURSING INTERVENTIONS

- Observe for signs and symptoms of myxedema coma: Hypotension, bradycardia, hypoventilation, acidosis, hypothermia, hyponatremia, hypocalcemia, cardiopulmonary arrest. This is a medical emergency.

- If myxedema coma occurs, support respirations and obtain arterial blood gases. Administer intravenous thyroid preparations as ordered, slowly to avoid heart failure. Intravenous glucose and steroids may also be ordered. Avoid fluid overload. Keep the patient warm but do not overheat.

- Avoid giving barbiturates, narcotics, sedatives, and anesthetics. This could result in death due to increased sensitivity.

- Attempt to prevent situations that may precipitate a myxedema coma: Stress, infections, cooling, trauma.

- Administer good skin care. Apply lotions to help keep the skin moist. Use mild soap for baths.

- Encourage the patient to change position at least every two hours to prevent decubitus ulcers. Use protective mattresses and pressure-relieving devices.

- Help the patient to avoid constipation and fecal impactions. Encourage a high-fiber diet with a liberal fluid intake. Attempt to increase level of activity.

- The goal of therapy is to increase the thyroid hormone level to normal. This is done slowly with close observations. Observe for signs and symptoms of thyroid overdose: Tachycardia, irritability, diaphoresis, headache, angina, heart failure, pulmonary edema, myocardial infarction.

- Assess and support the patient's psychosocial needs. Realize that this disease causes everything to slow down. Allow the patient to proceed at his/her own pace. Myxedema can cause mood swings, depression, and psychoses. Observe for suicidal tendencies. Arrange for a psychiatric or social service consultation. Reassure patient that with early hormone therapy he/she can expect the symptoms of myxedema to slowly disappear.

PATIENT AND FAMILY TEACHING

- Encourage the patient to slowly increase activity level and to get plenty of rest.
- Instruct patient in ways to avoid constipation and fecal impactions. Have dietician review foods which contain roughage. Advise liberal fluid intake daily, unless contraindicated.
- Stress the importance of lifetime thyroid hormone therapy.
- Instruct patient in signs and symptoms of thyroid overdose: Diarrhea, diaphoresis, tachycardia, heat intolerance, tremor, flushed face.
- Advise patient to report signs of thyroid overdose or ineffective treatment to physician.

HYPERTHYROIDISM (GRAVE'S DISEASE), THYROID CRISIS (STORM)

POTENTIAL PROBLEMS

Thyroid Crisis	Constipation
Heart Failure	Diarrhea
Coma	Heat Intolerance
Shock	Weakness
Pulmonary Edema	Tachycardia
Atrial Arrhythmias	Exophthalmos
Weight Loss	Psychosocial Problems

KEY NURSING INTERVENTIONS

- Observe for signs and symptoms of thyroid crisis or storm: Elevated temperature, tachycardia, dehydration, diarrhea, tachypnea, atrial arrhythmias, excessive irritability, delirium, confusion, psychotic behavior, pulmonary edema, shock.

- If thyroid crisis occurs, notify physician and arrange for transfer to ICU. Place the patient on an EKG monitor. Administer medications as ordered to help bring the patient to homeostasis: IV fluids, electrolytes, vitamins, iodine, propranolol, digitalis, antithyroids, sedatives, tranquilizers, steroids, diuretics, phenothiazines, vasopressors, antipyretics. Control temperature with cooling measures as ordered.

- Assess the patient and document signs and symptoms of chronic hyperthyroidism: Enlarged thyroid glands, anxiety, restlessness, tachycardia, palpitations, heat intolerance, diaphoresis, tremor, exophthalmos, weight loss, increased appetite, constipation, diarrhea, amenorrhea, atrial arrhythmias.

- Maintain a cool and tranquil environment. Eliminate excessive stimuli. Help the patient to avoid stressful situations.

- Encourage a liberal fluid intake if not contraindicated.

- Observe for signs and symptoms of toxic reactions from antithyroid drugs: Hypothyroidism, skin rash, urticaria, fever, agranulocytosis, increased susceptibility to infections.

- Provide a diet high in protein, carbohydrates, and vitamin B. Avoid foods and beverages that contain caffeine and other stimulants. Consult with hospital dietician.

- If the patient has exophthalmos (bulging of the eyes), instill eyedrops to keep the eyes moist. Have the patient sleep with the head of the bed elevated. The patient may need eye surgery to help relieve symptoms.

- See Thyroidectomy if surgery is indicated.

- Assess and support the patient's psychosocial needs. These patients can be easily excitable, irritable, aggressive, and exhibit bizarre behavior. This can be a difficult problem to deal with. Develop a care plan which may include providing diversional activities, setting limits on maladaptive behavior, and helping the patient gain insight into psychological problems. Arrange for a psychiatric or social service consultation as needed.

PATIENT AND FAMILY TEACHING

- If the patient is taking antithyroid medications, instruct him/her to report any signs and symptoms of infection: Fever, sore throat, or respiratory problems. Stress that infection may precipitate thyroid crisis along with dental procedures, fear, surgery and insulin reactions.

- Inform the patient and family of signs and symptoms of thyroid crisis, and to seek care at an emergency room if symptoms occur.

- Encourage the patient to wear a Medic Alert tag.

- If the patient has exophthalmos, demonstrate how to instill eye drops. Advise wearing sunglasses when outdoors.

- Encourage the patient to eat foods high in protein, carbohydrates, and minerals. Encourage a mentally and physically restful environment. Exercise should be in moderation.

THYROIDECTOMY

POTENTIAL PROBLEMS

Upper Airway Obstruction	Hypocalcemia
Hemorrhage	Hypothyroidism
Shock	Laryngeal Nerve Damage
Respiratory Problems	Psychosocial Problems
Thyroid Crisis	

KEY NURSING INTERVENTIONS

- Observe for and prevent postoperative complications (see Post-operative Care).

- Before surgery can take place, the patient must have normal thyroid levels and be in good condition. This is done with antithyroid drugs, iodine preparations, bed rest, proper diet, and alleviation of as much stress as possible. This process may take several months.

- This surgery is performed in close proximity to the trachea. Observe for signs and symptoms of upper airway obstruction: Restlessness, tachycardia, stridor, tachypnea, accessory muscle use, cyanosis, agitation. Report signs of obstruction to surgeon immediately.

- Keep cricothyrotomy or tracheostomy tray, suction equipment, and 1–2 grams of 10% calcium gluconate solution at the bedside.

- Assess patient's voice for nerve damage. Have patient say something every 30–60 minutes. Avoid excess talking which may prolong hoarseness. Usually hoarseness subsides in a few days.

- Observe for signs and symptoms of postoperative hemorrhage and shock: Blood-soaked dressings, hematemesis, tight dressings, hematoma to neck, diaphoresis, increased pulse, decreased blood pressure, restlessness, agitation.

- Prevent undue stress to suture lines. Maintain semi-Fowler's position for comfort. Avoid hyperextension and flexion of the neck. Maintain proper neck alignment by placing sand bags on both sides of the patient's head.

- Observe for signs and symptoms of hypocalcemia: Muscle spasms, twitching, tingling of lips, fingers, and toes; tetany; anxiety; seizures;

laryngospasm (see Hypoparathyroidism). Be prepared to administer calcium gluconate as ordered.

- Observe for signs and symptoms of thyroid crisis or storm: Elevated temperature (up to 106° F.), tachycardia, dehydration, diarrhea, tachypnea, atrial arrhythmias, excessive irritability, delirium, confusion, psychotic behavior, pulmonary edema, shock (see Hyperthyroidism).

- Encourage the patient to cough gently and deep breathe every hour to help prevent postoperative respiratory complications (see Postoperative Care).

- Assess and support the patient's psychosocial needs. Surgery involving the neck area can be very frightening. The patient may have a sore throat, hoarse voice, and be unable to move his/her head at first. Help the patient deal with these changes and assure him/her that these symptoms will go away as the neck muscles strengthen.

PATIENT AND FAMILY TEACHING

- See Preoperative Care.
- If a total thyroidectomy is performed, the patient will need lifetime hormone therapy (see Hypothyroidism).
- When allowed by the physician, begin to teach range of motion exercises to help strengthen neck muscles.
- Encourage the patient to keep scheduled visits to the physician to check thyroid levels.
- Instruct patient and family in correct thyroid medication administration.
- Describe the signs and symptoms of thyroid overdose or hyperthyroidism: Diarrhea, diaphoresis, tachycardia, heat intolerance, tremor, flushed face.
- Describe the signs and symptoms of hypothyroidism: Lethargy, apathy, edema, sensitivity to cold, dry skin and hair, forgetfulness, weight gain.
- Inform patient of signs and symptoms of hypoparathyroidism: Muscle spasms, irritability, tingling of fingers and toes, grimacing.
- Instruct patient to contact his/her physician immediately if any of these symptoms are noted.

HYPOPARATHYROIDISM

POTENTIAL PROBLEMS

Fluid and Electrolyte   Renal Calculi
  Imbalances   Dry Skin
Airway Obstruction   Pain
Arrhythmias   Cataracts
Tetany   Psychosis
Seizures   Psychosocial Problems
Brain Calcifications

KEY NURSING INTERVENTIONS

- Observe for signs and symptoms of fluid and electrolyte imbalances, especially hypocalcemia (see Fluids and Electrolytes).

- Observe for signs and symptoms of acute hypoparathyroidism, especially in patients who have had their thyroid or parathyroid glands removed: Sudden onset of muscle cramps; tetany; tingling of lips, fingers, and toes; anxiety; seizures; laryngospasm. This is a medical emergency because the patient may be unable to breathe.

- Keep cricothyrotomy or tracheostomy tray, suction equipment, and two ampoules of 10% calcium gluconate solution at the bedside.

- Assess the patient with chronic hypoparathyroidism for the following: Dry skin, brittle nails, weakness, lethargy, poor hair distribution, cataracts, arrhythmias, renal calculi, heart failure, personality changes, psychosis, mental retardation.

- Encourage fluids to 3000 cc per day unless contraindicated.

- Provide a diet high in calcium and vitamin D while low in phosphorus.

- Assess and support the patient's psychosocial needs. Patients who are having an acute attack of tetany will be in a panic state. Provide reassurance that these symptoms will disappear as soon as intravenous calcium is administered. Patients with chronic hypoparathyroidism may have personality changes ranging from mild mood swings to frank psychosis and mental retardation. Adjust nursing care appropriately. Arrange for a psychiatric or social service consultation, if necessary.

PATIENT AND FAMILY TEACHING

- Provide a list of foods that are high in calcium and vitamin D while low in phosphorus.
- See Thyroidectomy if surgery was performed.
- Instruct patient in the importance of follow-up visits for laboratory tests. Stress the fact that treatment is a lifelong process.

HYPERPARATHYROIDISM

POTENTIAL PROBLEMS

Hypercalcemia	Gastric Ulcers
Arrhythmias	Constipation
Dehydration	Muscle Weakness
Renal Pathology: Calculi,	Bone Deformities
Infection, Hypertension,	Pathologic Fractures
Renal Failure	Bone and Joint Pain
Psychosocial Problems	

KEY NURSING INTERVENTIONS

- Observe for signs and symptoms of fluid and electrolyte imbalances, especially hypercalcemia (see Fluid and Electrolytes).

- Observe for signs and symptoms of complications: Arrhythmias, kidney stones, dehydration, gastric ulcers, constipation, ileus, abdominal pain.

- Force fluids to 3–4 liters per day or as ordered.

- Maintain accurate intake and output. Strain urine if renal calculi are suspected.

- Encourage a diet which is low in calcium and high in phosphorus. Consult with hospital dietitian.

- Provide a safe environment to prevent accidental falls. Assist the patient when ambulating. These patients are susceptible to pathologic fractures.

- If the patient is on digitalis therapy, administer with caution. Hypercalcemia potentiates digitalis preparations. Avoid use of thiazide diuretics since they decrease renal excretion of calcium.

- Many patients are treated surgically by removal of one or more of the parathyroid glands. Observe for hypocalcemia and tetany postoperatively. Postoperative nursing care is similar to that for thyroidectomy (see Thyroidectomy and Hypoparathyroidism).

- Assess and support the patient's psychosocial needs. The patient may experience severe mood swings and depression due to high calcium levels. Observe for suicidal tendencies. Provide reassurance that with early surgical treatment, the patient may expect total recovery with the exception of irreversible side effects such as cataracts and kidney damage.

PATIENT AND FAMILY TEACHING

- Encourage the proper diet. Low calcium and high phosphorus preoperatively and usually high calcium and vitamin D postoperatively. Provide the patient with a food list.
- See Thyroidectomy and Hypoparathyroidism if surgery is performed.

ADDISON'S DISEASE (ADRENAL CORTICAL HYPOFUNCTION)

POTENTIAL PROBLEMS

Addisonian Crisis	Hyperkalemia
Renal Failure	Hypoglycemia
Dehydration	Infection
Hyponatremia	Shock
Hypotension	Psychosocial Problems
Arrhythmias	

KEY NURSING INTERVENTIONS

- Observe for signs and symptoms of fluid and electrolyte imbalances, especially hyperkalemia, hyponatremia, and dehydration (see Fluid and Electrolytes).

- Attempt to prevent situations that may precipitate an Addisonian crisis: Exposure to extreme temperatures, infections, overexertion, excessive vomiting or diarrhea, extreme emotional upsets, injury.

- Observe for signs and symptoms of an Addisonian crisis: Hypotension; weak pulse; tachycardia; cool, moist skin; nausea; vomiting; headache; changes in level of consciousness; elevation and then a drop in body temperature; shock; severe abdominal, back, and leg pain. This is a medical emergency.

- Usual treatment for Addisonian crisis includes the following: IV normal saline, IV hydrocortisone, oxygen, vasopressor drugs, plasma, possibly antibiotics if infection is present.

- Key nursing interventions during crisis include the following: Close monitoring of blood pressure, measuring of urine output hourly, protecting patient from physical and emotional stress, monitoring for overhydration, monitoring for steroid overdose (edema, hypotension, hypokalemia, paralysis, loss of consciousness, psychotic behavior).

- Observe for signs of hydrocortisone overdose: Hypertension, edema, weakness.

- Monitor blood pressure closely. Report decreasing blood pressure to physician.

- Weigh the patient daily. Observe for fluid retention.

- Provide a calm and quiet environment. Keep room warm and clean.
- Provide frequest rest periods to avoid overexertion.
- Observe for signs and symptoms of overcorrection of fluid and steroid therapy: Hypertension, pulmonary edema, bounding pulse, hypokalemia, hypernatremia, peripheral edema, changes in level of consciousness, weight gain.
- Usual diet is high carbohydrate and high-protein.
- Assess and support the patient's psychosocial needs. Addison's disease is difficult to diagnose because the signs and symptoms may be vague. The patient may become exhausted because of many tests and visits to different physicians. Once the disease is diagnosed, steroid therapy must be continued for a lifetime. Help the patient and family deal with physical, psychological, and lifestyle changes.

PATIENT AND FAMILY TEACHING

- See Steroid Therapy.
- Instruct the patient to report infections and increases in stress levels. The physician may need to increase the dosage of steroids.
- Emergency kits containing hydrocortisone may be needed. Check with physician.
- Inform patient of the advantages of an emergency identification bracelet and encourage obtaining one.
- Stress the importance of follow-up physician visits. Emphasize that treatment is a lifelong process.

CUSHING'S SYNDROME (ADRENAL CORTICAL HYPERFUNCTION)

POTENTIAL PROBLEMS

Hypokalemia	Pathologic Fractures
Alkalosis	Edema
Arrhythmias	Osteoporosis
Diabetes Mellitus	Skin Breakdown
Infection	Weakness
Hypertension	Back Pain
Hyperglycemia	Negative Nitrogen Balance
Congestive Heart Failure	Psychosocial Problems

KEY NURSING INTERVENTIONS

- Observe for signs and symptoms of fluid and electrolyte imbalances, especially hypokalemia (see Fluid and Electrolytes).

- Prevent infections by placing the patient in a private room. Use good hand washing technique. Restrict visitors with any type of infection, especially those with respiratory symptoms.

- Observe for signs and symptoms of any type of infection. These patients have a suppressed immune system. A severe infection may be present even though signs and symptoms are mild.

- Observe for signs and symptoms of diabetes mellitus. Prevent potential problems (see Diabetes Mellitus).

- Monitor the patient's blood pressure. Observe for hypertension and report to physician.

- Obtain daily weight. Assure accuracy.

- Protect patient from accidental falls. Use side-rails PRN.

- Provide good skin care. Use mild soaps and soft towels. Apply lotion to dry areas.

- Encourage the patient to rest frequently.

- Provide a diet rich in potassium and low in sodium. Consult with hospital dietician.

- Treatment is usually surgical depending upon the cause (see Hypophysectomy or Adrenalectomy).

- Assess and support the patient's psychosocial needs. Cushing's syndrome produces many physical changes such as a moon face, poor skin, buffalo hump, weight gain, and hypertension. In addition, these patients may have severe mood swings, depression, and psychosis. These changes are very disturbing to the patient and family. Observe the patient closely for suicidal tendencies. Arrange for a psychiatric or social service consultation as needed. Provide reassurance that with proper treatment these symptoms should subside.

PATIENT AND FAMILY TEACHING

- See Hypophysectomy, Adrenalectomy, and Steroid Therapy.
- See Preoperative Care.

PHEOCHROMOCYTOMA

POTENTIAL PROBLEMS

Paroxysmal and/or Chronic Hypertension	Sudden Blindness
	Electrolyte Imbalances
Stroke	Nausea
Cardiac Arrhythmias	Vomiting
Cardiac Failure	Psychosocial Problems
Hyperglycemia	

KEY NURSING INTERVENTIONS

- Check the blood pressure frequently. Observe for signs and symptoms of paroxysmal hypertension (sudden onset): Headache, diaphoresis, vertigo, dizziness, epistaxis, blurred vision, blindness, paresthesias, aphasia, unilateral muscle weakness, arrhythmias, pulmonary edema, cardiopulmonary arrest.

- Paroxysmal hypertension only responds to alpha adrenergic blocking drugs. Administer these drugs with caution. Monitor blood pressure constantly.

- Help the patient to avoid a hypertensive crisis. Provide a tranquil environment. Protect the patient from stressful situations. Avoid caffeine, cigarettes, and other stimulating agents.

- Usually, a 24-hour urine specimen is obtained for catecholamines and VMA. Check with your laboratory for collection procedure. Explain the procedure to the patient. Patient cooperation is essential in obtaining an accurate specimen.

- Once the diagnosis has been made and the blood pressure is under control, the physician will usually schedule the patient for removal of the tumor and/or adrenal glands (see Adrenalectomy).

- Assess and support the patient's psychosocial needs. Pheochromocytoma can produce severe physiological and emotional changes. Provide the patient with reassurance that symptoms usually disappear after surgery.

PATIENT AND FAMILY TEACHING

- Stress the importance of frequent rest periods and the avoidance of stressful situations.
- Instruct the patient to avoid stimulants such as coffee and tea.
- See Adrenalectomy.

ADRENALECTOMY

POTENTIAL PROBLEMS

Adrenal Crisis	Infection
Extreme Blood Pressure	Pain
Fluctuations	Hemorrhage
Shock	Psychosocial Problems

KEY NURSING INTERVENTIONS

- Monitor blood pressure frequently, especially for the first 24–48 hours postoperatively. Be prepared to administer intravenous fluids, vasopressors, and steroids for control of hypotension.

- See Abdominal Surgery.

- Observe for signs and symptoms of hemorrhage and shock: Abdominal pain, hematemesis, shoulder pain, abdominal rigidity, blood-soaked dressings, diaphoresis, altered mental status, decreased urine output, increased pulse, decreased blood pressure, restlessness, agitation.

- Observe for signs and symptoms of adrenal crisis: Hypotension; weak, thready pulse; tachycardia; diaphoresis; nausea; vomiting; muscle cramps; headache; altered mental status; elevation and then a drop in body temperature; shock.

- Prevent infections by placing the patient in a private room. Use good handwashing techniques. Restrict visitors with any type of infection, especially those with respiratory symptoms.

- Prevent postoperative complications (see Postoperative Care).

- Use strict aseptic technique when changing dressings.

- Attempt to prevent situations that may precipitate an adrenal crisis: Exposure to extreme temperatures, infections, overexertion, excessive vomiting or diarrhea, extreme emotional upsets.

- If both adrenal glands are removed, the patient will need lifetime corticosteroid therapy (see Steroid Therapy and Addison's Disease).

PATIENT AND FAMILY TEACHING

- See Preoperative Care.

- See Abdominal Surgery, Steroid Therapy, and Addison's Disease.

- Instruct patient and family in all procedures necessary to prepare patient for surgery.
- Emphasize the importance of reducing stress factors prior to surgery.

STEROID THERAPY

POTENTIAL PROBLEMS

Gastrointestinal Disturbances	Growth Suppression
Seizures	Glaucoma
Electrolyte Imbalances	Cataracts
Hypertension	Diabetes
Infection	Myopathies
Osteoporosis	Neuropathies
Thrombophlebitis	Psychosocial Problems

KEY NURSING INTERVENTIONS

- Observe for signs and symptoms of unacceptable side effects which should be reported to the physician: Nausea, vomiting, thirst, dizziness upon standing, abdominal pain, hematemesis, hypertension, hypokalemia, diabetes, glaucoma, osteoporosis, pathologic fractures, growth suppression, seizures, severe mood swings, anxiety, depression, or development of any type of infection.

- Observe for signs and symptoms of acceptable side effects that need not be reported unless they become a problem: Moon face, weight gain, edema, acne, polyuria, sleeping problems, fatigue, mild mood swings.

- Always check the *Physician's Desk Reference* for possible interaction with other medications which the patient might be taking.

- Steroids should be discontinued slowly in decreasing doses. Observe for signs and symptoms of steroid withdrawal: Lethargy, muscle weakness, anorexia, nausea, vomiting, diarrhea, constipation, hyperkalemia, hypotension, shock, adrenal insufficiency.

- Prevent infection. Some steroids suppress the immune system. Observe for signs and symptoms of infection in all areas of the body. Restrict visitors who have infectious disorders, especially those with respiratory infections. Use good handwashing techniques prior to patient contact.

- Observe open wounds for delayed healing response.

- Adminster PO steroids with milk or food to avoid gastric irritation.

- Administer IV steroids with caution. Steroids should be piggybacked into a flush line. Use an infusion pump for continuous drips. Check the flow rate frequently. If the IV needs to be changed for any reason, restart immediately.
- Assess and support the patient's psychosocial needs. Help the patient and family deal with the physical and psychological changes caused by steroids. Observe for severe psychological changes, especially depression and suicidal tendencies. Steroids alter the body's ability to deal with stress. Help the patient to avoid stressful or emotional situations.

PATIENT AND FAMILY TEACHING

- Explain the purpose of steroid therapy and the difference between acceptable and reportable side effects.
- Stress the importance of infection control. Instruct the patient to avoid crowded places and people with respiratory tract infections.
- Instruct the patient to inform the dentist and future medical personnel of current steroid therapy regime.
- Encourage the patient to wear a Medic Alert tag.
- Instruct patient in proper medication administration.

DIABETES INSIPIDUS

POTENTIAL PROBLEMS

Dehydration   Fluid and Electrolyte
Shock   Imbalance
                                         Psychosocial Problems

KEY NURSING INTERVENTIONS

- Diabetes insipidus may be due to a tumor, head trauma, or post neurosurgery (see Hypophysectomy).

- Observe for signs and symptoms of severe dehydration and shock: Dry mucous membranes, thirst, tachycardia, hypotension, poor skin turgor, oliguria.

- Keep the patient well hydrated. These patients may urinate 5–20 liters per day. This fluid needs to be replaced. Maintain accurate intake and output records.

- Administer vasopressin (antidiuretic hormone) as ordered. Hormone therapy may be temporary or need to be continued for a lifetime.

- Assess and support the patient's psychosocial needs. The need to drink and urinate this large volume of fluid may be very anxiety-producing. Provide reassurance that with hormone therapy these symptoms will subside.

PATIENT AND FAMILY TEACHING

- Stress the importance of maintaining continued lifetime hormone therapy, if indicated.

- See Hypophysectomy, if indicated.

- Reinforce explanation of pathology.

HYPOPHYSECTOMY

POTENTIAL PROBLEMS

Increased Intracranial   Pneumonia
    Pressure   Hypoglycemia
Hemorrhage   Thyroid Crisis
Addisonian Crisis   Meningitis
Diabetes Inspidus   Psychosocial Problems
Infertility

KEY NURSING INTERVENTIONS

- Observe for and prevent postoperative complications (see Postoperative Care and Craniotomy).

- Observe for signs and symptoms of hormone deficiencies:

  Adrenal Insufficiency—Dehydration, hyponatremia, hyperkalemia, hypotension, arrhythmias, hypoglycemia, weakness, anorexia, nausea, vomiting.

  Addisonian Crisis—Severe weakness; severe abdominal, leg, and back pain; high temperature followed by hypothermia; shock.

  Hypothyroidism—Sensitivity to cold temperatures, lethargy, dry hair and skin, weight gain, depression, apathy, edematous face.

  Diabetes Insipidus—Polyuria, polydipsia, urine specific gravity 1.001–1.006.

- Observe for signs and symptoms of fluid and electrolyte imbalances (see Fluid and Electrolytes).

- If the pituitary gland is completely removed, a complex lifetime hormone therapy is usually indicated. Administer these hormones with caution. Always check the *Physician's Desk Reference* for complications, side effects, and contraindications.

- Remember that hypothyroid patients are extremely sensitive to narcotics, barbiturates, and anesthetics. Administer these drugs with caution.

- Assess and support the patient's psychosocial needs. A hypophysectomy may be a frightening experience because it involves surgery that is close to the brain. The patient usually has to begin a lifetime of complex hormone therapy. Help the patient and family deal with these changes.

PATIENT AND FAMILY TEACHING

- Stress the importance of keeping scheduled visits to the physician, even when feeling good.
- Instruct the patient in proper administration of prescribed hormones, side effects, and signs and symptoms of imbalances, especially hypothyroidism, adrenal insufficiency, and diabetes insipidus.

DIABETES MELLITUS

POTENTIAL PROBLEMS

Hypoglycemia   Amputations
Diabetic Ketoacidosis (DKA)   Neuropathy
Hyperglycemic Hyperosmolar   Cerebrovascular Accident
  Non ketotic Coma (HHNK)   Lipodystrophies
Renal Disease   Infection
Heart Disease   Dehydration
Diabetic Retinopathy   Pain
Peripheral Vascular Disease   Cataracts
Foot and Leg Ulcerations   Psychosocial Problems

KEY NURSING INTERVENTIONS

- The goal in patient care of the diabetic is to maintain normal blood glucose levels. Keep complications to a minimum and help the patient learn as much as possible about this complex disease.

- Observe for signs and symptoms of acute potential problems:

  - *Hypoglycemia,* or insulin reaction, occurs when a meal is skipped after insulin injection, overdose of insulin, or excessive exercise. This is an emergency. Brain cells quickly die when sugar is not available.

    - *Signs and Symptoms:* Visual disturbances; low blood sugar levels; mental lethargy; stupor; coma; seizures; cool, moist skin; bradycardia; cardiac arrest.

    - *Treatment:* If the patient is awake, administer oral glucose solution. If the patient is not awake, administer IV dextrose as ordered or IM glucagon as ordered if unable to start IV. Always attempt to draw blood for analysis before administering sugar solutions as long as it does not lengthen the therapy.

  - *HHNK* occurs in nondiabetics, non-insulin-dependent diabetics, and comatose patients. It may be precipitated by stress, infection, total parenteral nutrition, poor oral intake of fluids.

    - *Signs and Symptoms:* High blood sugar levels; metabolic acidosis; thirst; nausea; vomiting; abdominal pain; flushed, dry skin;

dehydration; decreased level of consciousness; coma; hypotension; tachycardia; cardiac arrest.

- *Treatment:* This may include IV electrolyte solutions to correct severe dehydration and slow administrations of insulin to correct hyperglycemia. This condition has a 50% mortality rate.

- *DKA* occurs from prolonged hyperglycemia in which no insulin is present.

  - *Signs and Symptoms:* The same as those found in HHNK plus Kussmaul respirations, acetone breath, and ketosis.
  - *Treatment:* This may include subcutaneous insulin or IV insulin either in a bolus or a drip and IV sodium bicarbonate to correct severe metabolic acidosis. IV electrolytes may also be given.

- Assess the patient for signs and symptoms of long-term chronic complications: Poor vision or blindness, cardiac disease, kidney disease, neuropathies, skin breakdown, and peripheral vascular disease, especially in the feet.

- Administer insulin carefully. An order for insulin should include the strength and number of units, type of insulin, route and time to be given. Some physicians will order insulin on a sliding scale according to the amount of glucose found in the urine or blood. Always check the dosage with another nurse before administration. Keep a chart of rotating injection sites. Document time and location of injection.

- Attempt to prevent hypoglycemic episode. Check doses carefully. Make sure the patient adheres to special diet including snacks. Identify when the peak action of the last dose of insulin will be, and check on the patient more frequently during these times. Assure expedient delivery of meals and snacks.

  - **NOTE:** Exercise and skipping meals will potentiate the effect of insulin; illness, infection, stress, or surgery may cause a need for increased insulin.

- Protect skin from breakdown and pressure sores.

- Administer foot care daily. Soak the feet in a warm, mild soap solution. Avoid scalding of the feet by testing the water temperature yourself. Carefully pat the feet dry. Keep the skin moist with mild lotions or oils. Closely observe the feet for ulceration and infections. Never cut the toenails or remove calluses. Notify the physician if long nails become a problem. Instruct the patient to always wear slippers or shoes when out of bed to avoid foot injury.

- Prevent complications of immobility (see The Immobilized Patient).

- Assess and support the patient's psychosocial needs. The diabetic on a medical-surgical unit may have been hospitalized for many reasons. The patient may be newly diagnosed, out of control because of a complication, or coincidental to diabetes. Each patient will be in a different stage of coping with his/her illness. Carefully assess how the patient thinks and feels about diabetes. How has it or how will it affect his/her lifestyle? Identify the positive and negative coping mechanisms the patient has developed.

PATIENT AND FAMILY TEACHING

- Patient education is the single most important intervention the nurse can make for the diabetic regardless of how long the patient has had diabetes. Continue to assess what the patient already knows and what the patient needs to know. Assess the patient's anxiety level and willingness to learn (see Patient Education).
- Through a team effort, develop a well-written, mutually agreed upon care plan. Include all health care members.
- Refer the patient to the American Diabetes Association.
- Make use of hospital resources, including dietitians, pharmacists, books, pamphlets, audiovisual equipment and other teaching aids.
- Involve the family in patient care and teaching sessions.
- Reinforce explanation of pathology. Emphasize that diabetes is a systemic disease and not just a problem with blood sugar.
- Encourage the patient to wear a Medic Alert tag that identifies him/her as a diabetic.
- Begin to initiate patient teaching in the following areas: Disease process, signs and symptoms of hypoglycemia, DKA, other complications, foot care, diet, rest, exercise, medications, self-administered insulin injections, and the importance of continued follow-up medical care, blood and urine testing procedures.

RENAL SYSTEM

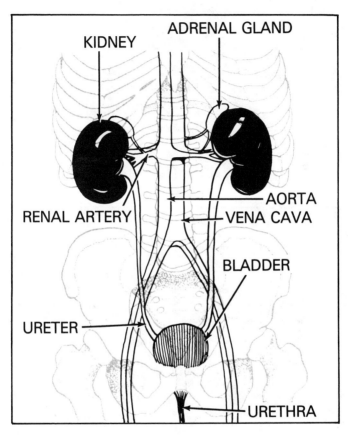

Urinary Organs

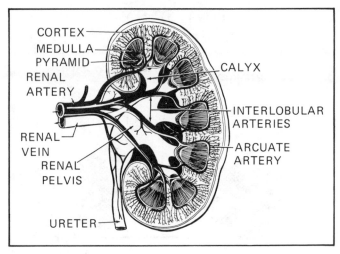

Coronal Section of Left Kidney

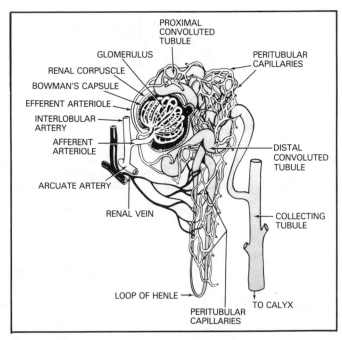

The Nephron Unit

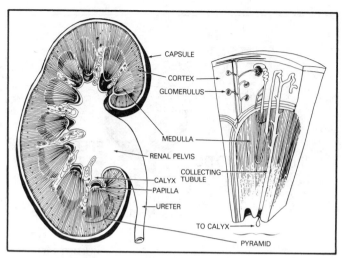

Coronal Section of Right Kidney

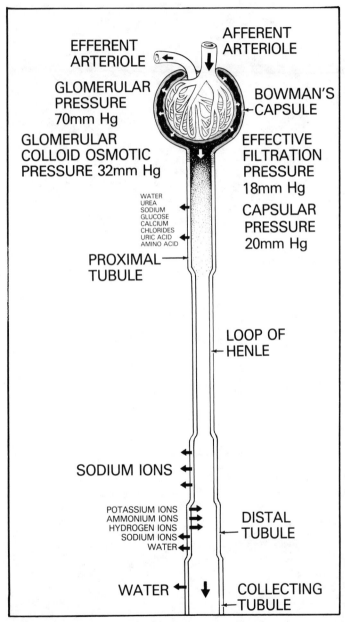

EFFERENT
ARTERIOLE

AFFERENT
ARTERIOLE

GLOMERULAR
PRESSURE
70mm Hg

BOWMAN'S
CAPSULE

GLOMERULAR
COLLOID OSMOTIC
PRESSURE 32mm Hg

EFFECTIVE
FILTRATION
PRESSURE
18mm Hg

WATER
UREA
SODIUM
GLUCOSE
CALCIUM
CHLORIDES
URIC ACID
AMINO ACID

CAPSULAR
PRESSURE
20mm Hg

PROXIMAL
TUBULE

LOOP OF
HENLE

SODIUM IONS

POTASSIUM IONS
AMMONIUM IONS
HYDROGEN IONS
SODIUM IONS
WATER

DISTAL
TUBULE

WATER

COLLECTING
TUBULE

The Nephron Unit

RENAL SYSTEM—PHYSIOLOGY SUMMARY

I. THE KIDNEYS

A. Filtration

The kidneys filter the blood to eliminate waste and reabsorb glucose, amino acids, electrolytes, and uric acid.

B. Structure

The kidneys are composed of microscopic units called nephrons.

C. Innervation

The kidneys are innervated by sympathetic nerves from T–4 to L–4.

D. Glomerular Filtration

1. The glomerular membrane of glomerular capillaries is approximately 100 to 1000 times more permeable than other capillaries.

2. Normally, the glomerular membrane is impermeable to plasma proteins.

3. Glomerular filtrate is the fluid filtered through the glomerular membrane.

4. Glomerular filtration is determined by glomerular pressure, Bowman's capsule pressure, plasma colloid osmotic pressure, renal blood flow rate, and glomerular membrane permeability.

5. Hydrostatic Pressure. High pressure in the glomerular capillary bed (60 to 70 mm Hg as opposed to 15 to 20 mm Hg in other capillaries) causes fluid to filter out of the glomerulus and into the Bowman's capsule.

6. Plasma Colloid Osmotic Pressure. As the plasma (minus plasma proteins) filters out into the Bowman's capsule due to hydrostatic pressure differential, the colloid osmotic pressure rises and stops further filtration.

E. Glomerular Filtration Rate

1. The glomerular filtration rate is the quantity of glomerular filtrate formed every minute (normally about 125 ml/min.).

2. Glomerular filtration rate *increases*:

   a) As glomerular capillary pressure increases.

   b) As renal blood flow rate increases.

   c) With mild constriction of the efferent arteriole (constriction of efferent arteriole around the peritubular bed raises the afferent arteriolar pressure in the glomerulus, causing increased filtration).

   d) As plasma colloidal osmotic pressure decreases.

3. Glomerular filtration rate *decreases*:

   a) As glomerular capillary pressure decreases.

   b) As renal blood flow rate decreases.

   c) With severe constriction of the efferent arteriole (blood flow rate will decrease, causing an excessive rise in plasma colloidal osmotic pressure).

   d) As plasma colloidal osmotic pressure increases.

   e) As the afferent arteriole constricts due to sympathetic stimulation.

F. Autoregulation of Glomerular Filtration Rate

1. Autoregulation is the ability of the kidney to maintain an effective glomerular filtration rate despite extreme rises in arterial pressure.

2. As arterial pressure rises, the afferent arteriole automatically constricts, allowing not more than a 15% to 20% increase in filtration rate.

G. Reabsorption and Clearance

1. Plasma filters across the glomerular membrane into the Bowman's capsule and passes through the tubules.

2. As it travels through the tubules, certain substances are reabsorbed back into the blood (glucose, amino acids, and proteins), and others are left or "cleared" (creatinine) to be excreted in urine.

3. Glucose is reabsorbed with water in the proximal tubule.

4. Nearly 99% of all sodium filtered is actively reabsorbed in the proximal, distal, and collecting tubules.

5. Sodium reabsorption is regulated by:

   a) Dietary intake (increased reabsorption with low intake and vice versa).

   b) Aldosterone excretion (see Endocrine System).

6. Potassium is reabsorbed in the proximal tubules and passively secreted in the distal tubules.

7. Calcium phosphate, uric acid, magnesium, chloride, and bicarbonate ions are reabsorbed by active transport.

8. Water is reabsorbed passively in the proximal, distal convoluted, and collecting tubules as a result of osmotic forces.

9. Water reabsorption in the distal and collecting portion of the nephron is also regulated by the osmolality of the extracellular fluid.

10. Water reabsorption is influenced by secretion of ADH (antidiuretic hormone) from the hypothalamus in response to increased osmolar concentration.

H. Tubular Secretion

Creatinine, potassium, hydrogen ions, and certain drugs are secreted into the tubules.

I. Urine

Is the end-product of glomerular filtration and reabsorption and is produced at approximately 1 ml/min.

J. Acid-Base Regulation

1. The kidney is the main organ of pH regulation.

2. In normal pH states, the kidneys secrete hydrogen and bicarbonate in equal amounts.

3. In acidotic states, the kidneys secrete hydrogen into the proximal, distal, and collecting tubules. Hydrogen ions bind with buffers such as bicarbonate, dibasic phosphate, and ammonia, and are excreted in the urine.

4. In alkalotic states, the kidneys reabsorb hydrogen ions; when the bicarbonate level is elevated, they excrete it in the urine.

K. Blood Pressure

1. When arterial blood pressure drops and the glomerular filtration rate subsequently falls, the kidneys release renin into the bloodstream.

2. Renin interacts with angiotensin I, synthesized by the liver, and is converted to angiotensin II in the lungs.

3. Angiotensin II acts on arterial smooth muscles to increase peripheral resistance and raise the blood pressure.

L. Other Functions

1. The kidneys synthesize 1,25-dihydroxy-cholecalciferol, which acts in the intestine to stimulate calcium absorption.

2. Erythropoietin, a glycoprotein which stimulates red blood cell production, is synthesized by the kidneys.

3. Nearly 20% of secreted insulin is removed by the kidneys and deactivated in the renal tubules.

4. The kidneys synthesize prostaglandins, used in a variety of ways by the body.

5. The kidneys generate energy necessary for their own functioning ability.

II. THE URETERS

The right and left ureters extend from the pelvis of the kidney to the posterior aspect of the bladder and serve to funnel urine into the bladder.

III. THE BLADDER

A. The Bladder

Serves as a reservoir for urine with a capacity of 300–400 ml.

B. Micturition

Occurs by voluntary control as distention stimulates stretch and tension receptors, causing the urge to urinate.

C. Parasympathetic Fibers

Carry impulses from the brain to the lumbosacral area, which stimulates the bladder.

IV. THE URETHRA

The urethra serves as passageway for urine to be eliminated from the bladder and the body. In the male the urethra also serves as the final path for the passage of semen.

RENAL SYSTEM ASSESSMENT

I. HISTORY

A. Past History of Renal or Urinary Problems

1. What type?
2. What therapy was utilized? Did it work?

B. Recent History

1. Problems with urination?

    a) Pain?
    b) Burning?
    c) Frequency?
    d) Hesitation?
    e) Itching?
    f) Incontinence?
    g) Stress incontinence?
    h) Change in color or amount?
    i) Presence of blood?

2. Fever, chills, sweating?
3. Skin changes?

    a) Pruritus?
    b) Rash?
    c) Frost?
    d) Dryness?
    e) Color?

4. Anorexia, nausea, vomiting, diarrhea?
5. Fluid and nutritional patterns?
6. Level of activity?

C. Dialysis

1. Presence of A-V shunt or fistula?
2. Type of dialysis used?
3. How long?

4. When was the last dialysation?

5. Ascertain if the patient produces urine.

D. Pain

Use PQRST mnemonic.

P—Provokes.   What makes the pain worse or better? What was the patient doing prior to the onset of pain?

Q—Quality.   Subjective description of pain by the patient. Use the patient's own words, i.e., burning, stabbing, pressure.

R—Radiation. Where is the pain located and does it radiate anywhere?

S—Severity.   Ask the patient to judge the pain on a scale of 1 to 10 with 10 being the worst pain ever felt.

T—Time.   How long has the patient had this pain? When did the pain begin and end?

E. Medications

1. List all medications, including over-the-counter drugs.

2. Allergies.

F. Nutrition

Describe a typical:

1. Breakfast.

2. Lunch.

3. Dinner.

4. Snacks.

II. BACKGROUND INFORMATION

A. Lab Values

Check for abnormal values.

1. Urine: Creatinine clearance, specific gravity, osmolality, chemistries, cultures.

2. Blood: Serum creatinine, BUN, osmolality, glucose, complete blood count, cultures, electrolytes.

B. Diagnostic Studies

Identify abnormal reports (KUB, IVP, nephrotomogram, renal angiography, renal biopsies, CAT scans, ultrasound, cystoscopy, radioactive venogram).

C. Fluid Status

Check intake and output records and daily weights.

D. Chart

Check chart for past relevant information.

III. ASSESSMENT

A. Inspection

1. Urine.

   a) Document the color, amount, clarity, odor, presence of blood, sediment, or bubbles.

   b) Check laboratory values for abnormalities.

2. Skin.

   Note the color. Check for presence of petechiae or bruising, frost or crystalline deposits, and edema.

3. Flanks.

   Inspect for masses, scars, lesions.

4. Fistulas or A-V shunts.

   Note the location. Never take blood pressure in affected extremity.

5. Urethra.

   a) Inspect the meatus for patency and presence of discharge.

   b) Note hygiene status of pubic and perianal area.

   c) Inspect for fistulas, tumors, lesions, and scars.

6. Catheters.

   Note the type, location, size, and quality of the draining urine.

7. Urinary diversion.

   a) If the patient has an ileal conduit, inspect the stoma for size, location, color, odor, and patency.

   b) Observe the peristomal skin for irritation.

B. Palpation

1. For right kidney palpation, place the patient supine. Stand to the right of the patient and place your left hand below the patient under the flank. Place your right hand just below the anterior costal margin and ask the patient to inhale. The lower pole of the right kidney should be palpable. Describe the kidney in terms of size, shape, presence of masses or tenderness.

2. The left kidney is rarely palpable.

3. Bladder.

   Palpate the bladder for distention and/or pain.

4. Fistulas or A-V shunts.

   Palpate for thrill, auscultate for bruit.

C. Percussion

Percuss gently with the fist over the costovertebral angle (CVA) for tenderness.

RENAL CALCULI

POTENTIAL PROBLEMS

Severe Pain   Renal Failure
Nausea and/or Vomiting   Urinary Tract Infection
Hematuria   Psychosocial Problems

KEY NURSING INTERVENTIONS

- Ascertain if the patient has any allergies, especially to IVP dye, iodine, shellfish, narcotics, and/or antibiotics.

- Obtain consent for IVP as ordered. This should be done prior to administration of narcotics.

- Control severe pain as ordered by IM or IV narcotics and/or moist heat to flank.
  NOTE: Observe for respiratory depression when large and/or frequent doses of narcotics are used.

- In order to find the cause of stones, strain all urine and send stones to the laboratory for analysis.

- Force fluids to at least 3000 cc/day. This will help facilitate spontaneous passage of calculi. Most stones will pass in this manner.

- Prepare the patient for possible diagnostic tests or surgery (IVP, cystoscopy, ureteral catheterization, ureterolithotomy, nephrectomy).

- Assess and support the patient's psychosocial needs. This is a very painful experience. Provide a low stimulus environment. Eliminate factors which may agitate the patient, i.e., visitors, bright lights, radios, televisions, frequent intervention.

PATIENT AND FAMILY TEACHING

- Instruct patient to continue to drink at least 2500 cc/day.

- Demonstrate how to strain the urine and to bring any collected stones to the physician after discharge.

- If the causative factor of stone formation is found while the patient is in the hospital, a special diet and/or medications may be prescribed. Make sure the patient and his/her family have a good understanding of this diet and the importance of medications. Approximately 20–30% of these patients will have recurrences of renal calculi. Most can be prevented if adherence to the medical regimen is followed.

ACUTE GLOMERULONEPHRITIS

POTENTIAL PROBLEMS

Cardiac Failure   Pulmonary Edema
Increased Intracranial   Psychosocial Problems
  Pressure
Renal Failure

KEY NURSING INTERVENTIONS

- Assess patient for signs and symptoms of cardiac failure: Muffled heart sounds, rales in lower lobes, elevated CVP, distended neck veins, dyspnea, edema in lower extremities.

- Observe for pulmonary edema: Severe dyspnea, orthopnea, tachycardia, bloody and frothy sputum, wheezing, bubbling chest sounds, cyanosis.

- Monitor patient for signs and symptoms of renal failure: Nausea, fatigue, oliguria or high output with dilute urine, edema, weight gain, weakness, hematuria.

- Assess patient for signs and symptoms of increasing intracranial pressure: Decreasing level of consciousness, bradycardia, widening pulse pressure, respiratory pattern changes, decreased or increased respiratory rate, headache, nausea, vomiting, pupillary changes, seizures.

- Protect patient from nosocomial infections. Wash hands with antimicrobial soap before and after patient care. Prevent exposure of patient to colds, flu, and upper respiratory diseases.

- Prevent complications of bedrest (see The Immobilized Patient).

- Have hospital dietician discuss special diet with patient (usually high carbohydrate, low protein, and low sodium).

- Encourage good dietary intake to prevent catabolism.

- Monitor fluid balance by obtaining daily weights and monitoring accurate input and output. Edematous parts should be measured and documented.

- If fluids are restricted, frequent oral hygiene and hard candies can relieve thirst.

- Check daily lab work for abnormal values or worsening trends.

- Provide frequent rest periods in daily schedule.
- Good hygiene is essential to prevent skin breakdown in edematous patients. Use sheep skins and egg crate mattresses.
- Assess and support patient's psychosocial needs. Prolonged bed rest with limited activity necessitates diversional, nonstressful activities to prevent boredom and frustrations. Independent patients may need help in assuming a dependent position. Allow as much self-care as possible. Be optimistic and hopeful, especially when the outcome is uncertain. Stress the importance of physical and mental rest in reducing hematuria and proteinuria.

PATIENT AND FAMILY TEACHING

- Stress the importance of preventing infections.
- Instruct patient in the importance of followup visits to the physician after discharge.
- Emphasize the need to follow prescribed diet.
- Discuss signs and symptoms of renal failure and instruct patient to contact the physician if they occur.

NEPHROSIS

POTENTIAL PROBLEMS

Renal Vein Thrombosis   Renal Failure
Pulmonary Emboli   Psychosocial Problems
Thrombophlebitis

KEY NURSING INTERVENTIONS

- Assess patient for signs and symptoms of renal vein thrombosis: Severe lumbar pain, renal enlargement, proteinuria, hematuria, oliguria, azotemia.

- Observe for signs and symptoms of pulmonary embolism: Sudden or gradual onset of severe chest pain, dyspnea, shortness of breath, cyanosis, neck vein distention, tachycardia, hypotension, arrhythmias, decreased lung sounds unilaterally, shock, depressed pO_2, increased pCO_2, cardiopulmonary arrest.

- Monitor for signs and symptoms of thrombophlebitis: Pain, redness and swelling of affected extremity; positive Homans' sign (pain in calf upon dorsiflexion of the foot).

- Assess patient for developing renal failure: Nausea, fatigue, oliguria or high output with dilute urine, edema, weight gain, weakness, hematuria.

- See Steroid Therapy, if indicated.

- Monitor daily laboratory reports for abnormalities and worsening trends.

- Protect patient from nosocomial infections. Wash hands with antimicrobial soap before and after patient care. Prevent patient exposure to colds, flu, and upper respiratory diseases.

- Monitor fluid balance with accurate intake and output, girth measurements, and daily weighing.

- Provide good skin care to prevent breakdown caused by edema.

- Prevent complications of bed rest (see The Immobilized Patient).

- See Anticoagulation Therapy, if indicated.

- Assess and support patient's psychosocial needs. Encourage diversional activities while on bed rest to relieve boredom. Recognize that the patient may have fears of renal failure and eventual dialysis. Discuss these fears and allow patient to express anxieties. Help patient to focus on medical regimen. Include family in care plan. Inform patient that physical discomforts such as nausea and fatigue contribute to depressed feelings.

PATIENT AND FAMILY TEACHING

- Have dietician discuss elements of prescribed diet (usually high protein, high calorie, and low sodium).

- If patient is receiving anticoagulant therapy, instruct in the need for care in shaving, monitoring stools for blood, carrying identification when discharged and proper drug administration.

- Stress the importance of activity limitations when severe edema is present.

- Advise patient to avoid contact and exposure to infections which may cause exacerbation.

ACUTE RENAL FAILURE

POTENTIAL PROBLEMS

Fluid Overload	Anorexia
Hyperkalemia	Nausea
Hyponatremia	Vomiting
Hypocalcemia	Diarrhea
Hypermagnesemia	Constipation
Hyperphosphatemia	Stomatitis
Acidosis	Pericarditis
Anemia	Uremic Encephalopathy
Secondary Infections	Platelet Dysfunction
Arrhythmias	Psychosocial Problems

KEY NURSING INTERVENTIONS

- Monitor laboratory values closely and observe patient for signs and symptoms of electrolyte imbalance:

  Hyperkalemia—Arrhythmias; EKG shows peaked T waves, wide QRS and ST depression; abdominal cramping; mental confusion; irritability; weakness; paralysis.

  Hyponatremia—Tachycardia, postural hypotension, personality changes, convulsions, coma.

  Hypophosphatemia and hypocalcemia—Muscle cramps, tetany, bronchospasm, tingling of fingers, toes, and lips.

  Hypermagnesemia—Depressed mental status, depressed respirations, hypotension, flaccid muscles, arrhythmias.

- Observe patient and arterial blood gases for metabolic acidosis: pH less than 7.35, bicarbonate less than 16, weakness, Kussmaul respirations.

- Monitor urine specific gravity. Observe for fixed values (usually 1.010) or increasing trends.

- Obtain accurate daily weights. Weigh patient in morning after voiding and before breakfast at the same time with same scale and same clothing.

- Monitor *all* intake and output carefully. Include foods high in water content and losses such as emeses, stools, and drainages. Document degree of perspiration and hyperventilation, also.

- Assess patient for signs and symptoms of hypovolemia: Dry skin and mucous membranes; thick, scanty saliva; elevated temperature; rapid, weak, thready pulse; rapid shallow respirations; orthostatic hypotension; narrow pulse pressure; weight loss.

- Assess patient for signs and symptoms of hypervolemia: Pitting edema over bony prominences; periorbital edema; rapid pulse; distended neck veins; increased CVP; dyspnea; tachypnea; moist rales; normal or hypertension; weight gain.

- Monitor IV intake carefully. Use microdrip tubing and a mechanical controller.

- Evaluate oral fluid intake for sodium, potassium, and protein content. Usually protein is restricted along with potassium and sodium, depending on laboratory values. Lemonade and cranberry juices are usually good because of their high sugar and low potassium and sodium content.

- Dietary regime usually consists of high carbohydrates, low protein and moderate fat, along with potassium and sodium restrictions. Encourage adequate intake. Prevent and treat nausea, anorexia, and stomatitis.

- Avoid antacids containing magnesium. Usually aluminum hydroxide is ordered to bind phosphates.

- Protect patient from secondary infections (respiratory, wounds, mouth, urinary tract). Perform good handwashing prior to patient contact. Encourage patient to turn, cough and deep breathe every 2 hrs.

- Observe patient for bleeding tendencies in skin, mucous membranes, urine, feces, and vomitus.

- If dialysis is performed, see Peritoneal or Hemodialysis for key nursing interventions.

- Assess and support patient's psychosocial needs. Be aware that physical discomforts associated with renal failure may affect patient's affect, morale, and attitude. Convey a hopeful, positive attitude. Be sympathetic in providing patient comfort measures.

PATIENT AND FAMILY TEACHING

- Instruct patient in all aspects of care.

- Discuss with family and visitors the need to protect patient from secondary infection.
- Have dietician review dietary allowances with patient.
- Explain physiological origins of altered psychological status of patient to family.

CHRONIC RENAL FAILURE

POTENTIAL PROBLEMS

Azotemia	Decubitus Ulcers
Hyperkalemia	Cardiac Tamponade
Hypocalcemia	Pericarditis
Hypermagnesemia	Edema
Hyponatremia	Anemia
Hypertension	Arrhythmias
Congestive Heart Failure	Bleeding Tendencies
Hyperphosphatemia	Anorexia
Metabolic Acidosis	Nausea
Ulcer Disease	Vomiting
Gastrointestinal Bleeding	Stomatitis
Peripheral Neuropathy	Gingivitis
Irritability	Renal Osteodystrophy
Seizures	Pruritus
Sensory Alterations	Infection
Hypervolemia	Drug Toxicity
Hypovolemia	Psychosocial Problems

KEY NURSING INTERVENTIONS

- See Peritoneal Dialysis or Hemodialysis.

- Monitor laboratory values closely and observe patient for signs and symptoms of electrolyte imbalance:

  Hyperkalemia—Arrhythmias; EKG shows peaked T waves, wide QRS and ST depression; abdominal cramping; mental confusion; irritability; weakness; paralysis.

  Hyponatremia—Tachycardia, postural hypotension, personality changes, convulsions, coma.

  Hypophosphatemia and Hypocalcemia—Muscle cramps; tetany; bronchospasm; tingling of fingers, toes, and lips.

  Hypermagnesemia—Depressed mental status, depressed respirations, hypotension, flaccid muscles, arrhythmias.

- Observe patient and arterial blood gases for metabolic acidosis: pH less than 7.35, bicarbonate less than 16, weakness, Kussmaul respirations.

- Monitor urine specific gravity. Observe for fixed values (usually 1.010) or increasing trends.

- Obtain accurate daily weights. Weigh patient in morning after voiding and before breakfast at the same time with same scale and same clothing.

- Monitor *all* intake and output carefully. Include foods high in water content and losses such as emeses, stools, and drainages. Document degree of perspiration and hyperventilation, also.

- Assess patient for signs and symptoms of hypovolemia: Dry skin and mucous membranes; thick, scanty saliva; elevated temperature; rapid, weak, thready pulse; rapid shallow respirations; orthostatic hypotension; narrow pulse pressure; weight loss.

- Assess patient for signs and symptoms of hypervolemia: Pitting edema over bony prominences, periorbital edema, rapid pulse, distended neck veins, increased CVP, dyspnea, tachypnea, moist rales, normal or hypertension, weight gain.

- Monitor IV intake carefully. Use microdrip tubing and a mechanical controller.

- Evaluate oral fluid intake for sodium, potassium and protein content. Usually protein is restricted along with potassium and sodium, depending on laboratory values. Lemonade and cranberry juices are usually good because of their high sugar and low potassium and sodium content.

- Avoid antacids containing magnesium. Usually aluminum hydroxide is ordered to bind phosphates.

- Observe for bleeding tendencies in skin, mucous membranes, urine, feces, and vomitus.

- Observe for changes in patient's sensorium.

- Assess patient for signs and symptoms of cardiac failure: Dyspnea, tachycardia, distended neck veins, cyanosis, pedal edema, rales, wheezes, fatigue.

- Prevent skin breakdown. Bathe patient with mild soap. Have patient turn and change position in bed every 1 to 2 hrs. Observe pressure areas for redness. Use of skin oils helps minimize pruritus.

- Assist patient with frequent oral care to prevent infections and minimize metallic taste.

- Observe for signs and symptoms of pericarditis: Chest pain may or may not be present; pericardial friction rub, tachycardia, fever.

- Monitor for developing cardiac tamponade: Diminished heart sounds, elevated venous pressure, distended neck veins, decreasing arterial pressure, narrowing pulse pressure, paradoxical pulse (a decrease of 10 mm Hg or more in systolic pressure with inspiration).

- Encourage and assist patient in changing position frequently to prevent tissue breakdown, especially when edema is present.

- Encourage patient to cough and deep breathe frequently to prevent infection.

- Assess pulse for rate, volume, and regularity. Weak pulse may indicate hypovolemia; bounding pulse may indicate hypervolemia; irregularities may indicate electrolyte imbalance.

- Assess respirations for rate, depth, and regularity. Rapid, *deep* respirations (Kussmaul) may indicate acidosis.

- Assess blood pressure for hypertension.

- Assess temperature closely. Look at hematocrit level and skin turgor if febrile for signs of dehydration.

- When fluids are not restricted, avoid fluid depletion which may cause uremia.

- Prevent catabolism by treating nausea and vomiting and attempting to stimulate appetite. Dietary regime varies depending on patient's laboratory values. Generally, diet consists of protein of high biologic value such as eggs, dairy products, and meat, which is usually restricted depending on blood urea nitrogen and creatinine values. Carbohydrates and fats are given to prevent catabolism, usually to total 35 kcal/kg/day. Sodium restriction is usually dependent on urine sodium excretion. Potassium is restricted based on serum potassium levels. Calcium is encouraged while phosphorus is restricted.

- Maintain seizure precautions as needed (see Seizure Disorders).

- Encourage activity only as tolerated. Provide frequent rest periods. Anemia, joint pain, and uremia may limit activity tolerance.

- Observe for signs of drug toxicity. Check the *Physician's Desk Reference* to see which of the patient's medications are excreted by the kidneys.

- Assess and support patient psychosocial needs. Allow time for patient to discuss fears and concerns. Assess changes in behavior carefully as indicative of metabolic changes. Inform family when these changes are a result of the disease. Maintain open communication with patient even when confused. Remember that patients with renal failure can become despondent and discouraged. Accept grieving behaviors and help patient progress through the stages.

PATIENT AND FAMILY TEACHING

- Have dietician teach patient about prescribed diet. Provide written materials to reinforce teaching.
- Discuss mental changes that occur with uremia with patient's family.
- Instruct family in the importance of preventing secondary infection in the patient.
- Explain all procedures to the patient, especially the importance of obtaining accurate daily weights and accurate intake and output.
- Reinforce the importance of maintaining good nutritional intake. Determine favorite foods and attempt to incorporate these into prescribed diet.

RENAL SURGERY

POTENTIAL PROBLEMS

Paralytic Ileus   Tube Dislodgement
Pulmonary Embolism   Obstructed Drainage Tubes
Shock   Infection
Hemorrhage   Pain
Pneumothorax   Psychosocial Problems
Atelectasis

KEY NURSING INTERVENTIONS

- See Preoperative and Postoperative Care.

- Observe for signs and symptoms of postoperative complications, especially the following:
  Hemorrhage and shock—Frank hematuria or bleeding from drainage tubes, excessive blood on dressings, increased pulse, decreasing blood pressure, diaphoresis, pallor, agitation, restlessness.
  Pneumothorax, atelectasis, pulmonary embolism—Sudden and severe chest pain, shortness of breath, dyspnea, tachypnea, diminished breath sounds unilaterally, cyanosis, cardiopulmonary arrest.
  Paralytic ileus—Nausea, vomiting, abdominal pain, distention, hypoactive bowel sounds.

- Prevent obstruction and infection of drainage tubes, i.e., nephrostomy tube, ureteral catheters, and urethral catheters by checking tubes for patency, maintaining accurate I&O, preventing tubes from kinking or pulling, observing the characteristics of the urine, irrigating only as ordered and using strict aseptic technique. Record output of each tube separately.

- Observe for signs and symptoms of tube dislodgement and report pain, absence of drainage, fever, chills, nausea, vomiting.

- Assess and support the patient's psychosocial needs. Because this surgery deals with the process of producing urine, the patient will probably be very anxious about the outcome. Help the patient and family deal with possible losses in body function.

PATIENT AND FAMILY TEACHING

- Explain the purpose and function of drainage tubes.

- Encourage fluid intake to at least 2000 cc/day.

- Upon discharge, inform the patient and family of signs and symptoms of complications (pain, hematuria, prolonged nausea or vomiting, dizziness, sweating, fainting, fever, pain, redness or swelling of incision, dysuria).

- If the patient is to go home with drainage tubes, dressings, or catheters, instruct and demonstrate their management. Assess the patient's and family's willingness and ability to do so.

- Have the patient avoid strenuous exercise, heavy lifting and dangerous activities until allowed by physician.

PERITONEAL DIALYSIS

POTENTIAL PROBLEMS

Perforated Bowel	Hyper/Hypoglycemia
Perforated Bladder	Protein/Vitamin Loss
Intraperitoneal Bleeding	Catheter Drainage Failure
Paralytic Ileus	Catheter Leakage
Arrhythmias	Catheter Infection
Peritonitis	Digitalis Toxicity
Reflex Bradycardia	Ascites
Hypo/Hypervolemia	Hypostatic Pneumonia
Hypocalcemia	Venous Thrombi
Hypokalemia	Pleural Effusion
Hypernatremia	Abdominal Pain
Hyperlipidemia	Psychosocial Problems

KEY NURSING INTERVENTIONS

Preparation

- Assemble and prepare necessary equipment using strict aseptic technique:
  - Peritoneal dialysis administration set, including catheter set, connecting tubing, and trocar set.
  - Additional medications (heparin, potassium chloride, antibiotics, lidocaine).
  - Skin preparation.
  - Sterile gloves.
  - Electrocardiographic monitor.
  - Dialysate solution (1.5% or 4.25% dextrose solution).
- Obtain consent per hospital policy.
- Have patient empty bladder.
- Warm dialyzing fluid to body temperature (37 degrees Centigrade).
- Obtain baseline vital signs and weight.
- Place patient in supine position for paracentesis.
- Reinforce explanation of the procedure to patient.

Procedure

- Assess and support patient's psychosocial needs. Approach patient in a calm and reassuring manner to allay fears and apprehensions. Be aware that uremia can induce changes in behavior similar to psychotic disturbances. Explain procedures with confidence and empathy for the patient's feelings. Paracentesis is a traumatic and invasive procedure which may be extremely frightening to the patient. As the procedure progresses, provide support and reassurance to help decrease anxiety.

- Assist physician with introduction of trocar and catheter, maintaining aseptic technique.

- Apply sterile dressing to catheter exit site.

- Connect catheter to administration set which has been cleared with dialysate.

- Instill dialysis solution by gravity over 5–10 mins. Prevent air from entering the system.

- After solution has infused, clamp tubing and allow to "dwell" in the peritoneal cavity for prescribed time (usually 30–45 mins.).

- Unclamp tube, lower solution bottles to the floor, and allow 10–20 mins. for drainage.

- Check vital signs frequently during the exchanges. Observe for hypotension indicative of hypovolemia and hypertension indicative of hypervolemia. Monitor electrocardiogram and pulse for irregularities indicative of hypokalemia.

- Repeat this cycle as prescribed (may vary from 12–36 hrs.).

- Monitor amount of return drainage closely. Maintain accurate intake and output records during dialysis. Records should include: The time of start and end of each exchange, amount infused and amount returned, number of exchanges, level of consciousness and vital signs with each exchange, medications added, and pre- and postdialysis weight.

- Observe for signs and symptoms of incomplete fluid recovery: Abdominal distention; complaints of fullness; less than 500 ml fluid recovery after several exchanges. Check tubing for kinks. Try repositioning patient from side to side and elevating head of bed. Gentle abdominal massage may also help. Prevent constipation which can cause fluid retention. Notify physician of inadequate drainage.

- Report persistent pain to physician.

- Monitor patient during infusion and dwell time for dyspnea. If dyspnea occurs, elevate head of bed, decrease infusion rate, help patient turn from side to side, and encourage deep breathing and coughing.

- Observe and document appearance of dialysate return. Blood-tinged return with initial outflow is normal. Cloudy return is indicative of infection. Report gross bleeding immediately. Normal return is clear and pale yellow. Amber return may indicate bladder perforation.

- Check catheter dressing frequently. Maintain dry dressing. Report leakage around catheter to physician.

- Prevent complications of bedrest (see The Immobilized Patient).

- Check on patient comfort during dialysis. Assist patient in changing positions. Provide nourishment during dialysate drainage. Discuss possible diversional activities to prevent boredom.

Following The Procedure

- Assess patient for signs and symptoms of peritonitis: Low-grade fever, abdominal pain with dialysate infusion, cloudy drainage, anorexia, malaise.

- Observe for hypoglycemia post dialysis: Palpitation, diaphoresis, confusion, agitation.

- Assess catheter exit site for infection: Tenderness, redness, drainage around the catheter.

- Change catheter dressing daily.

HEMODIALYSIS

POTENTIAL PROBLEMS

Dialysis Disequilibrium
   Syndrome
Cerebral Dyspraxia
Hemorrhage
Arrhythmias
Air Embolus
Hypo/Hypertension
Hypo/Hypernatremia
Hypokalemia
Hypercalcemia
Hypoosmolality
Hypo/Hyperthermia
Malnutrition
Arm Pain

Nausea/Vomiting
Hyperlipidemia
Iron Deficiency
Paradoxical Hypertension
Hemolysis
Transient Dyspnea
Pyrogenic Reaction
Water Intoxication
Anemia
Infection: AV Shunt
Clotting: AV Shunt
Pruritus
Separation of AV Cannulas
Psychosocial Problems

KEY NURSING INTERVENTIONS

Preparation

- Obtain and record accurate weight, blood pressure, pulse, respirations and temperature.

- Inform patient when dialysis is to be done. Answer questions and give reassurance to patient.

- Maintain accurate intake and output records for predialysis data base.

- Clarify with physician which medications are to be held predialysis.

- Obtain baseline laboratory data predialysis (phosphorus, magnesium, electrolytes, blood urea nitrogen, creatinine, hemoglobin, hematocrit, albumin).

Procedure

- Communicate frequently with dialysis nurse and assist as needed.

- Monitor vital signs closely.

- Assess and support psychosocial needs during dialysis. Recognize that psychiatric syndromes may be organic in nature and may subside as

BUN and creatinine decrease and electrolytes are balanced. Realize that the patient may feel threatened by loss of bodily functions, invasive procedures, loss of independence, and role disturbance. Help the patient develop a sense of trust with the health care team. Allow the patient to grieve. Let him know by your actions that grieving behaviors are accepted. Explain all steps of the dialysis procedure until patient is familiar and comfortable with it. Allow as many opportunities for independent activities as possible.

For hypotension:

- Suspect and investigate causes: Pre-existing hypovolemia, ultrafiltration, blood loss due to membrane leak or cannula separation, antihypertensive drugs, sedatives, tranquilizers, air embolism.

- Notify physician if hypotension persists. Ultrafiltration may be corrected by decreasing blood flow. Intravenous fluids may be used to increase blood pressure. Suspect pulmonary embolus or air embolus if hypotension is accompanied by chest pain and shortness of breath.

- Keep patient flat.

- Have normal saline and plasma expanders available for dialysis nurse.

- Check blood pressure frequently.

- *For hypertension:*

  - Suspect and investigate causes: Fluid overload, disequilibrium syndrome, anxiety, fear, apprehension, paradoxical hypertension due to drastic ultrafiltration, hypercalcemia.

  - Notify physician if unmanageable by dialysis (usually ultrafiltration will correct fluid overload etiology).

  - Check blood pressure frequently.

  - Assist dialysis nurse in obtaining antihypertensives as ordered.

  - Give intravenous normal saline as ordered for paradoxical hypertension.

- Identify patients at high risk for developing disequilibrium syndrome: Those with neurological disorders, those with severe azotemia (elevated BUN and creatinine), those receiving prolonged and vigorous dialysis.

- Assess patients for signs and symptoms of disequilibrium syndrome: Altered level of consciousness, muscle twitching, tachycardia, hypertension, tachypnea, nausea, vomiting, headache, agitation, convulsions, coma.

- *For Disequilibrium Syndrome:*

  - Notify physician when symptoms are identified.
  - Treatment by dialysis usually involves decreasing duration and flow rate of dialysis and dialyzing more frequently.
  - Be prepared to administer anticonvulsants as ordered.

- *For Nausea and Vomiting:*

  - Suspect and investigate possible causes: Hypotension, hypertension, disequilibrium syndrome, gastric erosion, anxiety, medications, hypercalcemia due to hard water syndrome, hemolysis, water intoxication.
  - Advise only small or no meals during dialysis.

- Assess patient for signs and symptoms of air embolus: Sudden onset of dyspnea, cough, cyanosis, respiratory arrest.

- *For Air Embolus:*

  - Stop dialysis and clamp blood line.
  - Turn patient to left side in Trendelenburg position.
  - Notify physician immediately.
  - Administer high concentration of oxygen as ordered.
  - Attempt to identify possible cause: Defective blood tubing, faulty blood line connections, air detector off or malfunctioning, displaced arterial needle.

- Monitor patient for signs and symptoms of hemolysis: Shortness of breath, chills, back pain, nausea, vomiting.

- *For Hemolysis:*

  - Notify physician when hemolysis suspected.
  - Discontinue dialysis immediately.
  - Usual laboratory studies are serial hematocrit and electrolytes, type and cross match.
  - Observe electrolyte values for rising potassium.
  - Watch for falling hematocrit.
  - Identify cause: Occlusion of blood pump, high dialysate temperature, copper contamination, improper dialysate preparation.
  - Monitor blood pressure frequently.

- Observe patient's temperature closely. Fever may be due to high dialysate temperature or pyrogenic reaction. Chilling may be due to cool dialysate temperature. Notify physician if fever persists after dialysis.
- Observe patient for signs and symptoms of electrolyte imbalances:
  - *Hypernatremia*—Headache, excess thirst, blurry vision, disorientation.
  - *Hyponatremia*—Muscle cramping.
  - *Hypokalemia*—Muscle weakness, ileus, cardiac arrhythmias.
  - *Hypercalcemia*—Weakness, lethargy, anorexia, vomiting, hypertension, burning of skin.
- Minimize risk of pulmonary infection by having patient turn, cough, and deep breathe during dialysis.
- Observe for signs and symptoms of water intoxication: Decreased level of consciousness, headache, nausea, vomiting, confusion, convulsions. Notify physician and identify cause (usually improper dialysate formula).

Following The Procedure

- Observe patient for postdialysis syndrome: Weakness, fatigue, dizziness, headaches, nausea, muscle cramps. Symptoms usually subside within 24 hrs.
- Keep affected extremity with AV shunt elevated 2–3 days post insertion. Weight-bearing is to be avoided 2–3 days post insertion of leg shunts.
- Prevent AV shunt infections by using aseptic technique when doing dressing changes and handling shunt. Cleaning should be done with dialysis. Change if dressing is wet. When necessary to enter T-tube, clean thoroughly with iodine preparation prior to puncture.
- Maintain proper cannula alignment of AV shunt by wrapping shunt dressings with gauze.
- Assess AV shunt for signs of clotting: Dark red color, absence of bruit, separation of serum and cells in cannula.
- Observe shunt for color and auscultate for bruit with vital signs and every hour post insertion × 24 hrs.
- Prevent shunt and fistula clotting. DO NOT:
  - Take blood pressure in affected extremity.
  - Start IV's in affected extremity.

- Draw blood specimens from affected extremity.
- Use constricting restraints near access site.

- Observe patient for signs and symptoms of infection: Persistent fever, reddened cannula exit sites, drainage from cannula exit sites, swollen access site.
- Assess for distal pulses, skin temperatures, and sensory changes in affected extremity. Sensory changes may be normal when fistula or shunt is new, while pulse deficit and cool extremity may indicate clot formation.
- Observe access site for bleeding. Slight oozing is normal post insertion. Report excess bleeding to physician.
- Keep cannula clamps on dressing at all times.
- Tape must be on bridges of shunt connections at all times to prevent disconnection.
- Apply shunt clamps immediately should separation occur. A loose tourniquet can be applied until medical help is obtained.
- Observe shunt sites frequently for 4–6 hrs. post dialysis for bleeding due to heparinization.
- Auscultate fistulas for presence of bruit with vital signs. Report absence of bruit to physician.
- Observe fistula site postoperatively for bleeding. Report excessive bleeding to physician.
- See Chronic or Acute Renal Failure.

URINARY DIVERSION: ILEAL CONDUIT, CUTANEOUS URETEROSTOMY, URETEROSIGMOIDOSTOMY

POTENTIAL PROBLEMS

Hemorrhage	Infection
Shock	Hematuria
Pulmonary Embolus	Intestinal Obstruction
Peritonitis	Skin Breakdown
Thrombophlebitis	Stoma Prolapse
Fluid and Electrolyte Imbalances	Pyelonephritis
	Ureteral Stricture
Paralytic Ileus	Psychosocial Problems

KEY NURSING INTERVENTIONS

- See Preoperative and Postoperative Care.

- Check chart to determine the reason for urinary diversion and plan care accordingly: Bladder cancer, pelvic cancer, trauma, birth defects.

- Observe for postoperative complications (see Postoperative Care).

- Check stoma frequently for complications: Excessive swelling or edema, cyanosis, bleeding.

- Inspect the skin around the stoma site for irritation and infection. Alkaline urine is very irritating. Keep urine acidic by administering ascorbic acid as ordered.

- Observe for fluid and electrolyte imbalances (see Fluid and Electrolytes).

- Properly apply and secure ileostomy or ureterostomy bag. Change appliance early in the morning before fluid intake. Remove old bag using adhesive solvent. Measure stoma each time bag is applied and cut bag ⅛ to 1/16 inch larger than stoma. Cleanse the skin and thoroughly remove all the old cement. Apply skin barrier. Apply cement to bag and place bag over the stoma, avoiding wrinkling where the adhesive touches the skin.

- Change bag as necessary, repeating above procedure usually every 5–7 days.

- Empty bag when less than half full. Connect to a drainage bag at night to facilitate continuous sleep.

- Control odor by increasing fluid intake, using deodorizing pills or white vinegar in the bag and avoiding odorous foods.

- Maintain reusable bags by removing all adhesive with solvent, wash the bag with detergent and soak it in vinegar or chlorine bleach for 5–10 minutes. Allow bag to dry before using.

- Assess and support patient's psychosocial needs. Anticipate problems associated with a change in body image and encourage discussion of feelings. Answer questions. Let the patient examine ostomy equipment preoperatively if ready. Help allay fears that the patient will have a drastic change in lifestyle. Inform the patient that sex, work, exercise, and most other activities may be resumed as soon as strength increases. Refer the patient to the United Ostomy Association and/or arrange for a visit by a patient with a similar ostomy. Realize that the patient may not want to look at the stoma or learn about stoma care immediately. A well integrated care plan, especially regarding patient teaching, is essential for patient progress.

- *FOR URETEROSIGMOIDOSTOMY:*

  - Postoperatively, the patient will have a rectal tube for urinary drainage. Prevent the tube from dislodgement or kinking by taping tube to buttocks and checking it frequently.

  - Inspect the perianal skin for irritation.

  - Avoid trauma to ureterosigmoid anastomosis by inserting rectal tube no more than 4 inches and by avoiding enemas, cathartics, and forceful irrigation.

  - Keep rectal tube inserted at night to facilitate continuous sleep.

- *FOR CUTANEOUS URETEROSTOMY:*

  - Use strict aseptic technique when inserting a catheter for dilatation to keep ureter patent.

  - Observe for ureteral stricture (abdominal or back pain, low urinary output).

PATIENT AND FAMILY TEACHING

- Attempt to involve significant other in patient care and discharge planning.

- Demonstrate proper stoma care, skin care and application of bags. Tell the patient to carry bags and cement at all times in case of problems.

- Encourage fluid intake to at least 2500 cc/day to help prevent ascending infections.
- Have the patient avoid heavy lifting and strenuous exercise until allowed by physician (usually for six months).
- Upon discharge, inform the patient and family of signs and symptoms of complications (cloudy or bloody urine, skin infection or irritation, graying of the stoma, bleeding at the stoma site, fever, chills, back or abdominal pain).
- Provide a list of companies or stores from which ostomy equipment may be purchased.
- If indicated, arrange through the physician for a home visit by an enterostomal therapist to continue patient care and teaching.

FOR URETEROSIGMOIDOSTOMY:

- Begin voiding/bowel training as soon as possible. Encourage voiding every 2–3 hours. With time the patient will eventually know the difference between the urge to void and the urge to defecate.
- Instruct the patient to avoid gas-forming food and air swallowing (gum chewing, carbonated drinks, and smoking). This causes flatus which, in turn, causes embarrassing stress incontinence.

RUPTURED BLADDER

POTENTIAL PROBLEMS

Peritonitis   Paralytic Ileus
Hemorrhage   Pain
Shock (Hypovolemic,   Infection
   Septic)   Psychosocial Problems

KEY NURSING INTERVENTIONS

- See Preoperative and Postoperative Care.

- Check chart to determine cause of bladder rupture and plan care accordingly (multiple trauma, pelvic fractures, accidental injury due to low abdominal or pelvic surgery).

- If rupture was due to trauma, do not insert urethral catheter until a retrograde urethrogram is done to rule out urethral trauma.

- Observe for signs and symptoms of postoperative complications, especially the following:

- *Hemorrhage and shock*—Frank hematuria or bleeding from catheters, excessive blood on dressings, increased pulse, decreasing blood pressure, diaphoresis, pallor, agitation, restlessness.

- *Peritonitis*—Severe, constant abdominal pain; decreased or absent bowel sounds; rigid abdomen on palpation; nausea; vomiting; fever.

- *Paralytic ileus*—Nausea, vomiting, abdominal pain, distention, hypoactive bowel sounds.

- After surgery there is usually a suprapubic and a urethral catheter in place. Prevent obstruction and infection of catheters by checking tubes for patency; maintaining accurate I&O; preventing tubes from kinking or pulling; observing the characteristics of the urine; maintaining a closed, sterile drainage system; recording the output of each tube separately.

- Assess and support the patient's psychosocial needs. Help the patient and family deal with changes in body image and body function.

PATIENT AND FAMILY TEACHING

- Explain purpose and function of suprapubic and urethral catheters.
- Encourage fluid intake of at least 2000 cc/day.
- Upon discharge inform patient and family of signs and symptoms of complications (increasing pain, fever, hematuria, sweating, fainting, low urine output, pain, redness, and swelling at incision site).
- If the patient is to go home with suprapubic catheter, instruct and demonstrate proper care.

NEUROGENIC BLADDER

POTENTIAL PROBLEMS

Autonomic Hyperreflexia   Renal Calculi
Hydronephrosis   Renal Failure
Urinary Tract Infection   Psychosocial Problems

KEY NURSING INTERVENTIONS

- Assess patient for signs and symptoms of autonomic hyperreflexia, a condition that may be due to bladder distention, skin pain, or visceral distention: Hypertension, bradycardia, headache, flushing, diaphoresis below level of lesion, blurred vision, nausea. This is a medical emergency. Notify physician immediately.

- *FOR AUTONOMIC HYPERREFLEXIA:*

  - Keep head elevated by maintaining semi-Fowler's position.
  - Monitor vital signs every 5 mins.
  - Catheterize patient as ordered.
  - Check patency of existing catheter.

- Prevent urinary tract infections by maintaining strict aseptic technique during catheterization and adherence to a catheter care program (see Indwelling Urethral Catheter).

- Prevent formation of renal calculi. Force fluids to 3000 cc/day. Encourage mobilization out of bed as much as possible.

- Observe for signs and symptoms of a full bladder when attempting bladder training: Perspiration, restlessness, cold hands and feet, anxiety, distention, voiding 25–50 cc more than one time per hour.

- When attempting bladder training, observe the following:

  - Encourage liberal fluid intake during the day.
  - Patient should attempt voiding at set intervals.
  - Assist initiation of voiding by applying pressure over abdomen, stretching the anal sphincter, stroking inner thighs and pubic area, or applying ice to these areas.
  - Catheterize immediately after voiding for residual.

- Gradually increase intervals to patient's tolerance.
- Observe for signs and symptoms of urinary tract infection: Fever, chills, hematuria, cloudy urine, malaise, nausea, vomiting, flank pain, dysuria, abdominal pain, pyuria.
- Document character and quantity of urine.
- Assess and support patient's psychosocial needs. Help patient cope with altered body image and self-concept changes. Emphasize patient's strengths. Maintain a steady and hopeful attitude when the prognosis is uncertain. Allow as much self-care and independence as possible. Include significant others in care plan.

PATIENT AND FAMILY TEACHING

- If teaching intermittent catheterization, emphasize the importance of good hand washing technique, cleaning catheter after the procedure with soap and water, or other recommended solution and maintaining catheters in a clean container.
- Stress the importance of performing intermittent catheterization at set intervals.
- Advise patient to take minimal fluids prior to bedtime.
- Teach the patient bladder training methods to stimulate micturition (see Key Nursing Interventions).

INDWELLING URETHRAL CATHETER

POTENTIAL PROBLEMS

Urinary Tract Infection   Catheter Obstruction
Reflux   Tissue Necrosis
Calculi   Tissue Breakdown
Bladder Spasms

KEY NURSING INTERVENTIONS

- Assess patient for signs and symptoms of urinary tract infection: Fever, chills, lower abdominal discomfort, hematuria, pyuria, malaise, nausea, vomiting, cloudy urine.

- Observe for signs and symptoms of catheter obstruction: Urinary output less than 30 to 50 cc per hour, bladder distention, feelings of fullness, diaphoresis, pain, anxiety, restlessness.

- Prevent tissue breakdown by taping catheter to inner aspect of thigh for females and to abdomen or upper anterior thigh for males.

- Do the following to prevent urinary tract infections: Maintain a closed catheter drainage system, administer perineal catheter care BID (preferably with antimicrobial solution), prevent retrograde flow of urine, encourage liberal fluid intake, keep drainage bag off the floor, clean catheter tubing with antiseptic solution away from the meatus.

- Keep drainage bag below level of bladder at all times.

- Do not allow patient to sit or lie on tubing.

- Whenever it is necessary to open the drainage system, maintain strict aseptic technique.

- Keep drainage tubing free of kinks and occlusions.

- Do not leave foreskin of males retracted after catheter care.

- When obtaining urine specimens, clean specimen port with antimicrobial solution and aspirate urine with sterile needle and syringe. Latex catheters may be punctured at a 45-degree angle but cautiously to prevent puncturing bulb inflation tube.

- Assess and support patient's psychosocial needs. Reassure patient that desire to urinate after insertion is normal.

PATIENT AND FAMILY TEACHING

- Instruct self-care patients in proper catheter care procedure.
- Stress the importance of adequate fluid intake.

REPRODUCTIVE SYSTEM

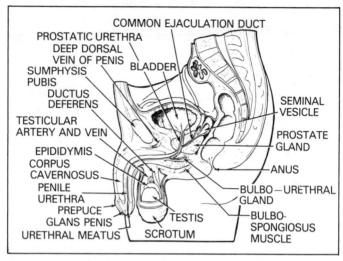

COMMON EJACULATION DUCT
PROSTATIC URETHRA
DEEP DORSAL
VEIN OF PENIS
BLADDER
SUMPHYSIS
PUBIS
DUCTUS
DEFERENS
SEMINAL
VESICLE
TESTICULAR
ARTERY AND VEIN
PROSTATE
GLAND
EPIDIDYMIS
CORPUS
CAVERNOSUS
ANUS
PENILE
URETHRA
BULBO—URETHRAL
GLAND
PREPUCE
GLANS PENIS
TESTIS
BULBO-
SPONGIOSUS
MUSCLE
URETHRAL MEATUS
SCROTUM

The Male Reproductive Organs

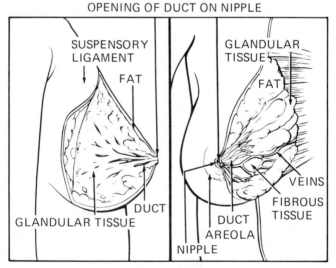

OPENING OF DUCT ON NIPPLE
SUSPENSORY
LIGAMENT
GLANDULAR
TISSUE
FAT
FAT
VEINS
FIBROUS
TISSUE
DUCT
DUCT
AREOLA
GLANDULAR TISSUE
NIPPLE

Internal and External Anatomy of the Breast

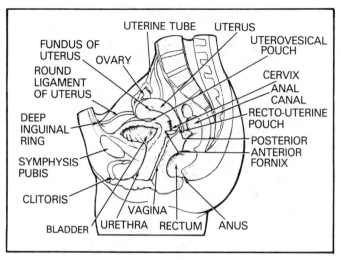

Mid-sagittal Section of Female Pelvis

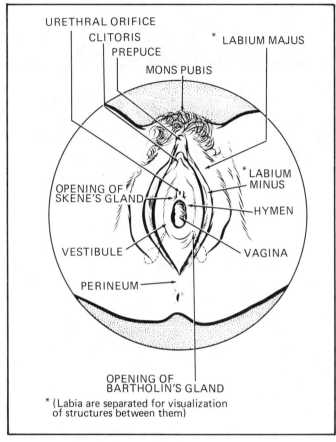

URETHRAL ORIFICE
CLITORIS
PREPUCE
MONS PUBIS
* LABIUM MAJUS
OPENING OF
SKENE'S GLAND
* LABIUM
MINUS
HYMEN
VESTIBULE
VAGINA
PERINEUM
OPENING OF
BARTHOLIN'S GLAND
* (Labia are separated for visualization
of structures between them)

Exterior Anatomy of Female Genitalia

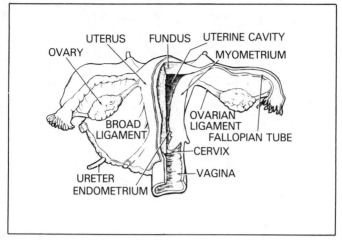

Female Reproductive Organs

REPRODUCTIVE SYSTEM— PHYSIOLOGY SUMMARY

I. THE MALE

A. <u>The testes</u>

Supported within the scrotum and produce:

1. Spermatozoa, the reproductive cells.
2. Sertoli's cells, which supply the spermatozoa with nutrients.
3. Leydig interstitial cells, which produce male androgen hormones (see Endocrine System).

B. <u>Spermatozoa</u>

Enabled to leave the testes through a series of tubules, the seminiferous tubules, which form the rete testes.

C. <u>The rete testes</u>

Open into the epididymis, which becomes the ductus deferens.

D. <u>The seminal vesicles</u>

Secrete a fluid which promotes sperm motility through a duct which joins the ductus deferens to form the ejaculatory duct.

E. <u>The ejaculatory duct</u>

Ejects sperm and seminal vesicle fluid into the urethra.

F. <u>The prostate gland</u>

Surrounds the proximal end of the urethra and secretes an alkaline fluid which aids in sperm motility.

G. <u>The Cowper's glands</u>

Secrete an alkaline fluid which is a constituent of semen.

H. <u>The penis</u>

1. The male organ for both urinary elimination and copulation.
2. With sexual stimulation, the arteries in the penis dilate, allowing blood to fill the cavernous spaces.
3. As the spaces fill and distend, blood is trapped as the veins become compressed, causing a firm erection.

II. THE FEMALE

A. The Mammary Glands

1. Breast development is controlled by estrogen and progesterone. Duct growth is stimulated by estrogen, and alveoli development is stimulated by progesterone.

2. Changes in breast tissue occur during menstruation (swelling of connective tissue) and pregnancy (areola darkens, the number of ducts increase, and the alveoli change).

3. Lactation is controlled by a rise in prolactin level after delivery. Lactation is maintained by suckling, which stimulates the anterior pituitary to secrete oxytocin. Oxytocin stimulates the cells surrounding the alveoli to contract, emptying milk into the ducts.

B. The Menstrual Cycle

1. The gonadotropins (FSH and LH) secreted by the anterior pituitary control the cyclical changes in the ovaries.

2. FSH stimulates development of graafian follicles, which begin to secrete estrogen.

3. FSH secretion increases from the first to the seventh day of the menstrual cycle.

4. Increasing estrogen levels during the proliferative phase cause the following:

   a) Suppression of FSH.

   b) Stimulation of LH secretion.

   c) Endometrial thickening.

   d) Proliferation of endometrial glands and cells.

   e) Endometrial water retention.

5. LH hormone causes the follicle to mature until the ovum is expelled at ovulation on the 14th or 15th day of the cycle.

6. Following ovulation, the follicle changes to become the corpus luteum.

7. LH stimulates the corpus luteum to secrete progesterone and a small amount of estrogen.

8. Increasing progesterone and estrogen levels during the secretory phase cause the following:

  a) Endometrial glands and arterioles to become coiled and grow longer.

  b) Endometrial gland secretion.

  c) Endometrial tissue to become vascular and edematous.

9. If pregnancy does not occur, the corpus luteum begins degeneration 22 to 24 days into the cycle.

10. With luteal degeneration, estrogen and progesterone secretion decrease, causing endometrial degeneration and menstruation.

11. The menstrual phase begins with the first day of menstruation and ends on the fourth or fifth day of the cycle.

12. Around the fifth day of the cycle, the anterior pituitary begins to secrete FSH and the cycle continues.

C. Menopause

1. The ovary functions for approximately 35 years after which the menstrual cycle stops, usually around age 45 to 50.

2. In menopause, the ovaries atrophy, and estrogen secretion decreases to the point where it can no longer inhibit the anterior pituitary's production of FSH and LH.

3. FSH and LH are then produced in large quantities, and estrogen production eventually ceases entirely.

REPRODUCTIVE SYSTEM ASSESSMENT

I. HISTORY (Male or Female)

A. Past history of reproductive system problems

1. What type?
2. What therapy was utilized? Did it work?

B. Recent History

1. Presence of discharge?

   a) Itching?

   b) Foul odor?

2. Sexual problems?
3. Fertility problems?
4. Urinary problems? (See Renal System Assessments.)

C. Contraceptives

Type of contraceptive used?

D. Pain

Use PQRST mnemonic.

P— Provokes.	What makes the pain worse or better? What was the patient doing prior to the onset of pain?
Q— Quality.	Subjective description of pain by the patient. Use the patient's own words, i.e., burning, stabbing, pressure.
R— Radiation.	Where is the pain located and does it radiate anywhere?
S— Severity.	Ask the patient to judge the pain on a scale of 1 to 10 with 10 being the worst pain ever felt.
T— Time.	How long has the patient had this pain? When did the pain begin and end?

E. Female

1. Menstrual history.

   a) Last menstrual period?

      b) Presence of dysmenorhea, menorrhagia, bleeding or spotting between periods, irregularity?

  2. Number of pregnancies, live births, abortions; eg: G III, P II, A I?

  3. Complications of childbirth?

  4. Type of delivery?

  5. Menopause.

      a) Last menstrual period?

      b) Presence of hot flashes, palpitations, sweating, bleeding, mood swings?

  6. Breasts.
    Drainage, nipple inversion, dimpling, lumps, pain?

F. Medications

  1. List medications, including over-the-counter drugs.

  2. Allergies.

G. Nutrition

Describe a typical:

  1. Breakfast

  2. Lunch

  3. Dinner

  4. Snacks

II. BACKGROUND INFORMATION

A. Lab Values

Check laboratory studies for abnormal values or worsening trends: Urine, blood, gram stains, cultures, pregnancy tests.

B. Diagnostic Studies

Identify abnormal reports of diagnostic studies.

C. Chart

Check old chart for past relevant information.

III. INSPECTION AND PALPATION

A. Male

1. Inspect and palpate the pubic area, penis, scrotum, testes for pain, swelling, size, shape, inflammation, ulcers, lesions, tumors, nodes, scars, symmetry, discharge, hernias, skin color, hair distribution, hygiene status, patency of urethra, presence of urinary catheters.

2. Transilluminate scrotum. Edematous fluid is translucent while blood is opaque.

B. Female

1. Inspect and palpate external structures of the vagina for pain, swelling, inflammation, bulging, growths, discharge, bleeding, and foul odor.

2. Perform or assist the physician with a speculum and bimanual examination. Observe the vaginal canal and cervix for inflammation, discharges, bleeding.

3. Palpate uterus and ovaries, noting size, shape, and area of tenderness.

4. Collect ordered specimens and send to laboratory (see Specimen Collection).

5. Inspect and palpate both breasts in a systematic order. With the patient standing and the arms at the side, observe the breasts for size, shape, symmetry, and condition of the nipple. Have the patient slowly raise the arms and then flex the pectoralis muscles. Observe for dimpling. Place the patient supine. Begin palpation at the nipple and proceed in a clockwise fashion out to the axilla. Describe any tumors in terms of location, size, shape, and movability.

DILATATION AND CURETTAGE, CONIZATION

POTENTIAL PROBLEMS

Perforated Uterus   Urinary Retention
Hemorrhage   Psychosocial Problems
Infection

KEY NURSING INTERVENTIONS

- Assess patient for signs and symptoms of hemorrhage and shock: Multiple saturated perineal pads (pads can be weighed for a more accurate estimate of blood loss); hypotension; tachycardia; rapid, shallow respirations; pale lips and tongue; pulse pressure of 20 mm Hg or less; restlessness.

- Monitor for signs and symptoms of perforated uterus: Shock, hemorrhage, severe pain unrelieved by analgesics, lower abdominal rigidity.

- Document number of perineal pads (and weight, if possible) and characteristics of vaginal drainage.

- Check for urinary retention: Absent voiding, bladder distention, voiding 25 to 50 cc more than one time per hour, complaints of fullness and discomfort, restlessness.

- If packing is present, avoid accidental removal. Instruct patient not to remove packing when voiding.

- Administer perineal care with antimicrobial solution or warm water after voiding and defecation.

PATIENT AND FAMILY TEACHING

- Advise patient to maintain vaginal rest until otherwise instructed by physician (no tub baths, sexual intercourse, douching).

- Instruct patient to refrain from excessive and strenuous activity (usually for one week).

- Advise patient to report signs and symptoms of infection: Elevated temperature, foul-smelling discharge, and severe pain unrelieved by analgesics.

- *FOR DILATATION AND CURETTAGE:*

  - Tell patient to expect mild vaginal drainage for several days and to report excessive vaginal bleeding (more than a normal menses).

- *FOR CONIZATION:*

  - Tell patient that pain lasting several days is normal postoperatively and that drainage may persist up to 8 weeks.

  - Stress that drainage lasting longer than 8 weeks should be reported to the physician.

VAGINAL HYSTERECTOMY, ANTERIOR/POSTERIOR COLPORRHAPHY

POTENTIAL PROBLEMS

Coronary Occlusion
Pulmonary Embolism
Hemorrhage
Shock
Sepsis
Lower Extremity
   Thrombophlebitis
Urinary Retention

Urinary Tract Infection
Paralytic Ileus
Intestinal Obstruction
Fistula
Bladder Injury
Psychosocial Problems

KEY NURSING INTERVENTIONS

- Assess perineal pads for excessive drainage frequently. (Pads can be weighed for a more accurate estimate of blood loss.) Report excessive bleeding immediately to physician.

- Monitor patient for signs and symptoms of shock: Cold, clammy skin; restlessness; oliguria or anuria; hypotension; tachycardia; rapid, shallow respirations; peripheral cyanosis; pale lips and tongue; pulse pressure of 20 mm Hg or less.

- Observe for signs and symptoms of pulmonary embolism: Chest pain, shortness of breath, dyspnea, tachypnea, tachycardia, cyanosis, cardiopulmonary arrest.

- Minimize the risk of pulmonary embolism and thrombophlebitis. Maintain low-Fowler's position and do not gatch the knees. Never massage the legs. Encourage foot and leg exercises while in bed. Mobilize patient frequently as ordered. Avoid crossing legs. Maintain antiembolism hose as ordered.

- Assess patient for signs and symptoms of thrombophlebitis: Pain, redness and swelling of affected extremity. Check for positive Homans' sign, which is pain in the calf upon dorsiflexion of the foot.

- Maintain a patent urinary catheter. Keep drainage bag in low position to prevent retrograde flow. Administer catheter care BID (usually with antimicrobial solution) (see Indwelling Urethral Catheter).

- If a suprapubic catheter is inserted, the patient can be assessed for urinary retention by the following: Clamp the suprapubic catheter and have the patient void; unclamp catheter and measure residual. Skin area around suprapubic catheter should be kept clean with antimicrobial solution.

- Observe for signs and symptoms of urinary retention post catheter removal: Absent voiding, bladder distention, voiding 25 to 50 cc more than one time per hour, complaints of fullness and discomfort, restlessness. Report to physician immediately.

- Check all four quadrants of abdomen for bowel sounds. Absent or diminished bowel sounds may be indicative of paralytic ileus and should be reported to the physician.

- *FOR VAGINAL HYSTERECTOMY:*

  - Avoid accidental removal of vaginal packing.

- *FOR ANTERIOR/POSTERIOR COLPORRHAPHY:*

  - Encourage frequent voiding (every 4 to 6 hrs.) after catheter is removed to prevent pressure on suture line.

- Assess and support patient's psychosocial needs. Recognize that the patient may have difficulty dealing with this loss and have alterations in her self-concept. Offer support and understanding of these feelings and create an open atmosphere conducive to free discussion of feelings.

PATIENT AND FAMILY TEACHING

- Advise the patient to maintain vaginal rest until otherwise instructed by physician (no tub baths, sexual intercourse, douching).

- Instruct patient to refrain from excessive and strenuous activity which may increase intra-abdominal pressure.

- Tell the patient to expect mild vaginal drainage for several days, fatigue, and occasional lower abdominal pains.

- Stress the importance of reporting persistent pain, bleeding, or voiding difficulties to the physician.

- Emphasize the importance of rest after discharge.

- Instruct patient to avoid sitting or standing for long periods and not to cross legs.

TOTAL ABDOMINAL HYSTERECTOMY, BILATERAL SALPINGO-OOPHORECTOMY

POTENTIAL PROBLEMS

Pulmonary Embolism   Infection
Hemorrhage   Urinary Retention
Shock   Pain
Thrombophlebitis   Constipation
Paralytic Ileus   Psychosocial Problems
Urinary Tract Infection

KEY NURSING INTERVENTIONS

- See Preoperative and Postoperative Care.

- Assess patient for signs and symptoms of hemorrhage and shock: Multiple saturated perineal pads; increased pulse; decreasing blood pressure; pallor; cool, clammy skin; restlessness; agitation.

- Assess patient for signs and symptoms of pulmonary embolism: Chest pain, shortness of breath, dyspnea, tachypnea, tachycardia, cyanosis, cardiopulmonary arrest.

- Observe for signs and symptoms of thrombophlebitis: Pain, redness, swelling of affected extremity and positive Homans' sign, (pain in calf upon dorsiflexion of the foot).

- Minimize risk of pulmonary embolism and thrombophlebitis by maintaining low-Fowler's position, avoiding gatching the knees, and never massaging the legs. Use antiembolism stockings and avoid crossing the legs and standing or sitting for long periods of time.

- Check for signs and symptoms of paralytic ileus: Hypoactive or absent bowel sounds, nausea, vomiting, abdominal pain.

- Document number of perineal pads used and characteristics of vaginal drainage.

- Observe for urinary retention after removal of urinary catheter: Absence of voiding, bladder distention, voiding 25–50 cc more than one time per hour, feeling of fullness or discomfort.

- Assess and support patient's psychosocial needs by facilitating movement through the grieving process. Inform patient that she may experience menopausal type symptoms such as crying, depression, nervousness, mood swings, etc. Assure her that this is normal and only temporary. Explain that because the uterus is removed, menstruation will cease. Anticipate and help the patient deal with problems surrounding cancer (if diagnosed), inability to bear children, hormone therapy, resuming sexual activity, self-perceived role changes, and problems in the home environment.

PATIENT AND FAMILY TEACHING

- Involve husband or significant other in patient care and discharge planning.

- Advise patient to maintain vaginal rest until otherwise instructed by physician (no tub baths, sexual intercourse, or douching); usually for 6–8 weeks.

- Have patient avoid strenuous exercise, heavy lifting, and standing or sitting for long periods of time.

- Instruct patient to report signs and symptoms of complications to physician: Chest pain, shortness of breath, pain or swelling of a lower extremity, fever, chills, dysuria, frequency, severe abdominal pain, dizziness, foul-smelling discharge, vaginal bleeding, and pain, redness or swelling of the incision.

- Tell patient to expect mild vaginal drainage for several days.

VULVECTOMY, LYMPHADENECTOMY

POTENTIAL PROBLEMS

Pulmonary Embolism
Myocardial Infarction
Hemorrhage
Shock
Thrombophlebitis
Poor or Absent Pedal and
   Popliteal Pulses

Cellulitis
Urinary Tract Infection
Wound Infection
Perineal Excoriation
Foot and Leg Edema
Psychosocial Problems

KEY NURSING INTERVENTIONS

- Assess patient for signs and symptoms of pulmonary embolism: Chest pain, shortness of breath, dyspnea, tachypnea, tachycardia, cyanosis, cardiopulmonary arrest.

- Observe for signs and symptoms of myocardial infarction due to emboli: Crushing, pressing, burning, aching chest pain; chest pain lasting longer than half an hour; retrosternal chest pain which may radiate to the anterior thorax, lower jaws, neck, shoulders and arms; dyspnea; diaphoresis; complaints of indigestion; arrhythmias.

- Observe for signs and symptoms of thrombophlebitis: Pain, redness and swelling of affected extremity. Check for positive Homans' sign, which is pain in the calf upon dorsiflexion of the foot.

- Maintain active suction as ordered for drainage.

- Monitor dressings for excessive bleeding. Change dressings frequently.

- Assess patient for signs and symptoms of shock: Cold, clammy skin; restlessness; oliguria or anuria; hypotension; tachycardia; rapid, shallow respirations; peripheral cyanosis; pale lips and tongue; pulse pressure of 20 mm Hg or less.

- Minimize the risk of pulmonary embolism and thrombophlebitis. Maintain low-Fowler's position and do not gatch the knees. Never massage the legs. Encourage foot and leg exercises while in bed. Mobilize patient frequently as ordered. Avoid crossing legs. Maintain antiembolism hose as ordered.

- Observe for urinary retention post catheter removal: Absent voiding, bladder distention, voiding 25 to 50 cc more than one time per hour, complaints of fullness and discomfort, restlessness.

- Administer catheter care with antimicrobial solution to prevent urinary tract infections.

- Perineum care usually consists of cleansing with warm antimicrobial solution or a 50/50 concentration of hydrogen peroxide and sterile saline. Administer perineum care after each voiding and defecation with prescribed solution.

- Heat lamp treatment is usually employed after perineum care.

- When sutures are removed, sitz baths are usually given with antimicrobial solution.

- Constipating medications (Lomotil, Paregoric) are frequently ordered postoperatively to avoid wound infection. Observation of regular bowel movements is necessary after these drugs are discontinued and a regular diet is resumed.

- Observe feet and legs for swelling. Monitor popliteal and pedal pulses for circulatory status.

- Assess and support patient's psychosocial needs. Include significant others in patient care plan. Alteration in body image is the greatest psychological hurdle for the patient. Intervention should focus on helping the patient cope. Create an open atmosphere that encourages discussion of feelings and opportunities to ask questions. Help the patient explore fears, anxieties, and frustrations.

PATIENT AND FAMILY TEACHING

- Instruct patient in the importance of rest and avoiding heavy lifting or strenuous activities after discharge.

- If wound irrigations, sitz baths, and dressing changes are necessary after discharge, instruct patient and significant other in aseptic principles of the procedure.

- Advise patient to contact the physician immediately if signs and symptoms of infection occur: Fever, chills, foul-smelling drainage, wound tenderness, redness and swelling.

- Discuss signs of urinary problems (retention, infection) and advise patient to contact the physician if such signs and symptoms occur.

MASTECTOMY

POTENTIAL PROBLEMS

Hemorrhage	Lymph Edema
Atelectasis	Frozen Shoulder
Infection	Psychosocial Problems
Pain	

KEY NURSING INTERVENTIONS

- See Preoperative and Postoperative Care.

- Check dressings for active hemorrhage and/or excessive constriction.

- Maintain Hemovac or other suction to drainage tubes.

- Check arm and hand of affected side for adequate circulation, sensitivity and motion.

- Do not take blood pressures, draw blood, or otherwise puncture the affected arm.

- Maintain a position of comfort while keeping the affected arm elevated above the heart. Do not turn patient to affected side.

- Initiate range of motion exercises (usually beginning the second day postoperatively). Develop a progressive exercise program. Consult a nursing text for a list of recommended exercises.

- Assess and support patient's psychosocial needs by performing a psychosocial assessment preoperatively. Provide a referral to the American Cancer Society's ''Reach to Recovery Program'' and to local support groups. Facilitate movement through the grieving process.

PATIENT AND FAMILY TEACHING

- Attempt to involve the husband or significant other in hospital care and discharge planning.

- Upon discharge, instruct patient to observe the incision and affected arm for signs and symptoms of infection: Pain, swelling, redness, red streaks, fever. These should be reported to the physician immediately.

- Demonstrate and provide a list of exercises.

- Inform patient of expected edema. This may be minimized by elevating the arm while sleeping, massaging the affected arm several times per day, and avoiding constrictive clothing.

- Stress the importance of avoiding injury to the affected arm. Never allow blood to be drawn or injections given. Avoid heavy lifting, extreme temperatures, burns, and puncture wounds.

- Demonstrate the use of a prosthesis. Provide a list of places at which to purchase them.

- Demonstrate breast self-examination and stress the importance of monthly examinations.

PROSTATECTOMY (TRANSURETHRAL, SUPRAPUBIC, RETROPUBIC, PERINEAL)

POTENTIAL PROBLEMS

Hemorrhage	Catheter Obstruction
Shock	Paralytic Ileus
Infection	Incontinence
Epididymitis	Constipation
Pneumonia	Psychosocial Problems
Pulmonary Embolus	Sexual Problems

KEY NURSING INTERVENTIONS

- See Preoperative and Postoperative Care.

- Identify type and location of surgery.

- Observe for signs and symptoms of hemorrhage and shock: Frank hematuria, excessive blood on dressings or from incision, increased pulse, decreasing blood pressure, diaphoresis, pallor, agitation, restlessness, catheter obstruction due to blood clot.

- Keep irrigation system patent by irrigating as ordered or just enough to keep urine a clear pink color. Maintain an accurate intake and output record that includes exact amount of irrigation solution used.

- Notify physician of clogged catheter and irrigate as ordered or with no more than 50 cc of normal saline.

- After catheter is removed, observe for urinary retention: Absent voiding, bladder distention, voiding 25–50 cc more than one time per hour, complaints of fullness and discomfort, restlessness.

- For perineal surgery do not administer enemas or take rectal temperatures to avoid agitation of the surgical wound.

- Assess and support patient's psychosocial needs by checking with physician to see how he expects the patient to function sexually after surgery. Total prostatectomy usually results in impotence. If impotence is not anticipated, sexual activity may be resumed in 6–8 weeks. Infertility usually results from retrograde ejaculation.

PATIENT AND FAMILY TEACHING

- Attempt to involve the wife or significant other in patient care and discharge planning.

- Explain the purposes of catheter and irrigation system.

- Inform patient that after the catheter is removed, he may experience dysuria, frequency, incontinence and/or urinary retention. The dysuria and frequency should subside in 2–3 weeks.

- Teach patient how to gain urinary control by doing perineal exercises 10–20 times per hour: Urinate as soon as the urge is felt, then stop the stream briefly and continue to void. Drink at least 2500 cc of fluid per day.

- Upon discharge instruct patient to observe for complications which are: blood in the urine, infection of the surgical site, infection of the urinary tract, and inability to void.

- Have patient avoid sitting for long periods, straining, or strenuous exercise which may contribute to increased bleeding.

TESTICULAR TORSION

POTENTIAL PROBLEMS

Pain	Urinary Problems
Nausea	Testicular Necrosis
Vomiting	Psychosocial Problems
Infection	

KEY NURSING INTERVENTIONS

- Keep patient NPO. Emergency surgery is usually performed with this condition.

- Assess arterial flow to testicle by auscultating with a Doppler every 30–60 minutes.

- To relieve pain and promote healing, maintain strict bed rest, elevate scrotum, and apply cool compresses or ice packs.

- Prevent urinary problems by monitoring intake and output, encouraging fluids up to 2500 cc/day, and checking urine for blood and clarity.

- Assess and support patient's psychosocial needs by informing patient that potency and fertility are not affected even if an orchiectomy must be performed due to necrosis. If the testicle is removed, a prosthesis may be implanted for aesthetic purposes.

PATIENT AND FAMILY TEACHING

- Involve wife or significant other in patient care and discharge planning.

- Explain the purpose of scrotal support is to promote healing and minimize pain.

ORCHIECTOMY

POTENTIAL PROBLEMS

Scrotal Edema   Vomiting
Pain   Psychosocial Problems
Cachexia   Elimination Problems
Nausea

KEY NURSING INTERVENTIONS

- See Preoperative and Postoperative Care.

- Check dressing for excessive bleeding or drainage.

- Prevent elimination problems by observing intake and output, catheterization if necessary, and administering laxatives or stool softeners as ordered.

- Plan patient care according to pathology. (Most orchiectomies are done due to malignant tumors but may also be done for nonmalignant pathologies.)

- Assess and support patient's psychosocial needs. Inform patient that if only one testicle is removed, sexual potency and fertility are not usually affected; oftentimes a prosthesis may be implanted for aesthetic purposes. Refer patient to the American Cancer Society or other local support groups, facilitating movement through the grieving process.

PATIENT AND FAMILY TEACHING

- Involve wife or significant other in patient care and discharge planning.

- Instruct patient to observe incision for signs and symptoms of infection: Pain, redness, swelling, red streaks, or fever.

- Explain and demonstrate self-examination of the testicle. Malignancy of the opposite testicle should be watched for.

- Encourage follow-up visits to detect possible early metastasis if malignancy was the pathology.

SENSORY FUNCTIONS

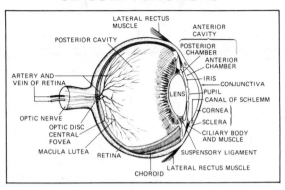

Mid-sagittal Section of Eyeball

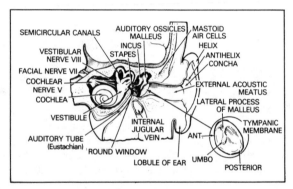

Outer, Middle, and Inner Ear

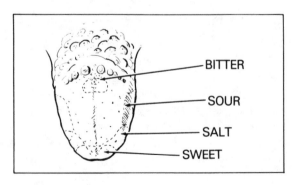

Taste Areas: Tongue

SENSORY FUNCTIONS—PHYSIOLOGY SUMMARY

I. SENSORY RECEPTORS

A. Pain

Pain sensation may be somatic, visceral or referred and is the result of stimulation of naked nerve endings (dendrites without myelin sheath and neurolemma).

B. Touch

Touch sensation is the result of stimulation of receptors called Meissner's corpuscles found in the dermis of the skin and mucous membrane of the tongue.

C. Pressure

Pressure sensation is caused by stimulation of Pacinian corpuscles.

D. Heat

Heat sensation is due to stimulation of Ruffini corpuscles.

E. Cold

Cold sensation is caused by stimulation of Krause end bulbs.

F. Proprioception

Proprioception of muscles, tendons and joints is due to stimulation of neuromuscular and neurotendinous spindles.

II. VISION

The sensation of vision occurs as a result of an image forming on the retina which is converted to nerve impulses and relayed to the brain.

A. Image Formation

1. Images are formed on the retina by the following:

   a) Refraction of light rays through the cornea, aqueous humor, lens and vitreous humor.

b) Accommodation of the lens which changes its curvature to allow focusing.

c) Constriction of the pupil which restricts the entrance of light rays to those which can be focused.

d) Convergence of both eyeballs which allows light rays to hit corresponding points of both retinas.

2. *Images formed on the retina*

Converted to nervous impulses by photoreceptor neurons called rods and cones.

3. *Cones*

Responsible for daylight and color vision. They are densely concentrated in the fovea centralis, which is a small part of the macula lutea.

4. *Rods*

Responsible for night vision and contain an extremely light-sensitive pigment called rhodopsin. Rods are absent from the fovea and are found in the periphery of the retina. The fovea centralis is the ''blind spot'' in night vision.

B. Neurological Conduction

1. As light rays strike the rods and cones, photochemical reactions occur which produce nerve impulses.

2. Impulses are conducted by neuron fibers which form the optic nerve.

3. The optic nerve fibers partially decussate at the optic chiasm. Optic nerve fibers from this point are called the optic tract and extend to the occipital lobe of the brain.

III. HEARING

The sensation of hearing occurs as a result of sound waves initiating nerve impulses which are conducted to the auditory area in the temporal lobe.

A. Sound Wave Transmission

1. Sound waves enter the ear through the external auditory canal.

2. The sound waves cause the tympanic membrane at the end of the canal to vibrate.

3. The vibrating tympanic membrane causes the malleus to move.

4. The vibrating malleus causes the incus and the stapes to vibrate.

5. The stapes vibrates against the oval window which produces sound waves in the perilymph.

6. From the oval window the sound waves travel up the scala vestibuli, through the cochlea, down the scala tympani, and against the round window.

B. Neurological Conduction

1. The sound waves cause movement of the basilar membrane which stimulates movement of the hair cells of the organ of Corti.

2. The hair movement initiates nerve impulses of the cochlear nerve which travel through the brain stem before reaching the temporal lobe.

IV. SMELL

The sensation of smell results from stimulation of olfactory nerve cells located in the mucosa of the nasal cavity.

V. TASTE

The sensation of taste results from stimulation of neural receptors in the papillae of the tongue, called taste buds.

A. Taste Receptors

1. There are four types of taste receptors:

   a) Sweet

   b) Sour

   c) Bitter

   d) Salt

2. Taste receptors transmit impulses to the taste center in the medulla.

B. Neurological Transmission

The medulla transmits impulses to the thalamus and cerebral cortex where the sensation is realized.

C. Flavors

Different flavors are produced as the four taste receptors combine in a variety of ways.

SENSORY ASSESSMENT

I. HISTORY

A. Past history of sensory problems

1. What type?
2. What therapy was utilized? Did it work?

B. Recent History

1. Blurred vision?
2. Flashing lights or spots?
3. Headaches?
4. Blindness?
5. Hearing loss?
6. Discharges?
7. Periodic inflammation?
8. Hay fever?
9. Difficulty in speech or swallowing?
10. Bleeding?
11. Vertigo?
12. Dizziness?
13. Tinnitus?

C. Past surgeries

D. Use of prostheses

1. Hearing Aids?
2. Contact lenses?
3. Glasses?
4. Dentures?
5. Partial plates?

E. Pain

Use PQRST mnemonic.

P—Provokes.   What makes the pain worse or better? What was the patient doing prior to the onset of pain?

Q—Quality.	Subjective description of pain by the patient. Use the patient's own words, i.e., Burning, stabbing, pressure.
R—Radiation.	Where is the pain located and does it radiate anywhere?
S—Severity.	Ask the patient to judge the pain on a scale of 1 to 10 with 10 being the worst pain ever felt.
T—Time.	How long as the patient had this pain? When did the pain begin and end?

F. Medications

1. List medications, including over-the-counter drugs.
2. Allergies.

G. Nutrition

Describe a typical:

1. Breakfast.
2. Lunch.
3. Dinner.
4. Snacks.

II. BACKGROUND INFORMATION

A. Lab Values

Check laboratory studies for abnormal values or worsening trends.

B. Diagnostic Studies

Identify abnormal results of diagnostic studies.

C. Chart

Check old chart for past relevant information.

III. ASSESSMENT

A. Eyes

1. Visual acuity.

      a) Snellen chart. Test each eye separately. If patient wears glasses, use them for acuity testing.

      b) Ability to read newspaper or fine print.

2. Inspect the iris, sclera, conjunctiva, cornea, lids, and periorbital area for moisture, symmetry, deformities, color, inflammation, redness, bleeding, protrusion, lesions, tumors.

3. Extraocular movements.

      a) Nystagmus: Lateral, vertical, circular.

      b) Strabismus.

4. Pupils (see Neurological Assessment).

5. Provide the physician with an ophthalmoscope for visualization of the anterior chamber and optic disc.

6. Gently palpate the periorbital area for lumps or tenderness.

B. Ears

1. Auditory acuity.

      a) Whispered sounds.

      b) Watch ticking.

2. Inspect the external ear (auricle) for lumps, lesions, wax, discharge, or blood.

3. Provide the physician with an otoscope for visualization of the canal and tympanic membrane.

4. Gently palpate the external ear and surrounding area for lumps or tenderness.

C. Nose

1. Inspect the nose and nostrils for patency, inflammation, discharge, or bleeding.

2. Provide the physician with nasal speculum or an otoscope for visualization of the nose internally.

3. Gently palpate the frontal and maxillary sinuses for lumps or tenderness.

D. Mouth

1. Inspect the mouth, lips, tongue, gums, hard palate, and teeth for hygiene, color, moisture, lumps, lesions, inflammation, redness, bleeding, missing teeth.

2. Provide the physician with a light source and a tongue blade for visualization of the mouth and throat.

3. With a gloved hand, palpate the above structures for lumps or tenderness.

EYE SURGERY

POTENTIAL PROBLEMS

Hemorrhage	Nausea
Pain	Vomiting
Infection	Sensory Deprivation
Injury	Psychosocial Problems

KEY NURSING INTERVENTIONS

- See Preoperative and Postoperative Care.

- Observe for signs and symptoms of postoperative complications: Excessive bleeding or drainage, sudden onset of eye pain, infection, restlessness, disorientation.

- Keep head of bed elevated or place in position as ordered by physician.

- Encourage frequent change of position. Usually the patient is allowed to turn to unaffected side. Stress the importance of deep breathing without coughing postoperatively. Coughing will increase intraocular pressure and is to be avoided.

- Prevent increased intraocular pressure by instructing the patient to avoid the following: Rubbing the eye, straining during bowel movements, coughing, sneezing, vomiting, bending over, sudden head movements, and emotional upsets. Administer antiemetics when nausea occurs. Vomiting is to be avoided.

- Keep call bell within reach. Instruct the patient to call nurse if needed and not to get out of bed alone.

- Maintain aseptic technique when changing dressings.

- Assess and support the patient's psychosocial needs. Eye surgery may be very anxiety-producing due to fear of sight loss. Depending on the patient's condition, most surgeries result in an improvement. Because one or both eyes will be patched after surgery, sensory deprivation may be a major problem. Observe for signs and symptoms: Restlessness, agitation, anger, depression, personality changes, thinking disturbances, hallucinations, disorientation, frank psychoses. Help prevent sensory deprivation by frequently orienting the patient to surroundings. Approach the patient from the unaffected side if eye is unpatched. Provide verbal and touch stimulation. Visit patient frequently. Encourage the family to visit often. If possible, place the patient in a room with an oriented patient.

PATIENT AND FAMILY TEACHING

- Instruct the patient to avoid increasing intraocular pressure (usually for six to eight weeks; see above).

- Inform the patient of signs and symptoms of complications: Bleeding, pain, infection, drainage, visual disturbances, loss of vision. Stress the importance of reporting these to the physician.

- Demonstrate the proper technique of instilling eye drops: Wash hands, pull lower lid down, look up, drop medication into cul-de-sac, close eye slowly, avoid rubbing or squeezing, and gently wipe off excess.

LABYRINTHITIS, MENIERE'S DISEASE

POTENTIAL PROBLEMS

Vertigo	Nystagmus
Nausea	Headache
Vomiting	Photophobia
Loss of Equilibrium	Psychosocial Problems
Tinnitus	

KEY NURSING INTERVENTIONS

- Provide a quiet, nonstressful environment. Usually a private, dark room away from a busy hallway is best.

- Assist the patient in getting out of bed and ambulating. Keep side rails up when in bed.

- Provide meals during periods of decreased nausea.

- Administer antiemetics, hypnotics, and tranquilizers as ordered. Observe for respiratory depression if strong or large dosages are used.

- Assess and support the patient's psychosocial needs. An acute attack causes extreme vertigo, nystagmus, nausea, vomiting, diaphoresis, tinnitus, hearing loss, and loss of equilibrium. The patient may be unable to sit, stand, or walk. Syncope may occur. This is a frightening and incapacitating experience. Stay with the patient during an acute attack. Help the patient to the floor or guide the patient back to bed and find a position of comfort. Provide reassurance that symptoms will cease.

PATIENT AND FAMILY TEACHING

- Explain the signs and symptoms to the family. Demonstrate how to best manage the patient during an acute attack.

- Instruct the patient to avoid sudden head movements, standing up quickly, and walking or driving if vertigo is present. Avoidance of alcohol, smoking, and high-salt diet is recommended.

EAR SURGERY

POTENTIAL PROBLEMS

Pain

Hearing Loss

Plugged Tube

Vertigo

Nausea

Vomiting

Infection, (mastoiditis, meningitis, chronic otitis media)

Psychosocial Problems

KEY NURSING INTERVENTIONS

- See Preoperative and Postoperative Care.
- Observe for signs and symptoms of complications: Bleeding, extreme vertigo, nausea, vomiting, tinnitus, hearing loss, gait disturbances, facial nerve injury, infection, extreme pain.
- Prevent infection by washing hands thoroughly before touching ears.
- Irrigate ears only as ordered. Avoid solutions that are too hot or cold. This may cause vertigo.
- Maintain bed rest and position in bed as ordered. Usually a frequent change of position will help facilitate drainage.
- Remove exudate from external ear using aseptic technique.
- Avoid using cotton or gauze in the ear unless otherwise ordered. This can obstruct the canal and prevent adequate drainage.
- Assess and support the patient's psychosocial needs. Explain that some vertigo may be expected. Assist the patient when changing position and ambulating.

PATIENT AND FAMILY TEACHING

- If tubes were inserted, explain their purpose. Instruct the patient to notify the physician when the tubes dislodge and fall out. Explain that this is to be expected.
- Demonstrate proper technique of instilling otic medications.
- Instruct the patient to avoid subsequent infections by avoiding people with upper respiratory tract infections, preventing water from entering the canal, never inserting objects into the ear, and thorough hand washing prior to touching.

INTEGUMENTARY SYSTEM

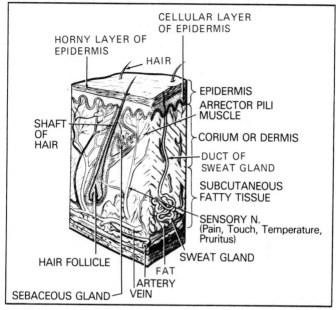

Anatomy of the Skin

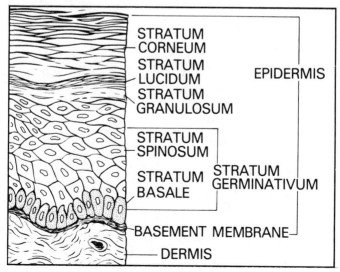

The Epidermal and Dermal Layers of the Skin

INTEGUMENTARY SYSTEM— PHYSIOLOGY SUMMARY

I. SKIN

A. The Epidermis

The epidermis is composed of five layers.

1. The Stratum Corneum is the outermost layer consisting of dead cells converted to the protein, keratin. This layer desquamates and is continually replaced.

2. The Stratum Lucidum lies beneath the stratum corneum and is one to two cells thick and is transparent.

3. The Stratum Granulosum is a 2- to 3-cell thick layer beneath the lucidum layer, containing granules in the cell's cytoplasm, and is involved in keratinization.

4. The Stratum Spinosum beneath the granulosum layer consists of many layers of irregularly shaped (prickly) cells.

5. The Stratum Germinativum is the deepest stratum containing the only epidermal cells that are capable of mitosis. New cells from this layer push upward into the outer layers until they eventually desquamate. This layer must be intact in order for the epidermis to regenerate. Melanocytes in the germinativum form melanin, the primary skin pigment. Excessive amounts of sunlight, adrenocorticotropic hormone (ACTH) and melanocyte-stimulating hormone (MSH) cause increased melanin production.

B. The Dermis

1. The dermis consists of two layers, the papillary, which is adjacent to the epidermis, and the reticular, which lies beneath the papillary and above the subcutaneous layer.

2. The dermis is composed of fibrous connective tissue, yellow elastic connective tissue, blood vessels, nerves, lymph vessels, hair follicles and sweat glands.

3. The dermis is attached to underlying tissue by subcutaneous tissue which is composed of areolar and adipose tissue.

II. GLANDS

A. Sebaceous Glands

Sebaceous glands secrete sebum, an oily substance from around hair follicles which keeps the hair and skin soft, prevents excessive water absorption, and heat loss.

B. Sweat Glands

Sweat glands are present in most parts of the skin.

1. Sweating functions to lower the body temperature.
2. Sweat consists of sodium chloride, urea, uric acid, amino acids, ammonia, sugar, lactic acid, and ascorbic acid.
3. Elevated blood temperature stimulates cerebral centers to initiate sweating.

III. SENSORY RECEPTORS

The skin contains sensory receptors to the sensations of pain, touch, temperature, and pressure (see Sensory Physiology Summary).

INTEGUMENTARY SYSTEM ASSESSMENT

I. HISTORY

A. Past history of integumentary problems

1. What type?
2. What therapy was utilized? Did it work?

B. Recent History

1. Presence of rash, hives, lumps, pimples, abscesses, boils, scaly or dry skin, mole or freckle changes?
2. Recent history of trauma: Bruising, open wounds, infection, burns, needle punctures?
3. Recent exposure to contagious diseases: Chicken pox; herpes simplex or zoster; athlete's foot; hand, foot and mouth disease; scabies; body lice?
4. Skin color changes?
5. Presence of itching?
6. Changes in hair growth patterns?
7. Changes in psychosocial patterns due to skin conditions?

C. Pain

Use PQRST mnemonic.

P—Provokes.	What makes the pain worse or better? What was the patient doing prior to the onset of pain?
Q—Quality.	Subjective description of pain by the patient. Use the patient's own words, i.e., Burning, stabbing, pressure.
R—Radiation.	Where is the pain located and does it radiate anywhere?
S—Severity.	Ask the patient to judge the pain on a scale of 1 to 10 with 10 being the worst pain ever felt.
T—Time.	How long has the patient had this pain? When did the pain begin and end?

D. Medications

1. List medications including over-the-counter drugs.
2. Allergies.

E. Nutrition

Describe a typical:

1. Breakfast.
2. Lunch.
3. Dinner.
4. Snacks.

II. BACKGROUND INFORMATION

A. Lab Values

Check laboratory studies for abnormal values or worsening trends.

B. Diagnostic Studies

Identify abnormal results of diagnostic studies.

C. Chart

Check old chart for past relevant information.

III. INSPECTION

Inspect the skin from head to toe for hygiene, color, presence of edema, vascular irregularities, scars, lesions, hair distribution, condition of nails, sensation.

A. Hygiene

Clean, dirty, odorous.

B. Color

Normal, pale, cyanotic, flushed, red, brown, jaundiced, uremic frost, alterations in pigment.

C. Edema

Dependent, pitting, non-pitting; describe location.

D. Vascular Irregularities

Ecchymosis, petechiae, dilated veins, spider angiomata, venous stars.

E. Scars

Describe in terms of location, size, type of trauma or surgery.

F. Lesions

Macule, papule, nodule, tumor, vesicle, ulceration, fissure, red streaks. Describe in terms of type, color, size, location, and distribution. Always inspect scars and lesions for signs and symptoms of infection.

G. Hair Distribution

Describe in terms of skin underneath and distribution.

H. Nails

Normal blanching and refill, clubbing, Beau's lines, paronychia, subungual hematoma, splinter hemorrhages.

I. Sensation

Paresthesias, numbness, tingling, areas of tenderness.

IV. PALPATION

Palpate the skin for pain, temperature, moisture, turgor.

A. Pain

Describe the location and condition of the skin surrounding the pain.

B. Temperature

Cool, normal, warm, hot.

C. Moisture

Wet, moist, normal, dry, oily.

D. Turgor

Normal, poor, tenting.

BURNS

POTENTIAL PROBLEMS

Pain
Fluid and Electrolyte
   Imbalance
Nutritional Problems
Shock
Respiratory Problems
Vascular Insufficiency
Contractures
Curling's Ulcer
Constipation

Negative Nitrogen Balance
Sepsis
Infection
Pressure Sores
Pneumonia
Pulmonary Edema
Paralytic Ileus
Psychosocial Problems

KEY NURSING INTERVENTIONS

- Initial treatment of burns usually consists of the following:

   - Removing all clothing and assessing extent of burn. If burn is due to chemicals, clothing should be handled carefully. Affected areas should be washed with clean, cool water to prevent further burning.

   - Applying cool saline dressings to burned areas for pain relief as ordered.

   - Keeping patient as warm as possible.

- Treatment varies with the extent of the burn. Document type of burn (thermal, chemical, electrical) and note the following: Areas of pain, redness, charring, blistering and sensory loss.

- Usual medical orders for more extensive burns which warrant hospitalization are the following:

- Strict isolation.

- Individualized IV therapy.

- Analgesics for pain.

- Nasogastric tube to intermittent suction and NPO.

- Foley catheter.

- Tetanus prophylaxis.

- Diagnostic studies (blood chemistry, complete blood count, arterial blood gases, urinalysis, myoglobin, type and crossmatch, chest x-ray, and electrocardiogram).

- Wound cultures.

- Antibiotic therapy.

- Weight daily.

- Topical cream applications.

- Intake and output.

- Hydrotherapy.

- Observe for signs and symptoms of fluid and electrolyte imbalance (see Fluids and Electrolytes). The potential for imbalance is proportional to the extent of the burn. Because of fluid shifts in the burn patient, IV therapy is more complex than for other conditions.

- Assess patient for signs and symptoms of shock: Thirst, restlessness, tachycardia, hypotension, oliguria, dry mucous membranes, agitation, delirium, seizures, coma.
  NOTE: Close observation is essential during the first 24 to 48 hrs. since the fluid shifts from the vascular space into the interstitial spaces during this time.

- Monitor patient for fluid overload after 2 to 4 days when fluid begins to return to the vascular space: Bounding pulse, neck vein distention, hypertension, increased CVP, difficulty breathing, and pulmonary edema.
  NOTE: Patients with good cardiac and renal functions usually compensate for this shift.

- Observe for negative nitrogen balance resulting from tissue destruction. Monitor daily weights, closely keeping in mind that initial weight gain will occur due to edema. Subsequent weight loss is due to diuresis and catabolism. Monitor hemoglobin, hematocrit, electrolytes and metabolites. High caloric intake is essential to counteract catabolism caused by tissue destruction.

- Observe for signs and symptoms of respiratory problems. Patients most likely to develop respiratory difficulty are those with inhalation burns, smoke inhalation, burns to the thorax, or any burn that keeps the patient bedridden. Signs and symptoms include: Tachypnea, dyspnea, cough, hoarseness, hemoptysis, cyanosis, altered level of consciousness, decreased pO_2, increased pCO_2, increased carbon monoxide levels. Administer oxygen as needed or prepare for endotracheal intubation and mechanical ventilation for severe respiratory distress.

- Observe for signs and symptoms of infection and sepsis: Excess drainage, foul-smelling discharge, redness at wound edges, fever, altered mental status, and positive wound and blood cultures.

- Observe burned extremities for signs and symptoms of decreased perfusion peripherally: Decreased or absent pulses, pain distal to burn, cyanosis, poor or absent capillary refill, decreased sensation and movement. This constitutes an emergency, and an escharotomy may have to be performed.

- Monitor accurate intake and output. Calculate IV and PO fluid intake carefully. Observe for oliguria or urinary output less than 30 cc/hr. Weigh the patient daily to assess fluid loss or retention.

- Insert nasogastric tube to low intermittent suction as ordered. Curling's stress ulcer is common in extensive burns. Test gastric asapirate for occult blood. Administer antacids as ordered. Once bowel sounds return, the nasogastric tube is usually removed.

- Advance diet slowly and as ordered. Consult with hospital dietician for high-protein diet.

- Maintain strict aseptic technique when doing dressing changes. Maintain reverse isolation as ordered (see Infection Control).

- Prevent contractures and complications of immobility. Splint burned extremities in position of function. Assist the patient in passive and active range of motion exercises. Encourage frequent change of position and ambulation as soon as possible. Attempt exercises when pain medications are at peak levels.

- Assess and support the patient's psychosocial needs. Begin psychosocial care as soon as possible. Assure the patient that pain will be controlled as much as possible. Pain is usually the severest initially and then diminishes. Extensive burns require long-term hospitalization and rehabilitation. Thus, an extensive care plan is essential. Develop a care plan involving the patient and entire health care team with realistic goals and expectations. Encourage the family to visit frequently. Provide creative diversional activities. Allow the patient as much control over the environment as possible. This will help fight boredom, depression, and sensory deprivation. Help the patient and family deal with changes in body image, lifestyle, role function. If burns are extensive and a long rehabilitation program is anticipated, involve a physical therapist or a rehabilitation team as soon as possible.

PATIENT AND FAMILY TEACHING

- Involve the family as much as possible in care planning.
- Explain daily routine, nursing care plan, and all procedures.
- Encourage the patient to do as much for him/herself as possible. An optimistic environment and attitude will maximize the best results.
- Instruct family and visitors in isolation procedures (if any).

DECUBITUS ULCERS, PRESSURE SORES

POTENTIAL PROBLEMS

Infection	Pain
Malnutrition	Psychosocial Problems
Subsequent Pressure Sores	

KEY NURSING INTERVENTIONS

- Decubitis ulcers are best treated by prevention. Identify patients who are most susceptible: Immobilized patients; postsurgical patients who have had prolonged anesthesia; those with poor circulation, impaired sensation, decreased hemoglobin and hematocrit, poor nutrition, edema, or pressure from casts, traction equipment, oxygen masks and cannulas. Decubitus ulcers may develop in only a few hours.

- Identify sites that are most likely to develop pressure sores: Bony prominences such as the occiput, vertebrae, elbows, ischial tuberosities, trochanters, sacrum, knees, heels, and ankles.

- Observe bony prominences for signs and symptoms of developing pressure sores: Redness, cyanosis, blistering, poor capillary refill, pain followed by anesthesia, or a break in the integrity of the skin.

- In general, to prevent ulcers from forming, promote good circulation to areas of increased pressure. Avoid prolonged periods in the same position. Keep the skin free of unnecessary moisture. Assure good nutritional intake.

- Once a decubitus ulcer has formed, promote healing and prevent others from forming.

- Turn the patient hourly or at least every two hours. Make use of as many positions as possible: Lateral, prone, and supine. Use pillows or foam wedges to help with position changes.

- Keep sheets dry and as wrinkle-free as possible. Check frequently for the presence of sweat, urine, and feces. Avoid use of plastic-type linen savers and uncovered plastic mattresses.

- Maintain good skin hygiene. Wash the patient daily with very mild soap. Use a gentle lotion. Massage lotion gently. This will help stimulate circulation on pressure areas.

- Make use of special pads and mattresses (i.e., egg crates, air mattresses, water beds, gelfoam pads, sheep skins, elbow and heel pads, Clinitron therapy if available).

- Encourage the patient to exercise as much as tolerated. Perform passive and/or active range of motion exercises twice per day.

- Assess the patient's nutritional status for adequate intake of calories, protein, vitamins and minerals.

- Avoid unnecessary stresses to the skin. Be careful not to shear skin when removing or placing the patient on a bed pan. Protect extremities and skin by using proper transfer techniques when moving the patient from bed to a wheelchair or gurney.

- Prevent infection of decubitus ulcers. Keep dressings clean and dry. Use aseptic technique when irrigating or changing dressings.

- Observe for signs and symptoms of infection of an ulcer: Redness, swelling, red streaks, swollen lymph nodes, fever, foul-smelling discharge.

- If a newly admitted patient arrives with a decubitus ulcer, document the following: Measured size, location, signs of infection, condition of the surrounding skin, and any evidence of developing ulcers.

- Once an ulcer develops, never place the patient on the affected side. This will only deepen the ulcer and begin to necrose deeper structures.

- Decubitis ulcers are treated with many different modalities, depending on the physician, hospital and the severity of the ulcer. Become familiar with the type of modalities being utilized on your patient. Treatments may include irrigation with special solutions, exposure to air, ultraviolet light, topical ointments, whirlpools, collagenase therapy, special dressings, debridement, hyperbaric oxygen therapy, IV antibiotics, drying agents, and surgical intervention.

- Assess and support the patient's psychosocial needs. Treatment of decubitus ulcers is slow and tedious. Help the patient and family deal with a prolonged hospital stay, pain, and changes in body image and lifestyle.

PATIENT AND FAMILY TEACHING

- Explain the purpose and stress the importance of frequent position changes, good skin hygiene and proper nutrition.

- If the patient is to go home or to an extended care facility, demonstrate to the patient and family how to best prevent decubitis ulcers from forming.

- Emphasize the fact that decubitis ulcers begin to develop in only a few hours, stressing the need to change position at least every two hours if not more frequently.

HERPES SIMPLEX AND ZOSTER

POTENTIAL PROBLEMS

Pain

Fever

Malaise

Itching

Infection

Dysuria

Dehydration

Postherpetic Neuralgia

Pneumonia

Facial, Optic, and Acoustic
 Nerve Involvement

Cross Contamination

Pyschosocial Problems

KEY NURSING INTERVENTIONS

- Herpes is often precipitated by other illnesses. Therefore, thorough history and accurate assessment is necessary.

- Herpetic lesions can be painful. Pain, itching, and inflammation may be relieved by analgesics; cool, moist compresses; antihistamines; topical steroids and systemic steroids. Caution: Steroids are usually not indicated when a secondary infection is suspected.

- For oral herpes, assess the patient's tolerance to PO intake. If the patient is dehydrated and unable to take PO fluids, intravenous therapy may be indicated.

- Observe lesions for signs and symptoms of infection: Redness, swelling, change in discharge, red streaks, fever.

- If a viral culture specimen is ordered, obtain appropriate culture media from the laboratory.

- Avoid spread of infection to others. Use thorough hand washing technique using antimicrobial soap before and after each patient contact. Apply dressings to draining lesions.

- See Infection Control for appropriate isolation measures.

- For herpes zoster, observe for complications depending upon location: Pneumonia; postherpetic neuralgia; optic, facial, and acoustic nerve involvement.

- Assess and support the patient's psychosocial needs. A herpes infection carries a very negative stigma due to recent publicity. Attempt to find out how the patient feels about this infection and what he/she knows about the disease. To help allay fears, provide as much information as possible. Inform the patient that the infections will probably recur but are usually less severe and decrease in frequency. Provide patient privacy and assure confidentiality of discussions and records.

PATIENT AND FAMILY TEACHING

- Demonstrate to the patient and family proper hand washing technique. Explain the importance of infection control.
- Instruct the patient to avoid contact with the eyes and any other open wounds.

MUSCULOSKELETAL SYSTEM

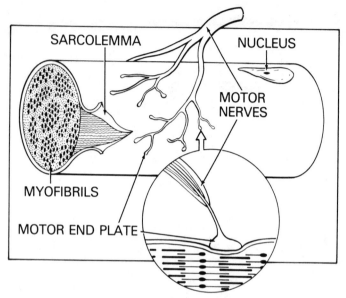

Motor Unit of Skeletal Muscles

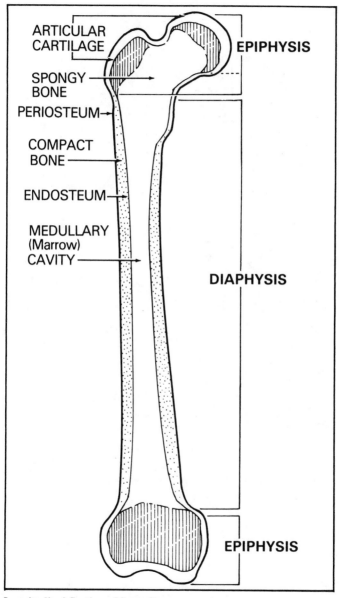

Longitudinal Section of Long Bone

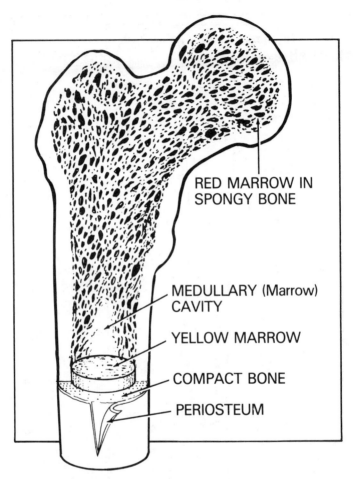

RED MARROW IN
SPONGY BONE

MEDULLARY (Marrow)
CAVITY

YELLOW MARROW

COMPACT BONE

PERIOSTEUM

Sagittal and Longitudinal Section of Long Bone

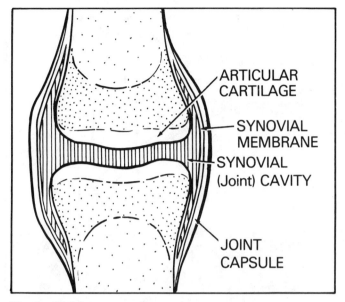

Diarthrotic Joint

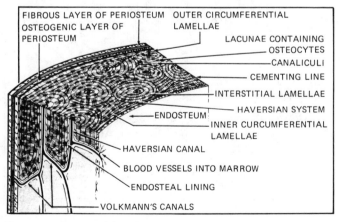

Haversion System of Compact Bone

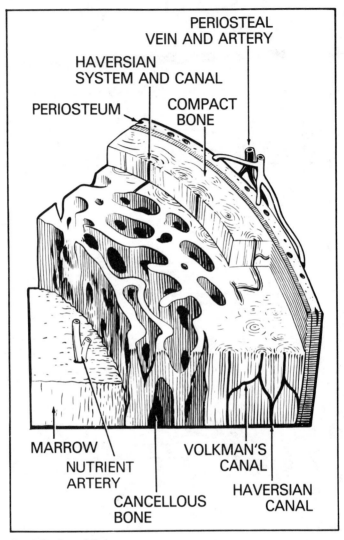

Cross Section of Bone

MUSCULOSKELETAL SYSTEM— PHYSIOLOGY SUMMARY

I. BONE FORMATION

Bone formation occurs through a process called ossification or osteogenesis.

A. Osteoblasts

The bone-forming cells, secrete mucopolysaccharides and collagen.

B. Mucopolysaccharides

Collect around osteoblast and collagen fibers and become fixed in it to form the bone matrix.

C. Calcification

Occurs as calcium salts are deposited in the matrix.

D. Bone deposition

Regulated by the extent of strain placed on the bone. Increased strain causes increased deposition.

II. BONE STRUCTURE

Calcified bone matrix is arranged in layers called lamellae. There are two types of bone, compact and cancellous.

A. Compact Bone

1. Compact bone is dense and strong with lamellae arranged in concentric layers.
2. The lamellae surround a canal containing blood and lymph vessels known as the haversian canal.
3. The lamellae are separated by spaces, the lacunae, which house mature bone cells, the osteocytes.
4. The lacunae communicate with the haversian canal by small canals called canaliculi.

B. Cancellous Bone

1. The large open spaces in cancellous bone are filled with red bone marrow.

2. Red bone marrow is composed of blood cells and the predecessors of red and white blood cells and platelets.

3. Adult bones containing red bone marrow are the ribs, vertebrae, sternum and pelvis.

4. Red bone marrow is present in the epiphyses of the humerus and femur most abundantly at birth and progressively diminishes through adulthood.

C. Long Bones

1. Long bones are composed of cancellous bone in the ends (epiphyses), compact bone in the shaft (diaphysis) an outer protective lining (periosteum), a cavity running lengthwise (medullary cavity), and an inner lining (endosteum).

2. Yellow marrow fills the medullary cavity of long bones and is connective tissue predominately made of fat cells.

3. Long bones comprise the femur, tibia, fibula, humerus, ulna, radius, and phalanges.

D. Short Bones

1. Short bones structurally are composed of inner cancellous bone with a thin outer covering of compact bone.

2. Short bones comprise the carpals and tarsals of the wrist and ankle.

E. Flat Bones

1. Flat bones structurally are composed of cancellous bone sandwiched between two layers of compact bone.

2. Flat bones comprise the cranial bones, ribs, scapula and part of the pelvis.

F. Irregular Bone

1. Structurally, irregular bones are the same as short bones but vary in shape.

2. Irregular bones comprise the vertebrae, sphenoid, ethmoid, sacrum, coccyx, mandible, and ossicles of the ear.

III. JOINTS

A. Types of Joints

There are three types of joints

1. Synarthroses—Nonmovable joints.

2. Amphiarthroses—Slightly movable joints.

3. Diarthroses—Freely movable joints which join bones with articular cavities enclosed by a capsule of cartilage that is reinforced with ligaments and cartilage that covers the ends of opposing bones. The capsule is lined by the synovial membrane which produces synovial fluid.

B. Synovial fluid

Provides nutrients for the cartilage and is a lubricant to minimize friction.

IV. MUSCLES

A. Striated Muscles

1. Striated or skeletal muscles are voluntary muscles comprised of multinucleated muscle cells, or fibers, and connective tissue.

2. Muscle fibers are found in bundles known as fasciculi, and groups of fasciculi are bound together to form a complete muscle.

3. Each muscle is encased by a sheath which contains blood, lymph, and nerve tissue.

B. Contraction

1. Motor nerve fibers innervate muscle fibers in varying ratios (1:10 muscle fibers in muscles governing fine movements to 1:150–200 muscle fibers in muscles governing gross movements. The group of muscles innervated by a single motor neuron is called a motor unit.

2. When nerve impulses reach the neuromuscular junction, acetylcholine is released, which increases the permeability of the muscle fiber membrane to sodium.

3. With the influx of sodium, the electrical potential of the muscle fiber changes, and it creates its own impulse at the neuromuscular junction.

4. With this impulse, calcium ions are released from the sarcoplasmic reticulum, a structure surrounding the muscle fibers.

5. Calcium ions initiate a series of muscle protein interactions which generate energy and cause muscular contraction.

6. Tonic contractions are continuous, partial contractions produced by relay contractions of small, scattered groups of muscles.

7. Isotonic contractions produce movements, while the muscle tension remains constant.

8. Isometric contractions do not produce movement, but the muscle tension increases.

9. Twitch contractions produce rapid, jerky movements. The muscle does not respond immediately to a single stimulus but responds a fraction of a second later and then relaxes.

10. Tetanic contractions are sustained contractions produced by a rapid succession of stimuli acting on a muscle.

11. Treppe (staircase phenomenon) is a twitch contraction that occurs with increasing strength in response to successive strength stimuli at a rate of 1 or 2 per second. A contracture eventually results.

12. Fibrillation is asynchronous contractions of individual muscle fibers which produce a flutter effect.

13. Convulsions are uncoordinated contractions of different muscles which are tetanic in nature.

C. Smooth Muscle

1. Smooth muscle differs from striated muscle in that the cell or fiber is single nucleated and is controlled by the autonomic nerve system.

2. Contraction of smooth muscles is somewhat similar to striated muscle; however, the nerve impulse is transmitted over the entire fiber and may pass from one fiber to another.

D. Cardiac Muscle

1. Cardiac muscle is striated involuntary muscle which is divided into two units called syncytia.

2. The walls and septum of the atria form one syncytium, and the walls and septum of the ventricles form the other.

3. Contraction occurs over an entire syncytium when one fiber of it is stimulated.

MUSCULOSKELETAL SYSTEM ASSESSMENT

I. HISTORY

A. Past history of musculoskeletal problems

1. What type?
2. What therapy was utilized? Did it work?
3. Previous admissions to hospital for similar symptoms?
4. History of past surgeries or amputations?
5. History of diabetes or systemic disease?

B. Recent history

1. Complaints of redness, swelling, weakness, spasms, cramps, deformities, contractures?
2. Mechanism of injury and precipitating events for traumatic injury?
3. Present level of activity? Difficulty performing activities of daily life?

C. Pain

Use PQRST mnemonic.

P— Provokes. What makes the pain worse or better? What was the patient doing prior to the onset of pain?

Q— Quality. Subjective description of pain by the patient. Use the patient's own words, i.e., Burning, stabbing, pressure.

R— Radiation. Where is the pain located and does it radiate anywhere?

S— Severity. Ask the patient to judge the pain on a scale of 1 to 10 with 10 being the worst pain ever felt.

T— Time. How long has the patient had this pain? When did the pain begin and end?

D. Medications

1. List medications, including over-the-counter drugs.
2. Allergies.

E. Nutrition

Describe a typical:

1. Breakfast.
2. Lunch.
3. Dinner.
4. Snacks.

II. BACKGROUND INFORMATION

A. Lab Values

Check laboratory studies for abnormal values or worsening trends.

B. Diagnostic Studies

Identify abnormal reports of diagnostic studies, i.e., X-rays, biopsies, fluid aspirations, bone scans, CAT scans, arthroscopy.

C. Chart

Check old chart for past relevant information.

III. INSPECTION

Generally inspect the patient for appearance, posture, type of gait (see Neurological Assessment), mobility, obvious deformities, level of activity.

A. Assistive Devices

Observe for use of canes, crutches, walkers, prostheses, wheelchairs. Check for presence of splints, casts, or traction.

B. Range of Motion

Inspect joints for full range of motion. Ask the patient to perform appropriate motions, i.e., Flexion, extension, pronation, supination, circumflexion, abduction, adduction (see Anatomical References).

C. Documentation

Documentation should include:

1. Presence of pain, symmetry, range of motion (in degrees).
2. Check muscles and bones for redness, swelling, size, shape, symmetry, contractures, hypertrophy, atrophy, scars.

IV. PALPATION

Palpate muscles, bones, and joints for pain, tenderness, heat, tumors, nodules, lesions.

A. Range of Motion

Perform passive range of motion and feel for resistance, grating, crepitation, symmetry, pain.

B. Muscle Strength

Compare muscle strength bilaterally.

C. Neurological and Circulation

Distal to any injury or pathology, check for sensation, skin color, and temperature, skin blanching, pulses, motion.

RHEUMATOID ARTHRITIS

POTENTIAL PROBLEMS

Gastrointestinal Ulceration and Bleeding	Blood Dyscrasias
Muscle Atrophy	Joint Pain
Muscle Spasms	Skin Breakdown
Contractures	Elevated Temperature
Anemia	Psychosocial Problems

KEY NURSING INTERVENTIONS

- While on bed rest, maintain therapeutic body alignment. Use one thin pillow under the head and no pillows under knees or affected joints. Assist patient to prone position for a half hour BID or TID. Use trochanter rolls, folded towels, and sand bags to prevent external rotation. Maintain supine position the greater part of each day. Use splints as ordered.

- Protect skin during heat or cold application treatments.

- Exercises should always be done after heat or cold application treatments.

- Avoid quick, jarring movements of extremities and handle joints carefully to avoid pain.

- Encourage patient to do prescribed exercises within the limits of patient's pain threshold (usually isometric, range of motion, and progressive resistive exercises).

- Encourage self-care activities within pain threshold.

- Avoid fatigue from excessive exercising. Encourage frequent, uninterrupted rest periods. More rest is necessary during acute phases.

- Administer gentle massage to muscles surrounding painful joints to help relieve pain. Never massage inflamed, painful joints.

- Observe for signs and symptoms of gastrointestinal bleeding: Dyspepsia; bloody vomitus; black, tarry stools.

- Prevent complications of bed rest (see The Immobilized Patient).

- Assess patient for untoward effects of medications:

  Salicylates—Ringing of ears, decreased hearing, nausea/vomiting, headache, dizziness, bleeding gums, acidosis, ataxia, slurred speech.

  Indocin—Nausea, vomiting, headache, anorexia, abdominal pain, diarrhea, depression, confusion, psychotic behavior, peptic ulcer.

  Butazolidin, Tandearil—Agranulocytosis, peptic ulcer, dermatitis, stomatitis, water and sodium retention, sore throat.

  Gold—Agranulocytosis, aplastic anemia, nephritis, dermatitis, purpura, stomatitis, bronchitis, hepatitis, photosensitivity, syncope, flushing, sweating, nausea, vomiting.

  Aralen, Plaquenil—Loss of vision, nausea, vomiting, rash, psychotic behavior, leukopenia, hair blanching.

  Adrenocorticosteroids—Exacerbation of rheumatoid symptoms.

  Motrin, Naprosyn, Nalfon—Nausea, vomiting, diarrhea, constipation, gastric distress, headache, dizziness.

  Cuprimine—Blood dyscrasias, rash, pruritus, anorexia, epigastric pain, nausea, vomiting, tinnitus, proteinuria.

- Assess and support patient's psychosocial needs. Recognize that preoccupation with the body and physical needs accompanies chronic illnesses and can become unhealthy. Anxieties may be reduced by self-care and occupational activities as well as psychiatric counseling. Emotional support from nurse and significant others can help reduce emotionally triggered exacerbations. Refer patient to the American Arthritis Foundation.

PATIENT AND FAMILY TEACHING

- Reinforce explanations regarding the nature of rheumatoid arthritis and warn patients about miracle cures promised by "quacks."

- Inform patient and family that emotional upsets can cause exacerbations and should be avoided.

- Advise patient against overexercising or excessive activity. Keep activity within pain threshold. If pain persists for several hours following exercises, modification of exercises should be made.

- Instruct patient not to massage painful joints which may aggravate inflammation.

- Stress the importance of good posture, preventing trauma to joints by gentle movements, avoiding tension on joints and avoiding obesity.

- Instruct patient and family in the use of assistive devices such as raised toilet seats, shower stools, etc.

- Emphasize proper administration of prescribed medications and the importance of reporting adverse side effects.
- Advise reporting black, tarry stools and continuous gastrointestinal disturbance to physician.

FRACTURED MANDIBLE

POTENTIAL PROBLEMS

Airway Obstruction	Pain
Aspiration	Constipation
Infection	Malnutrition
Nausea	Psychosocial Problems
Vomiting	
Hemorrhage	

KEY NURSING INTERVENTIONS

- See Preoperative and Postoperative Care.

- Assess patient for signs and symptoms of airway obstruction: Gurgling respirations, stridor, use of accessory muscles for respiration, cyanosis.

- Position patient on side with head elevated postoperatively.

- Keep wire cutters at bedside in an obvious place at all times.

- Maintain working suction at bedside at all times.

- Check with physician regarding permissible suctioning areas, especially when extensive oral and facial reconstruction is performed. Suction nasopharynx and oral cavity as indicated to prevent aspiration.

- Administer oral hygiene every one to two hours and PRN. Irrigation can be done using a syringe with tap water or saline. A cotton-tipped swab can be used to clean around the teeth. Lubricate lips to prevent drying.

- Encourage nutritional intake. Provide a straw as needed. Since the diet may become repetitive and lack bulk, consult the dietician for a varied liquid diet containing substances promoting regular bowel movements.

- Prevent complications of bed rest (see The Immbolized Patient).

- Assess and support patient's psychosocial needs. Recognize that the patient may be worried about body image and financial matters. If further reconstructive work is to be done, these worries may be compounded. Allow patient to participate in self-care activities and discuss diversional activities with the family. Include family or significant others in care and encourage visitors to boost patient's morale.

PATIENT AND FAMILY TEACHING

- Instruct patient and family in use of wire cutters prior to discharge and demonstrate their use.
- Stress the importance of maintaining good nutritional intake along with daily exercise to prevent constipation.
- Inform the patient of the importance of regular oral hygiene.

FRACTURED PELVIS

POTENTIAL PROBLEMS

Shock	Intra-abdominal Injuries
Hemorrhage	Paralytic Ileus
Fat Emboli	Infection
Thromboembolism	Pressure Sores
Ruptured Bladder	Pain
Iliac Vessel Trauma	Psychosocial Problems

KEY NURSING INTERVENTIONS

- Recognize early signs of impending shock: Tachycardia, normal or elevated blood pressure, tachypnea, good urine output, restlessness, apprehension.

- Assess patient for signs of progressive shock: Cold and clammy or warm and dry skin; pallor or cyanosis; rapid, weak, thready pulse; falling diastolic and systolic blood pressure; falling pulse pressure (usually less than 20 mm Hg); rapid, shallow respirations; impaired sensory perception; oliguria or anuria.

- Observe for signs and symptoms of pulmonary embolism: Dyspnea; substernal chest pain; tachycardia; cyanosis; restlessness; anxiety; hemoptysis; cough; syncope; EKG changes; fever, hypotension; cold, clammy skin; low pCO_2 and pO_2.

- Observe for signs and symptoms of fat embolism: Mental confusion, restlessness, apprehension, tachycardia, tachypnea, dyspnea, low pO_2.

- Monitor patient for signs and symptoms of intra-abdominal hemorrhage: Diminished or absent peripheral pulses, increasing abdominal girth, back pain, signs of shock, numbness, tingling and nerve pain, blood in stools.

- Assess for signs and symptoms of ruptured bladder: Pain in lower abdomen, hematuria, pelvic cellulitis, peritonitis.

- Recognize signs and symptoms of paralytic ileus: Absent bowel sounds, gastric and abdominal distention, inability to pass flatus.

- Maintain pelvic sling as ordered. Loosen only as ordered. Sling can be folded back over buttocks to use fracture bedpan. Administer skin care under sling QID. Use sheep skin to line sling.

- See Traction, if present.
- Encourage active range of motion exercises to extremities.
- Administer perineal care after defecation and BID using an antimicrobial solution.
- Prevent complications of bed rest (see The Immobilized Patient).
- Assess and support patient's psychosocial needs. Immobilization may cause frustration, irritability and dependent behaviors. Encourage participation in daily care and diversional activities. Include family or significant other in care. Maintain a positive attitude since recovery may take a long period of time.

PATIENT AND FAMILY TEACHING

- Instruct patient in contraindicated movements or positions.
- Explain the purpose and proper functioning of the sling or skeletal traction.

BUNIONECTOMY

POTENTIAL PROBLEMS

Pedal Edema	Pain
Infection	Psychosocial Problems

KEY NURSING INTERVENTIONS

- See Preoperative and Postoperative Care.
- Check and document circulation, color, and sensitivity of toes with vital signs.
- Elevate affected extremity on one to two pillows.
- Maintain food cradle to keep covers off toes.
- Apply ice packs as ordered.
- Encourage toe exercises as ordered (usually toe flexion exercises).
- Assist patient with ambulation using a walker or crutches as ordered.
- Prevent complications of bed rest (see The Immobilized Patient).

PATIENT AND FAMILY TEACHING

- Inform patient of future need for wide-toed and well-supported shoes.
- Instruct patient in safe use of walker or crutches.

TRACTION

POTENTIAL PROBLEMS

Pulmonary Embolus	Infection
Neurovascular Impairment	Traction Malfunction
Thrombophlebitis	Constipation
Pneumonia	Pain
Skin Breakdown	Psychosocial Problems

KEY NURSING INTERVENTIONS

- Observe for signs and symptoms of pulmonary embolism: Dyspnea; substernal chest pain; tachycardia; cyanosis; hemoptysis; cough; restlessness; anxiety; hypotension; cold, clammy skin; low pO_2 and pCO_2.

- Monitor patient for signs and symptoms of thrombophlebitis: Tenderness and redness over affected vein, edema, cyanosis or mottling, diminished pulses, positive Homans' sign (calf pain with dorsiflexion of foot) in affected extremity.

- Examine distal part of extremity in traction for coolness, swelling, paralysis, loss of sensation, and discoloration.

- Identify type of traction to be utilized. Prepare bed and traction equipment as much as possible before patient arrives.

- Assure proper function of traction equipment to assure a constant stretching force. Maintain pull of traction with the long axis of the bone. Assure freely hanging weights. Keep ropes and pulleys unobstructed from bed, linen, and other equipment. Keep ropes in wheel grooves of pulleys.

- Checks knots frequently. Make sure they are tight.

- Check for secure clamps.

- Maintain proper alignment of body and injured part.

- Traction adjustments are made by physician's orders only.

- Change patient's position every two hours and administer skin care. Follow physician's orders *exactly* regarding position changes. Use two people to assist patient in lifting. Provide skin care to all pressure points.

- Inspect skin at pin insertion sites, underneath skin traction, or underneath belts and straps for signs of infection, pressure sores, or irritation.
- Administer pin site care BID or as ordered. Apply cork or tape to ends of pins.
- Encourage and assist with passive and active range of motion and isometric exercises as ordered and tolerated.
- Avoid bumping bed or traction equipment.
- Prevent complications of bed rest (see The Immobilized Patient).
- Assess and support patient's psychosocial needs. Recognize that prolonged immobility becomes tiresome and monotonous and can frequently lead to disorientation in the elderly patient. Encourage self-care as much as possible and other diversional activities. Keep all articles within easy reach, especially the call light.

PATIENT AND FAMILY TEACHING

- Explain the purpose and proper functioning of traction.
- Inform patient of contraindicated movements or positions.
- Discuss diversional activities with patient and family.

CAST CARE

POTENTIAL PROBLEMS

Vascular Insufficiency
Nerve Compression/Damage
Volkmann's Ischemic
   Contracture
Tissue Necrosis
Thrombophlebitis
Psychosocial Problems

Infection
Pain
Itching
Pressure Sores

FOR BODY CAST

Cast Syndrome

KEY NURSING INTERVENTIONS

- Assess patient for signs and symptoms of vascular insufficiency and/or nerve compression in affected extremity: Increasing or unrelieved pain, blanching or cyanotic skin color in distal extremity, numbness or tingling feeling, diminished or absent pulse, cold skin temperature, paralysis or diminished motor function, swelling.

- Observe for signs and symptoms of developing Volkmann's contracture: Absent or diminished radial or pedal pulse, cyanotic skin color, swelling.

- Monitor patient for indications of pressure sores and tissue necrosis: Initial and severe burning pain over bony prominence which decreases as necrosis occurs, foul odor from cast, drainage through cast, hot area over lesion.

- While cast is wet, keep cast area uncovered but keep patient warm. Do not use heat lamps to dry cast. If cast dryer is used, keep at least 18 inches away from cast and move frequently. Handle moist cast with palms only. Prevent denting and avoid resting cast on hard surfaces while drying. Turn patient every 2–3 hours to promote uniform drying.

- Elevate extremity above the level of the heart. Support with pillows. Keep heel of foot off mattress.

- Pad rough cast edges with tape.

- Frequently check distal extremity skin color, temperature, sensation, motion, and vascular refill.

- When applying ice packs, place them beside the cast rather than directly on the cast.
- Document cast drainage, indicating date, time, size and color. Note enlarging areas.
- Observe for signs and symptoms of cast syndrome when patient is in a body cast: Prolonged nausea and repeated vomiting, abdominal pain, distention.
- Encourage and assist with prescribed exercises, usually isometric, quadriceps setting, gluteal setting, abdominal tightening, active and passive range of motion.
- Investigate all patient complaints, especially regarding pain.
- Prevent complications of bed rest (see The Immobilized Patient).
- Assess and support patient's psychosocial needs. Encourage as many self-care activities as possible to reduce tension, irritability, and depression. Discuss possible diversional activities with patient and family.

PATIENT AND FAMILY TEACHING

- Instruct patient to keep casted extremity elevated and to avoid getting cast wet.
- Instruct patient not to place any objects under the cast for scratching, and to avoid vigorous scratching under the cast with fingers.
- Explain the purpose of the stockinette and padding under the cast and the importance that these not be pulled out.
- Advise the patient to keep fingers and toes of affected extremity clean. A sock can be worn over the toes and cast to protect it.
- Instruct patient to inform physician if cast becomes excessively loose.
- Upon discharge, inform patient of signs and symptoms of vascular and nerve impairment in affected extremity and the importance of reporting these immediately to the physician.
- Demonstrate proper crutch walking if indicated.

LOWER EXTREMITY AMPUTATION

POTENTIAL PROBLEMS

Pulmonary Embolism	Stump Edema
Bronchopneumonia	Contractures
Hemorrhage	Phantom Pain
Necrosis of Incision Area	Severe Depression
Infection	Prosthesis Problems
Hematoma	Psychosocial Problems

KEY NURSING INTERVENTIONS

- See Preoperative and Postoperative Care.

- Observe for signs and symptoms of pulmonary embolism: Dyspnea, substernal chest pain; tachycardia; cyanosis; hemoptysis; cough; restlessness; anxiety; hypotension; cold, clammy skin; low pCO_2 and pO_2.

- Monitor for excessive bleeding. Keep tourniquet and sponge gauze at bedside in case of severe hemorrhage.

- Maintain active Hemovac or suction device and proper stump wrapping to prevent hematoma.

- Elevate stump up to 48 hours postoperatively and apply ice as ordered.

- Observe for necrosis of incision area.

- Prevent flexion contractures. Do not keep stump elevated for more than 48 hours postoperatively. Use trochanter roll to prevent external rotation and abduction. Assist with passive and active range of motion exercises TID. Help patient to prone position for several hours each day. Administer analgesics to relieve pain and prevent hip flexion.

- Observe for signs and symptoms of infection.

- Prevent complications of bed rest (see The Immobilized Patient).

- Work with Physical Therapy to reinforce teaching and encourage exercises.

- Assess and support patient's psychosocial needs. Allow patient time to work through the grieving process. Reinforce efforts made to cope with the loss. Allow as many self-care activities as possible to maintain feelings of independence and self-worth. Offer reassurance and empathy for complaints of phantom pain. Encourage patient to allow time for a complete prosthetic fit. Allow patient to express feelings of anger, fear and depression. Maintain a hopeful attitude. Include family or significant others in care. Include social worker and psychologist in care plan.

PATIENT AND FAMILY TEACHING

- If patient has emotional strength, begin patient teaching before surgery. Assist the patient and family in attaining realistic goals and expectations.
- Inform patient and family that phantom sensations are normal and may persist for awhile.
- Upon discharge, teach patient to observe for signs and symptoms of infection: Fever, chills, increased stump pain, incisional tenderness, increased stump edema, necrotic-appearing suture line, wound drainage.
- Emphasize the importance of daily stump inspection to alleviate skin irritation.
- Stress the importance of daily stump hygiene and the necessity of removing all soap. Irritating solutions and skin softeners are to be avoided.
- Stump stockings should be smooth fitting and discarded when torn.
- Advise patient to apply prosthesis immediately upon arising to prevent stump edema.
- Prosthetic care should include the following: Keeping inside socket clean, avoid adjusting prosthesis by self, and obtain professional help when problems arise.

TOTAL KNEE REPLACEMENT

POTENTIAL PROBLEMS

Fat Embolism	Edema
Thrombophlebitis	Flexion Contraction
Infection	Nerve Damage
Prosthesis Failure	Psychosocial Problems
Stress Fracture	

KEY NURSING INTERVENTIONS

- See Preoperative and Postoperative Care.
- Assess patient for signs and symptoms of fat embolism: Mental confusion, restlessness, apprehension, tachycardia, tachypnea, dyspnea, low pO_2.
- Monitor patient for signs and symptoms of thrombophlebitis: Tenderness and redness over affected vein, edema, cyanosis or mottling, diminished pulses, and positive Homans' sign (calf pain with dorsiflexion of foot) in affected extremity.
- Check circulation, sensitivity and motion of affected lower extremity and document.
- Keep Hemovac or suction device active, if present.
- See Cast Care if present.
- Elevate leg with pillow under ankle and apply ice as ordered.
- Maintain leg in extension to prevent flexion contracture.
- Prevent external rotation of affected extremity by using trochanter roll.
- Work with physical therapy to encourage prescribed exercises (usually isometric, quadriceps setting, then active straight leg raising and range of motion).
- Prevent complications of bed rest (see The Immobilized Patient).
- Assess and support patient's psychosocial needs. Patients with poor strength and physical ability may become easily discouraged with leg exercises. Offer encouragement and praise for all attempts made. Maintain a positive and hopeful attitude relating to prognosis.

PATIENT AND FAMILY TEACHING

- Instruct patient and family to observe activity limitations outlined by physician.

- Upon discharge, stress the importance of reporting signs and symptoms of infection: Fever, increased pain and tenderness, redness, swelling and drainage from incision area.

- Teach patient and family safe usage of canes, crutches, walkers or other assistive devices.

- Discuss the elimination of unsafe environmental conditions at home.

TOTAL HIP REPLACEMENT, HIP SURGERY

POTENTIAL PROBLEMS

Pulmonary Embolism	Infection
Shock	Urinary Retention
Fat Embolism	Pressure Sores
Thrombophlebitis	Constipation
Hemorrhage	Pain
Atelectasis	Confusion
Pneumonia	Psychosocial Problems
Dislocation of Prosthesis	

KEY NURSING INTERVENTIONS

- See Preoperative and Postoperative Care.

- Recognize early signs and symptoms of impending shock: Restlessness, apprehension, tachypnea, tachycardia, normal or elevated blood pressure, good urine output.

- Assess patient for signs and symptoms of progressive shock: Cold and clammy or warm and dry skin; pallor or cyanosis; dry mucous membranes; rapid, weak, thready pulse; rapid, shallow respirations; falling diastolic and systolic blood pressure; falling pulse pressure (usually less than 20 mm Hg); oliguria or anuria; hypothermia; impaired sensory perception; metabolic acidosis.

- Observe for signs and symptoms of pulmonary embolism: Dyspnea, substernal chest pain, tachycardia, cyanosis, restlessness, anxiety, hemoptysis, cough, syncope, EKG changes, fever, hypotension, cold and clammy skin, low pCO_2 and pO_2.

- Monitor patient for signs and symptoms of thrombophlebitis: Tenderness and redness over affected vein, edema, cyanosis or mottling, diminished pulses, and positive Homans' sign (calf pain with dorsiflexion of foot) in affected extremity.

- Assess patient for signs and symptoms of fat embolism: Mental confusion, restlessness, apprehension, tachycardia, tachypnea, dyspnea, low pO_2.

- Check circulation, sensitivity and motion of affected lower extremity and document.

- Observe for excessive bleeding. Check under buttocks for hidden drainage.

- Keep Hemovac or other suction device active if present.

- Follow physician's exact orders for positioning and moving patient. As ordered, turn patient to unaffected side every two hours. Support front and back of patient with pillows. Maintain secured abduction pillow when turning, if present.

- Maintain recumbent position to prevent hip flexion contractures. As ordered, elevate head of bed for short periods to provide comfort (usually not more than 45 degrees).

- Maintain affected leg in position as ordered (for hip pinning, usually elevated on one pillow, extended and with slight abduction; for total hip replacement and femoral head prosthetics, abducted with abduction pillow or several pillows between legs).

- Prevent external rotation of affected extremity by using trochanter roll.

- Work with Physical Therapy to encourage prescribed exercises (usually quadriceps, isometric, and range of motion).

- Maintain skin integrity and prevent complications of bed rest (see The Immobilized Patient).

- Use fracture pan for elimination.

- See Traction, if present.

- Assess and support patient's psychosocial needs, observe for confusion, especially at night and orient patient PRN. Encourage family or significant others to visit patient. Recognize that the patient may have unexpressed fears of pain, death, financial matters, being an invalid or a burden to the family. Encourage verbalization of fears. Allow patient as much control of activities and care plan as possible. Discuss ways of preventing sensory monotony and deprivation. Arrange for calendar and clock to be in patient's room near patient.

PATIENT AND FAMILY TEACHING

- Instruct patient and family to observe activity limitations outlined by physician.

- Discuss the elimination of unsafe environmental conditions at home.

- Teach patient and family safe usage of canes, walkers, or other assistive devices.

- Stress the importance of reporting signs and symptoms of infection: Fever, increased pain and tenderness, redness, swelling and drainage from the incision area.

- *FOR TOTAL HIP REPLACEMENT:*

  - Instruct patient to keep an abduction pillow between the knees when sleeping or lying down.

  - Advise patient to avoid the following: Crossing the legs, sitting for longer than one-hour intervals, hip flexion greater than 90 degrees, sitting in rocking and low chairs, extreme adduction, and internal rotation.

  - Contact Social Service to assist patient in obtaining a raised toilet seat and other assistive devices.

IV

FLUID AND ELECTROLYTE IMBALANCES

There are sixteen basic imbalances. Only twelve are discussed here. The other four are acid-base imbalances and are discussed in the arterial blood gas section. These imbalances are potentially-life-threatening. It is therefore important to identify patients who may succumb to these disturbances. It is also important to note that fluid and electrolyte imbalances rarely occur as a single imbalance.

I. PREDISPOSING IMBALANCE FACTORS

A. **Burns**

B. **IV Therapy**

C. **NPO**

D. **Nasogastric suction**

E. **Nasogastric feeding**

F. **Respiratory suctioning**

G. **Vomiting**

H. **Diarrhea**

I. **Chest tube drainage**

J. **Altered diet**

K. **Hemorrhage**

L. **Fever**

M. **Edema**

N. **Ostomies**

O. **Diuretic therapy**

P. **Hormone therapy**

Q. **Kidney disease**

R. **Liver disease**

S. **Congestive heart failure**

T. **Endocrine Disorders**

II. IMBALANCES

A. Hypovolemia

This loss of fluid from the vascular space may be caused by direct depletion, as in acute bleeding, or by a relative loss, such as vagal responses where the vascular space becomes enlarged.

1. Causes
   a) Hemorrhage, internal or external
   b) Diabetes insipidus
   c) Renal disorders
   d) Acute vagal responses
   e) Untoward reaction to nitroglycerin
   f) HHNK (hyperosmolar, hyperglycemic, nonketotic coma)

2. Signs and Symptoms
   a) Tachycardia
   b) Cool, moist skin
   c) Pallor
   d) Cyanosis
   e) Weak, thready pulse
   f) Hypotension
   g) Oliguria
   h) Postural hypotension
   i) Low central venous pressure
   j) Decreased level of consciousness

3. Laboratory

   Initially, hemoglobin and hematocrit remain the same but rapidly begin to decrease if bleeding continues.

4. Treatment

   Correction of underlying cause. Administration of isotonic IV fluids, blood, plasma, protein, or electrolyte solutions.

B. Hypervolemia

This excess of fluid in the vascular space is most commonly caused by overinfusion of IV fluids.

1. Causes

   Overinfusion of any IV solution at a rate greater than the renal system can handle.

2. Signs and Symptoms

   a) Bounding pulse

   b) Hypertension

   c) Pulmonary edema

   d) Neck and peripheral vein distention

   e) Peripheral edema

   f) Elevation of central venous pressure

   g) Cyanosis

3. Laboratory

   Decrease in hemoglobin, hematocrit, and BUN

4. Treatment

   Prevention is best. Check IV flow rate frequently. If hypervolemia occurs, diuretics, phlebotomy, dialysis, or rotating tourniquets may be implemented.

C. Plasma to Interstitial Shift

Normally, there is a 3:1 ratio of plasma to interstital fluid balance. This balance is upset when fluid flows out of the vascular space and into surrounding tissue. Serum protein is mainly responsible for the regulation of osmolality which determines shifting of fluids to and from compartments.

1. Causes

   a) Decreased water intake

   b) Hemorrhage

   c) Comatose patients given concentrated tubal feedings

   d) Severe vomiting or diarrhea

   e) Burns

   f) Gastric suctioning

   g) Crushing injuries

   h) Excessive sweating

   i) Fever

   j) Intestinal obstruction

   k) Draining fistulas or abscesses

   l) Liver or kidney disease

   m) Insensible respiratory loss as with mechanical ventilation or hyperventilation

   n) Extreme debilitation or illnesses

2. Signs and Symptoms

   a) Shock

   b) Tachycardia

   c) Cool, moist skin or hot, dry skin

   d) Weak, thready pulse

   e) Hypotension

   f) Oliguria

   g) Postural hypotension

   h) Low central venous pressure

   i) Poor skin turgor

   j) Dry mucous membranes

   k) Decreased level of consciousness

   l) Elevated temperature

3. Laboratory

   Elevation of hemoglobin, hematocrit and BUN

4. Treatment

   Correction of underlying cause. Administration of appropriate IV or PO fluids (usually dextrose with saline or dextrose with Ringer's lactate solution).

D. Interstitial to Plasma Shift

This imbalance may occur as a result of edematous fluid remobilization following a severe burn or crushing injury. It may also occur when infusion of hypertonic solutions upset serum osmolality and cause a shift.

1. Causes

   a) Severe burns

   b) Crushing injuries

    c) Excess infusion of blood, plasma, dextran, protein, or any other hypertonic solution

    d) Cortisone injections

    e) Kidney, liver, or heart disease

2. Signs and Symptoms

    a) Bounding pulse

    b) Hypertension

    c) Bradycardia

    d) Tachycardia

    e) Neck and peripheral vein distention

    f) Peripheral edema

    g) Central venous pressure elevation

    h) Weakness

    i) Polyuria

    j) Dyspnea

    k) Pulmonary edema

3. Laboratory

Decrease in hemoglobin, hematocrit, BUN, and hyponatremia

4. Treatment

Unless condition is severe and the heart, liver, and kidney functions are normal, no treatment is necessary. Excess fluid will be excreted. In compromised patients, treatment may include use of diuretics, phlebotomy, dialysis, or rotating tourniquets.

E. Hyponatremia

1. Causes

    a) Excessive sweating

    b) Excessive water intake

    c) Decreased salt intake

    d) Gastrointestinal suctioning with water intake

    e) Repeated no-sodium enemas

    f) Infusion of electrolyte-free solutions

    g) Adrenal insufficiency

    h) Congestive heart failure

    i) Renal failure

    j) Cirrhosis

    k) Excess ADH section

    l) Potent diuretics

    m) Near drownings in fresh water

    n) Burns

    o) Diarrhea

    p) Prolonged vomiting

    q) Diuretics

    r) Salt-losing renal disorders

    s) Hyperglycemia

    t) Hyperlipidemia

    u) Hypoproteinemia

    v) Starvation

2. Signs and Symptoms

    a) Headache

    b) Confusion

    c) Abdominal cramps

    d) Weakness

    e) Apathy

    f) Lassitude

    g) Irritability

    h) Apprehension

    i) Convulsions

    j) Oliguria

    k) Hyperactive reflexes

    l) Hypotension

    m) Poor skin turgor

3. Laboratory

Serum sodium level < 137 mEq/1
Serum chloride level < 93 mEq/1
Urine specific gravity < 1.010

4. Treatment

May include a decrease in water intake or increase in sodium intake in the diet. In more severe cases, infusion of half-normal, normal, or 5% sodium chloride solutions may be used.

F. Hypernatremia

1. Causes

   a) Decreased water intake

   b) Excess sodium intake

   c) Prolonged hyperventilation

   d) Prolonged watery diarrhea

   e) Steroid therapy

   f) Cushing's disease

   g) Comatose patients with low fluid intake

   h) Near drownings in salt water

   i) Diabetes insipidus or mellitus

   j) High-protein tube feeding

2. Signs and Symptoms

   a) Dehydration

   b) Poor turgor

   c) Dry membranes

   d) Warm, flushed skin

   e) Thirst

   f) Oliguria

   g) Temperature elevation

   h) Weakness

   i) Muscle pain

   j) Fever

3. Laboratory

   Serum sodium > 147 mEq/1
   Serum chloride > 107 mEq/1
   Urine specific gravity > 1.030

4. Treatment

   Correction of underlying cause, sodium-restricted diet, increase in PO fluids, diuretics, IV infusion of dextrose and water, followed by isotonic electrolyte solution.

G. Hypokalemia

1. Causes

   a) Decrease in potassium intake

   b) Diuretics

   c) Prolonged vomiting

   d) Diarrhea

   e) Burns

   f) Ulcerative colitis

   g) Fistulas

   h) Diabetic ketoacidosis

   i) Steroid therapy

   j) Cushing's disease

   k) Renal failure where potassium is excreted

   l) Congestive heart failure

   m) Aldosteronism

   Note: Low potassium potentiates digitalis preparations.

2. Signs and Symptoms

   a) Disturbed muscle function (gastrointestinal, skeletal, cardiac)

   b) Decreased reflexes

   c) Muscular irritability or weakness

   d) Speech changes

   e) Shallow respirations

   f) Thirst

   g) Paralytic ileus

   h) Abdominal distention

   i) Flatulence

   j) Irregular pulse

   k) Hypotension

   l) EKG shows flat T wave and presence of U wave. Cardiac arrest may occur.

3. Laboratory

   Serum potassium < 3.5 mEq/l

   Serum chloride < 98 mEq/l

4. Treatment

Increase in oral intake through diet or supplements. IV administration of no more than 80 mEq/1 and no faster than 10 mEq/hr.

H. Hyperkalemia

1. Causes

   a) Excessive oral intake

   b) Severe burns

   c) Crushing injuries

   d) Advanced kidney disease

   e) Adrenal insufficiency

   f) Excessive IV administration

   g) Hemorrhagic shock

2. Signs and Symptoms

   a) Irritability

   b) Confusion

   c) Nausea

   d) Abdominal cramping

   e) Diarrhea

   f) Flaccid muscles

   g) Oliguria

   h) Chest pain

   i) Hypotension

   j) EKG shows peaked T waves, wide QRS complexes, and ST depression. Cardiac arrest may occur.

3. Laboratory

   Serum potassium > 5.6

4. Treatment

   Decrease oral intake, Kayexalate enemas, IV administration of sodium bicarbonate, glucose, insulin, hemo- and peritoneal dialysis.

I. Hypocalcemia

1. Causes

   a) Vitamin D deficiency

   b) Diarrhea

   c) Draining wounds

   d) Pancreatitis

   e) Parathyroidectomy

   f) Burns

   g) Lactation

   h) Hypoparathyroidism

   i) Citrated blood administration

   j) Overcorrection of acidosis

   k) Renal failure

2. Signs and Symptoms

   a) Tingling of fingers, toes, lips

   b) Carpopedal spasm

   c) Muscle cramps

   d) Tetany

   e) Convulsions

   f) EKG shows prolonged QT interval. Arrhythmias may develop.

3. Laboratory

   Serum calcium < 4.5 mEq/1
   Sulkowitch urine test reveals no precipitation

4. Treatment

   Increase dietary intake of calcium and vitamin D, IV administration of a calcium preparation. Note: Do not administer IV calcium with saline. Saline causes calcium loss.

J. Hypercalcemia

1. Causes

   a) Vitamin D overdose

   b) Renal disease

   c) Hyperparathyroidism

    d) Parathyroid adenoma

    e) Prolonged immobilization

    f) Metastatic carcinoma

    g) Multiple myeloma

    h) Paget's disease

    i) Overuse of antacids

    j) Excess calcium intake

2. Signs and Symptoms

    a) Deep bone pain

    b) Pathologic fractures

    c) Flank pain

    d) Kidney stones

    e) Kidney infections

    f) Osteoporosis

    g) Lethargy

    h) Diarrhea

    i) Constipation

    j) Anorexia

    k) Nausea

    l) Vomiting

    m) Mental confusion

    n) EKG shows shortening of QT and QRS intervals

3. Laboratory

    Serum calcium > 5.8 mEq/l
    Increased serum phosphorus

4. Treatment

    Correction of underlying cause. Decrease oral intake of calcium, IV administration of isotonic saline, disodium phosphate, corticosteroids, sodium sulfate, and diuretics.

K. Hypomagnesemia

1. Causes

    a) Alcoholism

    b) Vomiting

    c) Low magnesium intake

    d) Malabsorption disorders

    e) Severe malnutrition

    f) Severe diarrhea

    g) Diabetic ketoacidosis

    h) Prolonged GI suctioning

    i) Diuretic therapy

    j) Hypoparathyroidism

    k) Pancreatitis

    l) Primary aldosteronism

    m) Post surgery patients

    n) Kidney disease

Note: Low magnesium potentiates digitalis preparations.

2. Signs and Symptoms

    a) Tetany

    b) Hyperactive reflexes

    c) Lethargy

    d) Hallucinations

    e) Confusion

    f) Irritability

    g) Nausea

    h) Vomiting

    i) Convulsions

    j) Tachycardic arrhythmias, artrial and ventricular in origin

    k) Hypotension

    l) Lidocaine-resistant ventricular arrhythmias

3. Laboratory

Serum magnesium < 1.4 mEq/l

4. Treatment

Increase in diet and IV administration of magnesium sulfate

L. **Hypermagnesemia**

1. Causes

    a) Excessive oral intake

    b) Overdose during replacement therapy

    c) Kidney disease

    d) Severe dehydration and oliguria

    e) Repeated enemas with magnesium sulfate

    f) Use of magnesium antacids with renal failure

2. Signs and Symptoms

    a) Lethargy

    b) Depressed respirations

    c) Warm sensation throughout the body

    d) Flushing

    e) Hypotension

    f) Flaccid muscles or paralysis

    g) Cardiac arrhythmias. Cardiac arrest can occur.

3. Laboratory

    Serum magnesium > 3.0 mEq/l

4. Treatment

    Decrease oral intake of magnesium, IV with 10% calcium gluconate. Patients with renal failure require dialysis.

V

ARTERIAL BLOOD GASES

I. PURPOSE

There are three main purposes for a physician ordering an arterial blood gas analysis:

A. <u>pH</u>

Evaluate acid-base balance (pH).

B. <u>pO_2</u>

Evaluate the efficiency of lungs to deliver oxygen to blood (pO_2).

C. <u>pCO_2</u>

Determine the ability of lungs to blow off waste (pCO_2).

II. BLOOD GAS NORMS

pH	7.35–7.45
pO_2	80–100 mm Hg
pCO_2	35–45 mm Hg
HCO_3	22–26 Eq/l
O_2 saturation	95% or greater
Base excess	$(-2) - (+2)$

III. EVALUATION

A. <u>pH</u>

Check pH for acidosis or alkalosis

B. <u>pCO_2</u>

Check pCO_2 for respiratory cause of altered pH

C. <u>HCO_3</u>

Check HCO_3 for metabolic cause of altered pH

D. Patient

Observe patient to see if his condition validates your analysis.

IV. RESPIRATORY ACIDOSIS

A. Causes

1. Chronic obstructive pulmonary disease
2. Airway obstruction
3. Pneumonia
4. Hemothorax
5. Cardiopulmonary arrest
6. Oversedation
7. Neuromuscular disorders
8. Pulmonary edema
9. Congestive heart failure
10. Hypoventilation on a respirator
11. Pulmonary embolus

B. Signs and Symptoms

1. Dyspnea
2. Wheezing
3. Hyperventilation
4. Disorientation
5. Tachycardia
6. Arrhythmias
7. Somnolence
8. Headache
9. Nausea
10. Diaphoresis

C. Laboratory

pH < 7.35
pCO_2 > 45 mm Hg

D. Treatment

Improve ventilation by bronchodilators, intermittent positive pressure breathing, *cautious* administration of oxygen, breathing exercises, mechanical ventilation. Administration of IV Ringer's lactate, IV sodium bicarbonate.

NOTE: Complications which can occur from treatment are as follows: Tetany, unconsciousness due to excess oxygen administration, and rebound respiratory alkalosis.

V. RESPIRATORY ALKALOSIS

A. Causes

1. Hyperventilation caused by anxiety or pulmonary embolus
2. Pain
3. Pregnancy
4. Severe anemia
5. Fever
6. Central Nervous System disorders
7. Head trauma
8. Brain surgery
9. Hypoxia resulting in hyperventilation
10. Hyperventilation on a respirator
11. Pulmonary fibrosis
12. Aspirin poisoning

B. Signs and Symptoms

1. Hyperreflexia
2. Positive Chvostek's sign (carpopedal spasm)
3. Muscular twitching
4. Rapid breathing
5. Numbness and tingling in hands and face
6. Dizziness

C. Laboratory

pH > 7.45

$pCO_2 < 35$ mm Hg

D. Treatment

Eliminate the cause of hyperventilation, neurological disorders, or aspirin poisoning. Ventilator settings should be re-evaluated and adjustments made.

VI. METABOLIC ACIDOSIS

A. Causes

1. Shock
2. Diabetic ketoacidosis
3. Renal failure
4. Fever
5. Hyperthyroidism
6. Severe diarrhea
7. Prolonged vomiting of intestinal contents
8. Dehydration
9. Starvation
10. Lactic acidosis
11. Diamox therapy
12. Ammonium chloride therapy
13. Pancreatic drainage
14. Uterosigmoidostomy
15. Boric acid ingestion
16. Aspirin poisoning
17. Liver diseases
18. Alcoholism
19. Paraldehyde therapy

B. Signs and Symptoms

1. Lethargy
2. Fruity breath
3. Disorientation
4. Weakness
5. Kussmaul respirations
6. Arrhythmias

C. Laboratory

pH > 7. 45

HCO_3 < 25 mEq/l

Hyperkalemia

D. Treatment

Administration of IV sodium chloride or Ringer's lactate solutions. IV sodium bicarbonate administration. Regular insulin is usually given to treat hyperkalemia.

NOTE: Complications which can occur from treatment are tetany and respiratory alkalosis.

VII. METABOLIC ALKALOSIS

A. Causes

1. Nasogastric suction
2. Severe vomiting of stomach contents
3. Diuretic therapy
4. Aldosteronism
5. Cushing's disease
6. Ingestion of strong alkalotic substances (baking soda, milk of magnesia)
7. Overdose of IV sodium bicarbonate to correct acidosis
8. Overinfusion of Ringer's lactate solution
9. Severe potassium deficiency

B. Signs and Symptoms

1. Lethargy
2. Disorientation
3. Confusion
4. Convulsions
5. Twitching
6. Shaking
7. Picking at sheets
8. Atrial tachycardia

9. Paralytic ileus
10. Depressed respirations with periodic apnea

C. Laboratory

pH > 7.45

HCO_3 > 29 mEq/l

Hypokalemia

D. Treatment

Correction of cause, administration of IV Ringer's lactate, 0.9% ammonium chloride, potassium

VI

IV THERAPY: PRINCIPLES AND GUIDELINES

I. PURPOSE OF IV THERAPY

A. Maintenance and Replacement

To maintain, replace, or prevent anticipated losses of blood, water, electrolytes, calories, proteins, fats, and vitamins that cannot be met adequately by oral intake.

B. Acid-base Balance

To restore acid-base imbalance.

C. Medications

To provide a route for IV medications.

II. COMMON CRYSTALLOID SOLUTIONS WITH INDICATIONS AND CONTRAINDICATIONS FOR USAGE

A. Dextrose Solutions

5% dextrose in water contains 5 gm of dextrose in 100 ml of water. Dextrose in water comes in 2.5, 5, 10, 20 and 50% concentrations.

1. Indications for Use

   a) Provides a medium in which to infuse drugs. Most drugs prepared for IV use can be administered in D_5W. There are a few exceptions. Therefore, the literature should be read before administration.

   b) Prevention of dehydration. 2.5% and 5% solutions are used. 5% dextrose is only isotonic in the bottle. The sugar is quickly metabolized, and the water rapidly leaves the vascular space.

   c) Nutrition. One liter of 5% dextrose solution contains only 170 calories. This prevents starvation ketosis and catabolism on a temporary basis. 20% and 50% dextrose solutions provide 680 and 1700 calories, respectively. When used with electrolytes, longer term nutrition may be achieved (see also Total Parenteral Nutrition).

d) Hypernatremia can be corrected if the cause is inadequate water intake or water loss due to vomiting and/or diarrhea. Infusion of the water decreases sodium concentration.

2. Contraindications

a) Never administer with blood. This causes hemolysis and agglutination.

b) D_5W should not be used as a maintenance solution. It can cause water intoxication and dilution of electrolytes.

c) Caution should be used in patients that cannot tolerate circulatory overload.

d) Higher glucose concentrations (10 to 50%) can cause dehydration and/or hyperinsulinism.

B. Sodium Chloride Solutions

Normal saline or 0.9% sodium chloride is an isotonic solution and contains 154 mEq of both sodium and chloride per liter.

1. Indications for Use

a) Most commonly used for infusion with blood and its components.

b) Hyponatremia.

c) Metabolic alkalosis. An increase in chloride ions causes a decrease in bicarbonate ions.

2. Contraindications

a) Use with caution in patients who already have sodium-retaining problems such as cardiac and renal patients.

b) Hypernatremia can result in patients who have normal sodium levels.

c) Acidosis can result since chloride ions cause a decrease in bicarbonate ions.

d) Hypokalemia can result since sodium causes potassium excretion.

C. 5% Dextrose and Hypotonic Saline (0.45% Saline and 0.2% Saline)

1. Indications for Use

   a) Most commonly used as initial hydrating fluid. It can be safely used without knowing the present electrolyte status of the patient.

   b) Commonly used for maintaining hydration in medical-surgical patients.

2. Contraindications

   a) Use with caution in edematous, cardiac, hepatic, or renal patients.

   b) Do not use with blood infusions.

D. Lactated Ringer's

Multiple electrolytes in concentrations that are close to normal plasma levels. Also contains lactate, which is a precursor of bicarbonate.

1. Indications for Use

   a) Commonly used as a fluid replacement for acute and mild blood loss. It is also used for replacement of fluids due to burns, vomiting, and diarrhea.

   b) Mild acidosis. The lactate ion is metabolized in the liver to produce bicarbonate.

   c) Can be used for blood administration in the absence of normal saline.

2. Contraindications

   a) Severe metabolic alkalosis or acidosis.

   b) Poor lactate metabolism, especially those with liver disease.

   c) Addison's disease. Potassium-free solutions are preferred.

   d) Use with caution in patients who have normal sodium levels.

III. COLLOIDS AND THEIR INDICATIONS

A. Purpose

1. Replace blood loss, acute or mild.

2. Increase the oxygen carrying capacity of the blood.

3. Restore clotting factors.

B. Whole Blood

1. In order for whole blood to be stored, it must contain preservatives. In addition, whole blood's composition changes while it is being stored. ACD, or acid citrate dextrose, is a common preservative. The acid prevents caramel formation of the dextrose after sterilization. Citrate inhibits clotting while the dextrose prolongs the life of the red blood cells. Whole blood with ACD can be stored for up to 21 days. The following changes occur with stored blood: The oxygen carrying capacity is reduced; the potassium level rises sharply; and the clotting ability quickly drops. Be sure to check the expiration date. Make sure fresh whole blood is used for massive transfusions, newborns, and when clotting factors are needed.

2. Indications for Use

   a) Acute blood loss from trauma or ruptured vessels.

   b) Cardiac surgery. Blood is needed to prime the heart-lung machine.

   c) Newborn infants with hemolytic anemia.

C. Packed Cells

1. Most of the plasma is removed from whole blood to obtain packed cells. Packed cells are about one-half the volume of whole blood but still maintain the same oxygen carrying capacity. Packed cells have less excess sodium and potassium than whole blood.

2. Indications for Use

   a) Patients who have normal blood volume but still need blood.

   b) Patients who cannot tolerate more volume, especially those with cardiac conditions.

c) Patient with hepatic disease who cannot tolerate excess citrate.

d) Patients who cannot tolerate excess sodium and potassium.

D. Frozen Blood

1. All the plasma is removed, leaving only the red blood cells (RBC's), which can be frozen and stored for three years. Before infusion the cells are thawed and washed. Advantages of frozen blood are as follows: No antibodies are left; incidence of hepatitis is very low; there are very few white cell antigens; it has a long storage time; and it has a low viscosity for rapid administration.

2. Indications for Use

a) Transplant patients.

b) Patients who have high risk for hepatitis.

c) Indications similar to packed cells.

E. Plasma

1. This is the fluid that remains after the RBC's have been removed. It can be stored for long periods of time, depending on the type of plasma. Plasma can be liquid, freeze-dried, or fresh frozen. Disadvantages of plasma are as follows: Hepatitis can still be transmitted; it must be compatible with the recipient's cells.

2. Indications for Use

a) Burn patients.

b) Hypovolemic patients.

F. Human Albumin

1. Albumin is obtained from plasma. It comes in a 25% solution. Advantages of albumin are as follows: No risk of hepatitis; it can be diluted in crystalloid solutions; untoward reactions are rare.

2. Indications for Use

a) Patients with hypoalbuminemia (kidney and liver conditions).

b) Similar to plasma.

G. Dextran

1. This is a synthetic plasma substitute. Advantages are as follows: No storage problem, no risk of hepatitis, and untoward reactions are rare.

2. Indications for Use

   a) Burn patients

   b) Hypovolemic patients

   c) Patients with hypoalbuminemia

H. White Blood Cells

1. All the red blood cells and 80% of the plasma have been removed. Disadvantages are as follows: Causes a febrile reaction, severe chills, disorientation and mild hypertension. Administer with caution. Must be compatible with recipient's cells.

2. Indications for Use

   Granulocytopenia that is not responsive to antibiotics.

I. Platelets

1. Platelets have been extracted from the plasma and then resuspended in 50 cc of plasma. These units must be constantly agitated prior to administration to prevent agglutination and be given rapidly. Platelets are also packed in multiunit packs which are administered the same as blood but at a faster rate.

2. Indications for Use

   a) Thrombocytopenia.

   b) Decreased platelet count.

   c) Abnormal platelets.

IV. ASSESSMENT OF THE PATIENT RECEIVING IV THERAPY

In assessing the patient who is receiving IV therapy, the nurse must understand the disease process of the patient and the rationale behind the therapy.

A. Urinary output

Indicative of arterial pressure and glomerular filtration. It should always be within normal parameters. Normal output is 50 ml/hr. Oliguria or anuria is less than 30 ml/hr.

B. Central venous pressure

Gives an indication of blood volume. Normal CVP is 5 to 10 cm of H_2O. Low values may indicate hypovolemia. Higher values may indicate circulatory overload and congestive heart failure.

C. Vital sign changes

Note trends in blood pressure, pulse, respirations, and temperature. Check vital signs frequently. Check postural vital signs if hypovolemia is suspected.

D. Weight

A sudden gain or loss in weight is usually fluid related. Weigh the patient daily as ordered or PRN at the same time each day. A gain or loss of 1 kg is equivalent to a gain or loss of 1 liter of body fluid.

E. Neck vein distention

Normally neck veins will fill and distend when the patient is supine. If not, hypovolemia may be present. Neck veins should empty when the head of the bed is elevated to 45 degrees and above. If not, circulatory overload or congestive heart failure may be present.

F. Edema

Excess fluid inside the interstital compartment. This is never normal. Common places for edema are the lungs, liver, abdomen, sacrum, feet, and extremity of infusing IV.

G. Intake and output

Essential to any patient receiving IV therapy. It should be very accurate. Extreme differences should be noted and explained.

V. BLOOD ADMINISTRATION PROCEDURE

NOTE: This section is only a guideline. Your particular hospital procedure manual should be reviewed and followed.

A. Type and Crossmatch

The patient's blood should always be typed and crossmatched to the donor's blood. Make sure blood samples have been drawn and sent to the laboratory.

B. Patient Identification

Blood bank personnel, the nurse accepting, and the nurse administering the blood should check the following:

1. Name and hospital number of patient.
2. Blood group of donor and blood group of patient with blood groups on blood container.
3. Blood numbers on receipt with blood numbers on container.
4. Expiration date.
5. Have the patient verbally identify himself.

C. Documentation

Blood receipt or release form particular to your hospital should be signed by blood bank personnel and the RN accepting the blood. The nurse's notes should contain the times of initiation and cessation of infusion along with any untoward or adverse reactions.

D. Inspection

Visually inspect blood prior to administration for abnormal color or gas bubbles which may indicate bacterial growth. Look for clumping and clotting. Do not administer if these changes are noted.

E. Administration

1. Blood should be administered no later than thirty minutes after the time that it leaves the blood bank. If blood cannot be administered in this time, *do not* store in the unit refrigerator. Check with blood bank to return blood.
2. If blood is to be warmed, always use a hospital-approved blood warmer. Never use room temperature or hot water.
3. The unit of blood should be gently mixed by inverting it once or twice prior to administration.
4. A sterile pyrogen-free 170-micron filter should be used and changed after two units have infused to prevent clogging.

5. To initiate infusion, use an isotonic solution such as normal saline. Never use 5% dextrose in water, hypertonic, or hypotonic solutions. These will cause hemolysis or shrinkage of the red blood cells.

6. An 18-gauge needle or larger should be used.

F. Blood Pumps

Blood pumps are used to speed or maintain an infusion rate, especially with small-bore needles. Blood pumps should be ordered by the physician and used with caution since chances of an air embolism, fluid overload, and citrate toxicity are greatly increased.

G. Vital Signs

Vital signs including temperature should be taken just prior to administration for baseline values. Vital signs should also be taken during and after blood has been infused.

H. Observation

Constant observation for at least the initial five minutes with a slow drip rate is imperative because most symptoms of fatal reactions occur early. The nurse must have knowledge of blood and its components. The nurse is responsible for knowledge of and observation for adverse transfusion reactions. With most adverse reactions, the transfusion should be discontinued, IV kept open with normal saline, vital signs taken, the physician notified, the blood bank notified, the blood container saved, and proper documentation made in the chart.

VI. COMPLICATIONS OF IV AND BLOOD COMPONENT THERAPY

A. Adverse Reactions Specific to Blood Transfusions

1. Hemolytic Transfusion Reaction

a) Cause
Infusion of incompatible blood, causing rupture of red blood cells in the bloodstream.

b) Signs and Symptoms

(1) Low back pain.

(2) Leg pain.

(3) Tightness in chest.

(4) Shortness of breath.

(5) Shock.

c) Treatment

(1) Discontinue infusion.

(2) Notify physician.

(3) Frequent vital signs.

(4) Treat shock.

(5) Save blood bag and notify blood bank.

d) Prevention

(1) Carefully identify blood bag and receipt.

(2) Always check the patient's identification and blood type of the patient and donor.

2. Febrile Reaction

a) Cause
Imbalance or agglutination of white blood cells. Occurs in patients who have had massive transfusions of 30 units or more.

b) Signs and Symptoms

(1) Rapid rise in temperature.

(2) Chills.

(3) Headache.

(4) Low back pain.

(5) Nausea, vomiting.

(6) Shock.

c) Treatment

(1) Discontinue infusion.

(2) Frequent vital signs.

(3) Notify physician.

(4) Save blood bag and notify blood bank.

(5) Treat symptomatically.

   d) Prevention

      (1) Close observation of massive transfusion patients.

      (2) Administration of frozen blood—white blood cells have been removed.

3. Citrate Toxicity

   a) Cause

      (1) Rapid infusion of ACD blood.

      (2) Can occur in patients with liver or renal impairment. The liver metabolizes citrate ions. If liver metabolism is poor, the citrate ions combine with calcium ions, causing a calcium deficit.

   b) Signs and Symptoms

      (1) Muscle cramps, tetany.

      (2) Tingling of fingers and toes.

      (3) Convulsions.

      (4) Hypotension.

      (5) Cardiac arrest.

   c) Treatment

      (1) Discontinue infusion.

      (2) Notify physician.

      (3) Treat symptomatically.

      (4) Save blood bag and notify blood bank.

      (5) Treat shock.

   d) Prevention

      (1) Careful inspection of blood bag prior to administration.

      (2) Check for discoloration and/or gas bubbles.

B. Adverse Reactions from IV Therapy

1. Anaphylaxis

   a) Cause
   An extreme sensitivity to drugs or blood.

b) Signs and Symptoms

    (1) Flushing of skin with or without itching. Feeling of warmth.

    (2) Hives or rash.

    (3) Abdominal cramping or nausea.

    (4) Feeling of thickening of tongue or throat.

    (5) Respiratory difficulty with or without wheezes.

    (6) Shock.

c) Treatment

    (1) Discontinue infusion.

    (2) Notify physician.

    (3) Administer ordered drug therapy: Epinephrine, antihistamines, steroids.

    (4) Treat shock.

d) Prevention

    (1) Check chart and verbally ask patient for allergies.

    (2) Make frequent checks initially when administering blood.

2. Circulatory Overload

a) Cause

    (1) Rapid infusion.

    (2) Excess infusion.

b) Signs and Symptoms

    (1) Neck vein distention.

    (2) Headache.

    (3) Increased blood pressure.

    (4) Increased central venous pressure.

    (5) Shortness of breath, dyspnea.

    (6) Pulmonary edema, rales.

    (7) Shock.

c) Treatment

    (1) Discontinue infusion but keep IV open.

    (2) Notify physician.

(3) Place patient in sitting position to facilitate better breathing.

(4) Treat shock.

d) Prevention

(1) Identify patients prone to fluid overload, i.e., infants, elderly, and patients prone to congestive heart failure.

(2) Use 500-cc bottles or less on above patients.

(3) Periodically check infusion rate.

3. Air Embolism

a) Cause.

(1) A fast, large bolus of air from a blood pump.

(2) A leak in the IV tubing.

(3) The IV bottle runs dry and a new bottle is added without checking for air in the tubing.

b) Signs and Symptoms

(1) Chest pain.

(2) Shortness of breath.

(3) Shock.

c) Treatment

(1) Immediately place patient on left side in Trendelenburg position.

(2) Notify physician.

(3) Correct IV tubing malfunction.

(4) Treat shock.

d) Prevention

(1) Replace bottles before they are empty.

(2) Tightly close off unused tubing in Y-type tubing.

(3) Make sure air is out of tubing before starting infusion.

(4) Use blood pumps with caution.

4. Thrombophlebitis

a) Cause

 (1) Infection at site.

 (2) Clot formation.

 (3) Overuse of vein.

 (4) Large bore catheters.

 (5) Infusion of irritating solutions, i.e., hypertonic glucose, strong acids or alkalies, potassium preparations, chemotherapeutic drugs, barbiturates.

b) Signs and Symptoms

 (1) Pain at site.

 (2) Redness at site and along vein.

c) Treatment

 (1) Discontinue infusion.

 (2) Choose another site, if ordered.

 (3) Initially apply cool compresses for pain relief, then warm compresses to facilitate healing.

d) Prevention

 (1) Use larger veins for irritating solutions.

 (2) Frequently inspect site.

 (3) Use smaller bore catheters whenever possible.

5. Infection

a) Cause
Contamination of site from poor aseptic technique, fluid contamination, or infection from other source in patient.

b) Signs and Symptoms

 (1) Pain and redness at injection site.

 (2) Fever.

 (3) Malaise.

 (4) Shock.

c) Treatment

   (1) Change IV site.

   (2) Keep catheter, tubing, and bottle for possible culturing.

   (3) Apply warm compresses to local infection.

   (4) Obtain blood cultures and administer antipyretics and antibiotic therapy when ordered.

d) Prevention

   (1) Employ strict aseptic technique.

   (2) Use smaller catheters.

   (3) Change IV site, tubing, and IV bottle per hospital policy.

   (4) Frequently check IV site.

   (5) Check IV bottle for clarity, cracks, and vacuum.

6. Infiltration

a) Cause

   (1) Rupture of vein.

   (2) Dislodging of catheter from vein.

b) Signs and Symptoms

   (1) Edema at site, cool to touch.

   (2) Dependent edema in extremity.

   (3) Pain at site.

   (4) Slowing or stoppage of fluid.

   (5) Irritating solutions can cause necrosis of surrounding tissue.

c) Treatment

   (1) Discontinue infusion.

   (2) Notify physician, especially if irritating solution used.

   (3) Apply warm compresses.

   (4) Restart infusion, if ordered.

d) Prevention

(1) Anchor catheter securely.

(2) Frequently check IV site, especially immediately after starting IV.

(3) Properly splint extremity.

VII. TOTAL PARENTERAL NUTRITION—TPN

A. Principles

Total parenteral nutrition, or hyperalimentation, is used when nutritional needs cannot be met through oral intake. The main purpose is to prevent gluconeogenesis or conversion of protein to calories instead of synthesis of tissue. TPN also provides essential electrolytes, amino acids, vitamins, and othe trace elements needed for cellular life.

B. Indications for Use

1. Nasogastric ineffectiveness.

2. Hyperemesis.

3. Chemotherapy, radiotherapy.

4. Cerebrovascular accidents.

5. Anorexia nervosa.

6. Gastrointestinal rest.

   a) Acute inflammatory bowel disease.

   b) Gastrointestinal fistula.

   c) Major bowel resection.

   d) Intestinal obstruction.

7. Acute renal failure.

8. Any patient demonstrating large nitrogen losses, such as burn patients or metastatic cancer patients.

C. Physician Responsibilities

1. Placement of central venous catheter.

2. Chest x-ray after placement.

3. Baseline laboratory studies before TPN. These should include the following: Complete blood count, elec-

trolytes, chemistry panel, creatinine, magnesium, triglycerides.

4. Monitoring laboratory studies after initiating TPN. These should include the following: Daily glucose levels for one week; three times per week: Glucose, creatinine, BUN, electrolytes; once a week: Complete blood count, magnesium, chemistry panel, partial thromboplastin time.

5. Solution order should be rewritten everyday after evaluation of laboratory studies. All TPN orders should include the following:

    a) Base solution with rate of administration, total volume in 24 hrs., and percent of dextrose.

    b) Caloric content.

    c) Nitrogen content or protein equivalent.

    d) Additives and electrolytes per 1000 ml, including but not limited to:

       Potassium chloride

       Sodium chloride

       Potassium phosphate

       Magnesium sulfate

       Calcium gluconate

       Calcium acetate

       Sodium acetate

       Potassium acetate

       M.V.I.

       Folic acid

       B-complex with Vitamin C

       Insulin

       Heparin

D. Nursing Responsibilities

1. Explanation of procedure to patient to reduce anxiety. This should include:

    a) Principles and reasons for TPN.

    b) Discussion of catheter insertion procedure.

    c) Importance of clean, dry dressings.

    d) Purpose of infusion pump and purpose of alarm.

    e) Reasons behind daily monitoring of blood, urine, and weight.

2. Daily monitoring

    a) Vital signs with temperature every 4 hrs.

    b) Fractional urine or chemstrips every 6 hrs.

    c) Strict intake and output.

    d) Daily weights.

    e) IV rate within 20% of orders.

    f) Dressing and tubing changes per hospital procedure.

    g) Other monitoring as ordered by physician.

3. Precautions

    a) Infusion rate should be constant. Check flow frequently. Bottles tend to run behind. Never speed up an infusion more than 10%. It is best to simply readjust the schedule of bottles.

    b) Catheter should never be irrigated by the nurse. The physician should be notified of catheter malfunction.

    c) Never push or piggyback medications through TPN lines. Always use peripheral lines.

    d) If TPN is no longer indicated, the physician's orders should include a gradual decrease of infusion to wean the patient. This will prevent an insulin reaction.

    e) If solution is to be discontinued suddenly due to untoward reaction or bottle breakage, always hang a 10% dextrose solution. If catheter cannot be used, hang a 10% dextrose solution peripherally.

    f) Always save the bottle, tubing, and catheter if infection occurs. These items may be cultured and appropriate treatment started.

    g) Close monitoring of the patient is essential. Untoward reactions include those of peripheral IV therapy. Reactions tend to be more severe because of solution concentration and central placement of catheter.

    h) The nurse should know signs and symptoms of hyper- and hypoglycemia.

VIII. RATE CALCULATION

A. Method One

Drops/min = $\dfrac{\text{Total Vol. to be Infused} \times \text{Drip Chamber Drops/ml}}{\text{Total Infusion time in Minutes}}$

Example: Physician's order states to administer 1000 cc of 5% dextrose in water each 8 hrs. The nurse decides to use a drip chamber which has 15 drops/ml.

$$\frac{1000 \times 15}{480} = 31.25 \text{ or } 30 \text{ drops/min.}$$

B. Method Two

1. First calculate milliliters per hour if not already given. This is done by dividing the amount to be given by the time to be given.

Examples:

ml		hrs.		ml/hr/ (approximate)
1000	÷	8	=	125
1000	÷	12	=	83
1000	÷	24	=	42
100	÷	0.5 (30 mins.)	=	200
50	÷	0.33 (20 mins.)	=	150
50	÷	0.25 (15 mins.)	=	200

2. Next, select the drip chamber size.

   a) Blood tubing—10 drops/ml—Use for blood administration.

   b) Macrodrip—15 drops/ml—Use for giving larger volumes of fluid. Any rate over 80 ml/hr. should have a macrodrip drip chamber.

   c) Minidrip—60 drops/ml—Use for slower drip rates, children, elderly, people prone to congestive heart failure, and for administering piggyback medications.

3. Once the drip chamber size is selected, convert ml/hr. to drops/min. by dividing the number of ml/hr. by six (6) for the blood tubing or by four (4) for the macrodrip. No

conversion number is needed for the microdrip because ml/hr. directly converts into drops/min.

Examples: gtt/min.

ml/hr.	Blood Divide cc/hr by 6	Macro Divide cc/hr by 4	Micro cc/hr = gtt/min.
42	7 gtt/min.	10 gtt/min.	42 gtt/min.
83	14 gtt/min.	21 gtt/min.	83 gtt/min.
125	21 gtt/min.	31 gtt/min.	125 gtt/min.
150	25 gtt/min.	37 gtt/min.	150 gtt/min.
200	33 gtt/min.	50 gtt/min.	200 gtt/min.

VII

DIAGNOSTIC PROCEDURES

Because diagnostic procedures are essential to effective management of medical problems, it is of the utmost importance to assure that the patient is properly prepared prior to the procedure. Nursing intervention following diagnostic procedures is important in preventing and treating complications.

This chapter focuses on general and specific nursing interventions for radiography, radionuclide, ultrasound, thermography, endoscopy, and special procedures based on what is most widely practiced. It must be stressed that individual hospital procedures and policies must always be observed in preparing patients for tests.

A. GENERAL NURSING INTERVENTIONS

The following interventions apply to all diagnostic procedures:

KEY NURSING INTERVENTIONS

Preparation

- Inform patient of the date and time of scheduled procedure.
- Reinforce physician's explanation of the procedure. Instruct patient regarding the procedure if no previous explanation has been given. Stress importance of patient's cooperation.
- Instruct patient to remove all jewelry and metal within the examining field. (Lock valuables in hospital safe.)
- Have patient void prior to procedure, unless procedure calls for full bladder.
- Dress patient in hospital gown without metal snaps.
- Obtain written consent per hospital policy.
- Check for and document on front of chart all allergies, especially to iodine, seafood and contrast dyes. Notify Radiology or physician of allergies.
- Assess and support patient's psychosocial needs. Use active listening skills while patient verbalizes fears and concerns. Reassure patient that all members of the health care team are concerned for the safety and

welfare of the patient and will be supportive in all aspects of the patient's care.

Following the Procedure

- Check for other scheduled procedures and subsequent interventions before resuming previous diet.
- FOR NUCLEAR MEDICINE PROCEDURES:
  - Observe injection area for hemorrhage.
  - Observe for delayed allergic reaction.

B. RADIOGRAMS (X-RAYS)

- **BARIUM ENEMA**

KEY NURSING INTERVENTIONS

Preparation

- Provide low-residue diet 2–3 days prior to test.
- Clear liquids for lunch and supper prior to test (no dairy products).
- Force fluids unless contraindicated.
- NPO after midnight prior to test.
- Administer cathartic in the afternoon the day prior to test.
- Administer tap water enemas the evening prior to test.
  NOTE: Pathological conditions such as ulcerative colitis and active gastrointestinal bleeding may prohibit intensive bowel preparation. Check with physician for desired bowel preparation.

Following the Procedure

- See Barium Swallow.
- Resume medications as ordered.

- **BARIUM SWALLOW**

KEY NURSING INTERVENTIONS

Preparation

- NPO after midnight prior to test.
- Hold antacids as ordered only.

Following the Procedure

- Administer cathartic and/or enema.

- Document quality of stool for 2–3 days.
- Force fluids unless contraindicated.

• CHOLANGIOGRAM, INTRAVENOUS

KEY NURSING INTERVENTIONS

Preparation

- Order low-residue diet the day prior to test.
- Order simple fats with evening meal (milk, cream, butter, eggs).
- No food after evening meal.
- Keep the patient NPO after midnight prior to test.
- Provide fluids as ordered.
- Obtain written consent.
- Check for and document on front of chart allergies to iodine, seafood, and contrast dyes. Notify Radiology of allergies.
- Administer cathartic and/or enemas.

Following the Procedure

- Observe injection site for signs of hemorrhage and infection.
- Observe for delayed allergic reaction.
- Encourage fluids to eliminate contrast unless contraindicated.

• CHOLANGIOGRAM, T-TUBE

KEY NURSING INTERVENTIONS

Preparation

- NPO after midnight prior to test.
- Obtain written consent.
- Check for and document on front of chart allergies to iodine, seafood, and contrast dyes. Notify Radiology of allergies.

Following the Procedure

- Observe for delayed allergic reaction.
- Reconnect T-tube to drainage system.
- Maintain a sterile dressing over T-tube site if T-tube is removed.

• CHOLECYSTOGRAM, ORAL

KEY NURSING INTERVENTIONS

Preparation

- Order high-fat lunch and fat-free dinner the day prior to test.
- NPO after evening meal except for small amounts of water.
- Check for and document on front of chart allergies to iodine, seafood, and contrast dyes.
- Notify physician of above allergies before administering contrast tablets.
- If no allergy, administer contrast tablets 2–3 hrs. after evening meal (usually iopanoic acid) tab 1 q 15–20 mins. × 6 doses with minimal water per hospital policy.
- Notify Radiology and physician if reaction to contrast occurs: Cramps, nausea, vomiting, diarrhea.
- Administer cleansing enema (tap water) the morning of the test.

Following the Procedure

- Resume pre-test medications.
- Encourage fluids unless contraindicated.

• HYSTEROSALPINGOGRAM

KEY NURSING INTERVENTIONS

Preparation

- Check for and document on front of chart allergies to iodine, seafood, and contrast dyes. Notify Radiology of allergies.
- Administer laxative evening prior to test.
- Administer suppository or enema morning of test.
- Inform patient that occasional cramping is normal during the procedure.

Following the Procedure

- Provide perineal pad.
- Observe for signs of infection.

- Reassure patient that cramps and nausea will subside if present. Report to physician if discomfort continues.
- Vaginal discharge is normal 1–2 days after the procedure.

• INTRAVENOUS PYELOGRAM

KEY NURSING INTERVENTIONS

Preparation

- Encourage fluids unless contraindicated.
- Provide no food after evening meal prior to test.
- Keep patient NPO after midnight prior to test.
- Administer cathartic and/or enemas.
- Obtain written consent.
- Check for and document on front of chart allergies to iodine, seafood, and contrast dyes. Notify Radiology of allergies.

Following the Procedure

- Observe injection site for signs of hemorrhage or infection.
- Observe for delayed allergic reaction.
- Encourage fluid intake unless contraindicated.

• MYELOGRAM

KEY NURSING INTERVENTIONS

Preparation

- Maintain NPO as ordered (usually for 4–8 hrs. prior to test).
- Obtain written consent for lumbar puncture or as ordered.
- Check for and document on front of chart allergies to iodine, seafood, and contrast dyes. Notify Radiology of allergies.
- Administer cleansing enemas.
- Inform patient of tilting position changes which will occur during the procedure in order to move dye.

Following the Procedure

- Identify contrast media used. If isophendylate (non-water soluble) is used, keep patient flat for 24 hrs. If metrizoate sodium (water soluble) is used, keep head elevated 60 degrees and do not lie flat for 8 hrs. If dye was not removed, keep head elevated 30–45 degrees for 8 to 12 hrs. or as ordered.

- Do neurologic checks and vital signs every 30 mins. × 4, then every 4 hrs. × 24 hrs.
- Encourage PO fluids to eliminate dye unless contraindicated.

• NEPHROTOMOGRAM

KEY NURSING INTERVENTIONS

Preparation

- Administer cathartic and/or enema the evening prior to test.
- No food may be taken after evening meal prior to test.
- The patient must remain NPO after midnight prior to test.
- Check for and document on front of chart allergies to iodine, seafood, and contrast dyes. Notify Radiology of allergies.
- Obtain written consent.
- Encourage fluids the evening before test unless contraindicated.
- Inform patient that a feeling of warmth or salty taste in the mouth is normal when dye is injected.

Following the Procedure

- Observe injection site for signs of hemorrhage and infection.
- Monitor intake and output for 24 hrs.
- Observe for delayed allergic reaction.
- Encourage fluids to eliminate contrast unless contraindicated.

• UPPER GASTROINTESTINAL AND SMALL BOWEL SERIES

KEY NURSING INTERVENTIONS

Preparation

- Provide low-residue diet for 2–3 days prior to test.
- NPO and no smoking after midnight prior to test.
- Hold medications after midnight prior to test only as ordered. (Check with physician.)
- Provide cathartic and enema (tap water or saline) the evening prior to procedure.

Following the Procedure

- See Barium Swallow.
- Resume medications as ordered.

- **VOIDING CYSTOURETHROGRAM**

KEY NURSING INTERVENTIONS

Preparation

- Catheterize patient as ordered.
- Give clear liquid breakfast the morning of examination.
- Check for and document on front of chart allergies to iodine, seafood and contrast dyes. Notify Radiology of allergies.

Following the Procedure

- Monitor intake and output for 24 hrs.
- Document quality of urine for 24 hrs.
- Force fluids unless contraindicated.
- Observe for delayed allergic reaction.
- Assess patient for signs and symptoms of urinary tract infection: Dysuria, cloudy urine, frequency, fever.

C. CAT SCAN

KEY NURSING INTERVENTIONS

Preparation

- Maintain NPO only as per policy or doctor's orders (frequently 4 hrs. prior to test).
- Obtain written consent.
- Check for and document on front of chart allergies to iodine, seafood, and contrast dyes. Notify Radiology of allergies.
- Explain the importance of lying perfectly still during the procedure.

Following the Procedure

- Observe incision area for hemorrhage if contrast was used.
- Observe patient for delayed allergic reactions.
- Encourage fluids to eliminate contrast unless contraindicated.

D. NUCLEAR MEDICINE

• BONE SCAN

KEY NURSING INTERVENTIONS

- Instruct patient to force fluids after injection of tracer and until scan is done.
- Nursing personnel should wear gloves when handling urine after injection is given.

• CISTERNOGRAM OR RADIOISOTOPE MYELOGRAM

KEY NURSING INTERVENTIONS

- See Myelogram.

• GALLIUM-67 SOFT TISSUE IMAGING SCAN

KEY NURSING INTERVENTIONS

- Maintain stool precautions post scan.

• LUNG SCAN

KEY NURSING INTERVENTIONS

- Check for and document on front of chart allergy to technetium. Notify Nuclear Medicine if present.

• RADIOISOTOPE CHOLANGIOGRAM (PIPIDA)

KEY NURSING INTERVENTIONS

- No food may be eaten 2 hrs. prior to test per policy.
- Maintain stool precautions post scan.

• RENAL FLOW DTPA

KEY NURSING INTERVENTIONS

- Maintain urine precautions post scan.

- **RENOGRAM**

KEY NURSING INTERVENTIONS

- Hold antihypertensives as ordered by physician.
- Maintain urine precautions post scan.

- **THALLIUM REST TEST**

KEY NURSING INTERVENTIONS

- No food may be eaten after evening meal prior to test per policy or doctor's orders.
- Patient may have fluids.

- **THALLIUM STRESS TEST**

KEY NURSING INTERVENTIONS

- No alcohol or smoking is allowed 24 hrs. prior to test.
- A light breakfast may be given prior to test or NPO per policy or doctor's orders.

- **THYROID SCAN WITH I-131**

KEY NURSING INTERVENTIONS

- No food may be eaten prior to ingestion of capsule.
- Patient may have fluids.
- Maintain urine precautions post scan.

- **THYROID SCAN WITH TECHNETIUM-99m**

KEY NURSING INTERVENTIONS

- Maintain urine precautions post scan.

E. ULTRASOUND

- **GALLBLADDER AND BILIARY ULTRASOUND**

KEY NURSING INTERVENTIONS

Preparation

- Order fat-free meal the evening prior to test.

- No food may be eaten after evening meal.
- NPO after midnight prior to test.

Following the Procedure

- Cleanse remaining lubricant from skin.
- Observe injection site for hemorrhage if sincalide was given.

• LIVER/SPLEEN/PANCREAS ULTRASOUND

KEY NURSING INTERVENTIONS

Preparation

- NPO after evening meal per policy or doctor's orders.

Following the Procedure

- Cleanse remaining lubricant from skin.

• PELVIC ULTRASOUND

KEY NURSING INTERVENTIONS

Preparation

- Force fluids to fill bladder.
- Instruct patient not to void.
- Inform patient that during the procedure a tap water enema and/or catheterization may be necessary. (Explain these procedures to patient.)

Following the Procedure

- Cleanse remaining lubricant from skin.
- Allow patient to void.

F. ENDOSCOPY

• COLONOSCOPY

KEY NURSING INTERVENTIONS

Preparation

- Provide clear liquid diet as ordered (usually 48 hrs. prior to procedure).

- Cleanse bowel per hospital routine (laxatives and water or sodium biphosphate enemas).
- Obtain written consent.
- Inform patient that "gas" pains are normal during the procedure.

Following the Procedure

- Observe for signs of bowel perforation: Malaise, rectal bleeding, abdominal pain and distention.
- Check vital signs every 30 mins. $\times$ 4, then every 4 hrs. $\times$ 24 hrs.

• ENDOSCOPIC RETROGRADE CHOLANGIOPANCREATICOGRAPHY (ERCP)

KEY NURSING INTERVENTIONS

Preparation

- No food after evening meal prior to test.
- Obtain written consent.
- Check for and document on front of chart allergies to iodine, seafood, and contrast dyes. Notify Radiology of allergies.

Following the Procedure

- Observe for signs and symptoms of bacteremia: Fever, chills, hypotension, upper left quadrant pain. Report to physician if present.

• ESOPHAGOGASTRODUODENOSCOPY

KEY NURSING INTERVENTIONS

Preparation

- Maintain NPO as ordered (usually 12 hrs. prior to test).
- Administer pre-test medications as ordered (usually atropine sulfate).
- Obtain written consent.
- Remove dentures and glasses.
- Inform patient that test will not be painful but may be uncomfortable due to gagging. Speech will not be possible when the tube is passed.

Following the Procedure

- Check vital signs every 15 mins. $\times$ 4, then every 4 hrs. $\times$ 24 hrs.

- Observe for signs of perforation: Pain with swallowing, neck movements, respirations, torso movements in back and abdomen, dyspnea, and cyanosis.

- Maintain NPO until gag reflex returns.

• PROCTOSIGMOIDOSCOPY

KEY NURSING INTERVENTIONS

Preparation

- Maintain clear liquid diet without fruit juices (usually 48 hrs. prior to procedure).

- Patient may have a light breakfast the morning of the test.

- Administer bowel preparation as ordered (usually tap water or sodium biphosphate enemas).

- Obtain written consent.

- Assist patient to knee-chest or left lateral Sims position.

- Assemble equipment including specimen containers (culture tubes, slides with jar containing 95% ethyl alcohol, and a jar with 10% formalin).

Following the Procedure

- If specimen was taken, observe for excessive bleeding. Monitor vital signs every 30 mins. × 4, then every 4 hrs. × 24 hrs.

- Observe for signs of bowel perforation (see Colonoscopy).

G. MISCELLANEOUS PROCEDURES

• ANGIOGRAPHY, CEREBRAL

KEY NURSING INTERVENTIONS

Preparation

- See Angiography/Venography.

- Obtain baseline vital signs, neurologic checks, and level of consciousness.

Following the Procedure

- Do neurologic checks with vital signs every 15 mins. × 4, then every 1 hr. × 4, and then every 4 hrs. × 24 hrs.

- Observe for complications associated with use of carotid artery and report to physician: Dysphagia, respiratory insufficiency, disorientation, weakness and numbness in extremities, transient ischemic attack.
- If femoral artery is used, keep affected leg straight for 12 hrs. Check temperature, color, sensation, and pulse for signs of occlusion.
- If brachial artery is used, keep affected arm immobile for 12 hrs. Check temperature, color, sensation, and pulses in extremity for signs of occlusion.
- Maintain absolute bed rest for 12–24 hrs. or as ordered.

• ANGIOGRAPHY/VENOGRAPHY

KEY NURSING INTERVENTIONS

Preparation

- Maintain NPO as ordered.
- Obtain written consent.
- Check for and document on front of chart allergies to iodine, seafood, and contrast dyes. Notify Radiology of allergies.
- Administer pre-procedure medications as ordered.

Following the Procedure

- Observe incision area for hemorrhage. Apply pressure should bleeding occur. (Sandbags may be used.)
- Check temperature, color, sensation, and pulse in affected extremity for signs of occlusion.
- Observe patient for delayed allergic reactions.
- Observe extremity for signs of infection: Redness, swelling, pain, tenderness.
- Maintain activity restrictions as ordered (usually 12 hrs.).
- Encourage fluids unless contraindicated.

• ARTHROGRAM

KEY NURSING INTERVENTIONS

Preparation

- Maintain NPO as ordered only.
- Check for and document on front of chart allergies to local anesthetics, contrast dyes, iodine and seafood. Notify Radiology of allergies.

- Obtain written consent.
- Shave and prepare areas only as ordered.

Following the Procedure

- Maintain joint rest for 12 hrs. or as ordered.
- Apply ice to joint unless contraindicated.
- Observe for increased swelling and crepitation 1–2 days post procedure and report to physician.
- Observe patient for delayed allergic reactions.
- Support affected extremity on a pillow.
- Observe for signs of infection.
- Medicate for pain.

• ELECTROENCEPHALOGRAPHY

KEY NURSING INTERVENTIONS

Preparation

- Hold medications only as ordered. (Usually anticonvulsants, barbiturates and tranquilizers are held 5 hrs. prior to test).
- For a sleep electroencephalogram, limit sleeping time to 4–5 hrs. the night prior to test.
- If test is done in patient's room, keep a padded tongue blade and oral airway at bedside.
- Have patient wash his/her hair the evening prior to test.

Following the Procedure

- Check with physician about resuming medications that were previously held.
- Wash patient's hair.

• THERMOGRAPHY—CERVICAL/THORACIC/LUMBAR

KEY NURSING INTERVENTIONS

Preparation

- Instruct patient not to smoke 4–6 hrs. prior to procedure.

Following the Procedure

- Patient may resume smoking.

• PNEUMOPLETHYSMOGRAPHY

KEY NURSING INTERVENTIONS

Preparation

- Remove contact lenses.
- Administer eye drops as ordered.

Following the Procedure

- Instruct patient not to rub eyes or wear contact lenses for 2 hrs. post procedure or as otherwise ordered.
- Observe for signs of corneal abrasion: Complaints of pain and photophobia.

H. SPECIAL PROCEDURES

ABDOMINAL PARACENTESIS

POTENTIAL PROBLEMS

Shock   Hepatic Coma (in Liver
Infection   Disease)
Hypovolemia   Psychosocial Problems

KEY NURSING INTERVENTIONS

Preparation

- Obtain written consent.
- Check for and document on front of chart the patient's allergies to local anesthetics and sedatives.
- Explain procedure to the patient.
- Order equipment (paracentesis tray, sterile gloves, drapes, local anesthetics, abdominal binder, skin prep tray, specimen bottles, collection bottle or bucket). Set up equipment using aseptic technique.
- Have patient void prior to procedure.
- Obtain baseline vital signs.

Procedure

- Assist patient to position as desired by physician, which may be one of the following: Fowler's or sitting on edge of bed with feet and arms supported on overbed table.
- Assist physician in preparing patient and organizing equipment.
- Check vital signs during procedure. Observe for signs of shock: Hypotension; tachycardia; pallor; weak, thready pulse; tachypnea.
- Stay near patient to provide reassurance and support. Keep patient informed of what is happening.
- Apply sterile dressing over needle site.

Following the Procedure

- Check vital signs every 15 mins. × 4, then every hour × 4, then every 4 hrs. × 24 hrs. or as ordered.

- Observe abdomen for leakage from insertion site, subcutaneous emphysema, and scrotal edema when checking vital signs and PRN.

- Document volume of fluid removed along with description of color and viscosity.

- Assist patient to position of comfort and maintain bedrest as ordered.

- Send specimens to laboratory (see Specimen Collection).

- Observe for signs and symptoms of infection: Fever; abdominal pain; purulent drainage, redness, and tenderness at puncture site.

- Observe for signs and symptoms of hypovolemia: Tachycardia; cool, moist skin; pallor; cyanosis; weak, thready pulse; hypotension; oliguria; postural hypotension; low CVP; decreased level of consciousness.

BONE MARROW ASPIRATION AND BIOPSY

POTENTIAL PROBLEMS

Hemorrhage   Pain
Infection   Psychosocial Problems
Injury to organs beneath
  bone

KEY NURSING INTERVENTIONS

Preparation

- Explain procedure to the patient.

- Obtain a written consent.

- Obtain necessary equipment: Bone marrow aspiration or biopsy needles, syringes, skin prep, 1% lidocaine, sterile towels, sterile gloves. Check with laboratory for specimen collection containers.

- Check chart to be sure coagulation studies have been completed, i.e., prothrombin time, partial thromboplastin time, platelet count, blood type and crossmatch. Check laboratory values for abnormal results and notify physician.

- Assess and support the patient's psychosocial needs. This can be a frightening experience. Reassure the patient that you will be there during the procedure. The physician may order a sedative if the patient is too anxious or uncooperative.

- Obtain baseline vital signs.

Procedure

- Place the patient in the appropriate position depending upon biopsy sight, i.e., sternum, iliac crest, lumbar vertebrae.

- Assist the physician in preparing the puncture site and organizing the equipment. Maintain aseptic technique.

- Stay with the patient during the procedure. Instruct patient not to move, which could cause injury to organs underneath the bone.

- After the physician has removed the needle, place a sterile dressing over the puncture site and apply firm direct pressure.

- Keep the patient on bed rest for 24 hours or as instructed by the physician.

Following the Procedure

- Take vital signs frequently.
- Send specimens to laboratory as soon as possible.
- Observe for signs and symptoms of hemorrhage: Blood-soaked dressings, hematoma over bone area, pain, diaphoresis, increased pulse, cyanosis, decreased blood pressure, agitation, restlessness.

BRONCHOSCOPY

POTENTIAL PROBLEMS

Airway Obstruction	Arrhythmia
Laryngeal Spasm	Trachea Perforation
Bronchospasm	Pneumonia
Pneumothorax	Sore Throat
Hemorrhage	Psychosocial Problems
Pain	

KEY NURSING INTERVENTIONS

Preparation

- Prepare patient for surgery (see Preoperative Care).
- Obtain written consent.
- Have patient void prior to procedure.
- Record baseline vital signs and respiratory assessment.
- Document all allergies on front of chart.
- Reinforce explanation of procedure.

Following the Procedure

- Prevent postoperative complications (see Postoperative Care).
- Assess respiratory system with postoperative vital signs.
- Observe for signs and symptoms of airway obstruction: Stridor, panic, agitation, decreased breath sounds, cyanosis, tachypnea, tachycardia, decreased tidal volume, use of accessory respiratory muscles.
- Keep working suction equipment at bedside.
- Keep oral and nasal airways available.
- Maintain semi-Fowler's position for conscious patient.
- Maintain side-lying position with elevated head for unconscious patient.
- Keep emergency tracheostomy tray at bedside × 24 hrs.
- Maintain NPO until gag reflex returns and as ordered (usually 2 to 6 hrs.).

- Report unrelieved bronchospasm to physician.
- Assess patient for signs and symptoms of pneumothorax: Sudden, severe chest pain; dyspnea; tachypnea; tachycardia; diminished or absent breath sounds; hyperresonance on affected side.
- Observe for signs and symptoms of trachea perforation: Subcutaneous emphysema, around neck and face, dyspnea.
- Observe sputum for frank bleeding. Slight blood-streaked sputum is normal for several hours.
- Provide ice collar to reduce pain.

CARDIAC CATHETERIZATION

POTENTIAL PROBLEMS

Myocardial Infarction	Thrombophlebitis
Arrhythmias	Bleeding at Injection
Cardiac Tamponade	Site
Pneumothorax	Anaphylaxis
Pain	Psychosocial Problems

KEY NURSING INTERVENTIONS

Preparation

- See Preoperative Care.
- Obtain written consent.
- Check for patient allergies, especially to dyes, iodine and seafood. Document per hospital procedure.
- Patients are usually NPO for 8 hrs. prior to procedure or as ordered.
- Document baseline vital signs, height, weight.
- Assess all peripheral pulses and document quality (see Vital Sign Assessment, Pulse).
- Reinforce explanation of procedure and clarify any questions. Inform family or significant other of waiting area location.
- Assess and support psychosocial needs. Inform patient that a local anesthetic will be used and that he/she should experience little pain. Emphasize the importance of patient cooperation in following physician instructions to hold breath and cough. Tell patient that the procedure will be done on a special table that will turn patient laterally at various times.

Following the Procedure

- See Postoperative Care.
- Monitor vital signs frequently as ordered and PRN. Assess for arrhythmias and hypotension and report immediately to physician.
- Observe for bleeding at the puncture site. If bleeding occurs, apply pressure and notify physician. Occasionally, a sandbag will be placed on site for several hours.

- Assess peripheral pulses and compare to pre-procedure baseline. Report diminished or absent pulses which were previously present.

- Usually patient is kept on strict bed rest for 12 hrs. post procedure. If the groin was used as access site, keep affected leg straight at groin. If arm was used, keep affected arm immobilized as ordered.

- Discuss with physician the use of warm moist compresses to relieve pain at puncture site.

- Observe for signs and symptoms of pneumothorax: Sudden, severe chest pain; dyspnea; tachypnea; tachycardia; diminished or absent breath sounds; hyperresonance on affected side.

- Assess affected extremity for signs and symptoms of thrombophlebitis: Tenderness and redness over affected vein, edema, cyanosis, mottling, diminished pulses, positive Homans' sign (pain in calf with dorsiflexion of foot) in affected extremity.

- Observe for signs and symptoms of myocardial infarction: Steady, severe chest pain unrelieved by nitrates; diaphoresis; pallor; hypotension; dyspnea; nausea; vomiting; tachycardia or bradycardia; anxiety.

- Observe for signs and symptoms of cardiac tamponade: Decreased systolic pressure, narrow pulse pressure; tachycardia; pulses paradoxus (pulse becomes weaker during inspiration); distant heart sounds; dyspnea; orthopnea; cyanosis; restlessness; diaphoresis; distended neck veins. Report immediately to physician.

LAPAROSCOPY

POTENTIAL PROBLEMS

Hemorrhage   Post Anesthesia Problems
Infection   Pain
Perforated Viscus   Psychosocial Problems
Mild Metabolic Acidosis

KEY NURSING INTERVENTIONS

Preparation

- See Preoperative Care.
- Explain procedure to patient.
- Obtain a written consent.
- Ascertain whether the patient has any allergies to medications and document on front of chart.
- Keep the patient NPO for 8–12 hrs. prior to procedure.
- Have the patient void prior to procedure.
- Obtain baseline vital signs.
- Assess and support the patient's psychosocial needs. Since this procedure often involves visualization of the reproductive organs, the patient will probably be very anxious. Provide reassurance and attempt to clarify any questions the patient may have.

Following the Procedure

- See Postoperative Care.
- Take vital signs frequently.
- Observe for signs and symptoms of hemorrhage: Blood-soaked dressings, abdominal pain, shoulder pain, diaphoresis, cool skin, increased pulse, decreased blood pressure, agitation, restlessness, firm abdomen.
- Observe for signs and symptoms of perforated viscus: Abdominal pain, guarding, firm abdomen, decreased bowel sounds, fever, shock.
- Observe for signs and symptoms of metabolic acidosis (see Arterial Blood Gases). Depending on what is to be performed, the surgeon may

inject 3 to 4 liters of CO_2 into the abdominal cavity for better visualization. If a significant amount of CO_2 is retained post procedure, the patient may have mild acidosis.

LIVER BIOPSY

POTENTIAL PROBLEMS

Hemorrhage   Pain
Peritonitis   Psychosocial Problems
Pneumothorax

KEY NURSING INTERVENTIONS

Preparation

- Explain procedure to patient.

- Obtain a written consent.

- Obtain necessary equipment: Liver biopsy needle, syringe, 1% lido-caine, skin prep, sterile towels or drape, dressings, sterile gloves, extra pillow. Check with laboratory for specimen collection containers.

- Check the chart to be sure coagulation studies have been completed, i.e., prothrombin time, partial thromboplastin time, platelet count, blood type and crossmatch. Patients with liver conditions may have a tendency to bleed. Check laboratory values for abnormal results and notify physician.

- Keep the patient NPO in case surgery is indicated post procedure.

- Practice special breathing technique used in the procedure: Inhalation, exhalation, then holding the breath for 15 secs.

- Administer sedatives 30–60 mins. pre procedure as ordered.

- Assess and support the patient's psychosocial needs. This can be a frightening experience. Reassure the patient that you will be there during the procedure. Explain that with the patient's cooperation, there is little risk of complications. If the patient is too anxious or uncooperative, notify the physician. The procedure may have to be cancelled to avoid injury.

- Obtain baseline vital signs.

Procedure

- Assist the patient to position desired by physician, which may be supine or left lateral position with right arm abducted.

- Assist the physician in preparing the puncture site and organizing the equipment. Maintain aseptic technique.
- The physician will instruct the patient when to inhale and exhale, then to hold his/her breath. The biopsy needle will then be inserted and removed. This will take 5 to 10 secs. Stay with the patient and provide reassurance.
- After the physician has removed the needle, place a sterile dressing over the puncture site.
- Place the patient in a right lateral position with a pillow under side to control bleeding. Instruct the patient to remain there for two hours. Bed rest should be maintained for 12 hrs.

Following the Procedure

- Take vital signs frequently.
- Send specimens to the laboratory as soon as possible.
- Observe for signs and symptoms of pneumothorax: Shortness of breath, chest pain, decreased breath sounds unilaterally, tachypnea, tachycardia.
- Observe for signs and symptoms of hemorrhage: Blood-soaked dressings, abdominal pain, shoulder pain, diaphoresis, increased pulse, cyanosis, decreased blood pressure, agitation, restlessness.
- Observe for signs and symptoms of peritonitis: Abdominal pain, fever, nausea, vomiting, shortness of breath, tenderness, firm abdomen.

LUMBAR PUNCTURE

POTENTIAL PROBLEMS

Respiratory Failure	Infection
Damage of Intervertebral Disk	Headache
	Bleeding
Leakage of Cerebrospinal Fluid	Brain Herniation
	Psychosocial Problems

KEY NURSING INTERVENTIONS

Preparation

- Obtain written consent.

- Obtain baseline vital signs and neurological assessment.

- Explain the importance of patient cooperation in positioning. Inform patient of side-lying position with knees pulled toward chin.

- Have patient void prior to procedure.

- Prepare necessary equipment before procedure: Lumbar puncture set; preparation solution; sterile gloves, Xylocaine, 1–2% with and without epinephrine, syringe, 25-gauge needle, medications as ordered.

- Maintain aseptic technique in setting up equipment.

- Assess and support patient's psychosocial needs. Inform patient that the injection of anesthetic may be a little painful and that during the procedure he/she may experience the feeling of pressure and possibly some brief pain down the legs or in the hips. Emphasize that this is normal and that cooperation in maintaining correct positioning is essential.

Procedure

- Position patient laterally with back near edge of the bed. Place a pillow under head. Assist patient in bringing knees up to the chest and flexing the head as much as possible.

- Communicate with patient during procedure to reduce anxiety. Promote relaxation by talking calmly and reassuring patient frequently. Be near patient.

Following the Procedure

- Apply sterile dressing to puncture site.
- Return patient to supine position with head flat. Keep head flat as ordered (usually 12–24 hrs.) and on strict bed rest.
- Instruct patient in the importance of recumbency in preventing headache.
- Take specimens to laboratory *immediately*. Assure tubes are labelled with correct sequence (No. 1, No. 2, No. 3, etc.) and patient identification. If infectious pathogens are suspected in cerebrospinal fluid, take isolation precautions in handling tubes and label appropriately.
- Obtain vital signs and document patient's response to procedure.
- Observe for signs of herniation by monitoring vital signs and neurologic checks frequently. Report respiratory difficulty, changes in motor function, pupillary reactions, and loss of consciousness immediately to physician.

RENAL BIOPSY

POTENTIAL PROBLEMS

Hemorrhage   Pain
Infection   Psychosocial Problems
Pneumothorax

KEY NURSING INTERVENTIONS

Preparation

- Explain procedure to the patient.

- Obtain a written consent.

- Contact radiology department for scheduling and arranging the necessary equipment if appropriate. Renal biopsies are usually done under fluroscopy for better visualization.

- Check the chart for completion of appropriate laboratory studies, i.e., prothrombin time, partial thromboplastin time, platelet count, blood type and crossmatch, blood urea nitrogen, creatinine, urinalysis, urine cultures. Check laboratory values for abnormal results and notify physician.

- Keep the patient NPO in case surgery is indicated post procedure.

- Inform patient that he/she may have to hold his/her breath when needle is inserted.

- Assess and support the patient's psychosocial needs. Reassure the patient that this is a safe procedure and that cooperation is necessary.

- Obtain baseline vital signs.

Procedure

- Assist the patient in assuming the prone position. A pillow or sandbag may be placed under the abdomen to help straighten the spine.

- Assist the physician in preparing the puncture site and organizing the equipment. Maintain aseptic technique.

- The physician will instruct the patient to hold his/her breath each time tissue samples are taken. Stay with the patient and provide reassurance.

- After the physician has removed the needle, place a sterile dressing over the puncture site and apply firm direct pressure.

Following the Procedure

- Leave the patient in a prone position for 30 mins. Maintain strict bed rest for 24 hrs. Instruct the patient to avoid strenuous activity for at least two weeks or as instructed by the physician.
- Take vital signs frequently.
- Send specimens to the laboratory as soon as possible.
- Encourage a liberal fluid intake of at least 3000 cc/day.
- Observe for signs and symptoms of hemorrhage: Blood-soaked dressings, progressive hematuria (a small amount of blood in the urine may be considered normal), flank pain, shoulder pain, diaphoresis, increased pulse, cyanosis, decreased blood pressure, agitation, restlessness.
- Observe for signs and symptoms of pneumothorax: Shortness of breath, chest pain, decreased breath sounds unilaterally, tachypnea, tachycardia.

SYNOVIAL FLUID ASPIRATION

POTENTIAL PROBLEMS

Infection   Psychosocial Problems
Pain

KEY NURSING INTERVENTIONS

Preparation

- Obtain written consent.

- Administer sedatives or analgesics as ordered.

- Check for and document on front of chart patient's allergies to local anesthetics, iodine and seafood.

- Reinforce explanation of the procedure.

- Obtain necessary equipment (usually spinal needle, syringes, alcohol swabs, iodophore prep, sterile saline). Order sterile specimen containers, tubes for culture, cytology, clot and glucose. Check with laboratory for required additives (usually EDTA or heparin for cytology, potassium oxalate for glucose, heparin for crystal).

- Have patient void prior to procedure.

- Prepare joint area as ordered.

Following the Procedure

- Observe for increasing swelling and crepitation 1 to 2 days post procedure and report to physician.

- Observe for signs and symptoms of infection: Redness, tenderness, edema, purulent drainage, fever.

- Maintain appropriate isolation if infection is suspected (see Isolation and Infection Control).

- Support affected limb on pillow.

- Maintain joint rest for 12 hrs. or as ordered.

- Apply ice to affected joint for 24–48 hrs. unless contraindicated.

THORACENTESIS

POTENTIAL PROBLEMS

Shock	Infection
Pain	Pneumothorax
Tension Pneumothorax	Psychosocial Problems
Mediastinal Shift	

KEY NURSING INTERVENTIONS

Preparation

- Explain procedure to patient.
- Obtain written consent.
- Check for and document on front of chart allergies to local anesthetics and sedatives.
- Order equipment (thoracentesis tray, local anesthetics, 50-cc syringe, 17-gauge aspirating needle, three-way stopcock, sterile tubing, hemostats, sterile specimen tube and collection container, sterile towels, skin prep, sterile dressing).
- Have patient void prior to procedure.
- Obtain baseline vital signs and respiratory assessment.

Procedure

- Assist patient to position desired by physician which may be one of the following:

  Sitting on edge of bed, feet supported on stool and arms supported on bedtable; lying in bed with head of bed elevated 30 to 45 degrees; sitting in chair backwards with arms supported on back of chair.

- Assist physician in preparing puncture site and organizing equipment. Maintain aseptic technique.
- Stay with the patient to provide reassurance and support. Keep patient informed of what is happening.
- Check vital signs during procedure.

- Observe patient for the following:

  Pallor, cyanosis, weakness, diaphoresis, tachypnea, chills, coughing, nausea. Report to physician.

- Apply sterile pressure dressing over puncture site.

Following the Procedure

- Check vital signs every 15 mins. $\times$ 4, then every hour $\times$ 4 and then every 4 hrs. $\times$ 24 hrs. or as ordered. Assess chest sounds with vital signs.

- Send specimens to laboratory (see Specimen Collection). If infection is suspected, take isolation precautions.

- Assist patient to position of comfort. (Usually patient is positioned to recumbent with puncture side up to prevent seepage.)

- Observe for signs and symptoms of shock: Hypotension; weak, rapid, thready pulse; tachypnea; pallor; cool, moist skin.

- Assess patient for signs and symptoms of pneumothorax: Sudden, severe chest pain; dyspnea; tachypnea; tachycardia; diminished or absent breath sounds; hyperresonance on affected side.

- Observe for signs and symptoms of reaccumulation of fluid: Hemoptysis, persistent coughing, dyspnea, cyanosis, subcutaneous emphysema.

- Assess patient for mediastinal shift: Cardiac distress, pulmonary edema.

- Monitor patient for signs and symptoms of infection: Fever, pleuritic pain, purulent drainage, redness and tenderness at puncture site.

- Observe for fluid and electrolyte imbalances (see Fluid and Electrolytes).

- Observe for signs and symptoms of tension pneumothorax: Decreased breath sounds unilaterally, tachypnea, chest pain, shortness of breath, tracheal deviation, distended neck veins, hypotension.

APPENDIX A

PATIENT EDUCATION

Patient education is one of the msot responsible functions of nursing. The nurse must be a good communicator, have knowledge of the subject matter, and understand the basic mechanisms of learning in order to be effective. This section presents a review of patient education guidelines in order to enhance the nurse's teaching skills.

I. PRIOR TO INSTRUCTION

A. Learning Barriers

1. Assess the patient for possible learning barriers

    a) High anxiety due to illness or other personal and/or social problems. (The acute stage of illness is a poor time to begin teaching.)

    b) The environment (lack of privacy, noise, room temperature, etc.).

    c) Mental, physical or emotional handicaps or inabilities (Attention span, memory, vision, hearing, coordination, etc.).

    d) Cultural barriers (language, customs, etc.).

    e) Educational background (intellectual abilities, reading skills, etc.).

    f) Past experiences.

    g) Socioeconomic class.

    h) Value systems.

    i) Attitudes related to illness.

    j) Lack of support systems. (Family, friends, significant others.)

2. Remove as many barriers within your control before beginning instruction.

B. Learning Needs Assessment

1. Assess what the patient desires to know.
2. Assess what the patient already knows about the subject.
3. Determine what the patient needs to know.

II. THE INSTRUCTION PROCESS

A. Plan

1. Establish goals with the patient based on what the patient *desires* to know and what the patient *needs* to know. Write these down for the patient to review periodically.
2. Arrange for significant others to be included in teaching sessions when possible.
3. Plan the order of information to be taught according to the needs of the patient. Begin with what the patient is most anxious about or desires most. This will remove barriers to learning other material.

B. Teach

1. Select a variety of methods and learning devices

   a) Written materials.
   b) Audiovisual aids.
   c) Discussion.
   d) Role models.
   e) Demonstrations.

2. Use language and terms the patient can understand.
3. Allow time for questions. Provide an open atmosphere that encourages the patient to ask questions.
4. If unsure of an answer to a question, tell the patient you are unsure but you will obtain the answer from a knowledgeable source.
5. Give the rationale behind the facts to increase understanding.
6. Restate information in different words if it is not understood.
7. Use other resources such as dieticians, pharmacists, etc.

8. Set time limits for each session to prevent overloading the patient with too much information. Short sessions lasting around 15 minutes are preferred.

9. Provide reading material suitable for the patient's reading ability.

10. Correct with kindness and gentleness.

11. Provide a list of referrals such as home health agencies, organizations, etc.

III. EVALUATING INSTRUCTIONS

To determine if the goals have been met, evaluate the patient's understanding of the instruction. Have the patient repeat the information presented, and give return demonstrations of skills taught.

IV. COMMUNICATION TO HEALTH CARE TEAM

A. Documentation

Document material taught and patient's response in the nurse's notes and on all teaching forms.

B. Verbal Communication

Communicate patient's progress and learning needs in report, case conferences, and physician conferences.

SAFETY

In the delivery of quality patient care, the nurse is responsible for protecting the patient, visitors, other hospital personnel and herself from harm. This section presents guidelines of safety practice related to drug administration, patient, nurse, environmental, radiation and electrical safety.

I. DRUG ADMINISTRATION SAFETY

A. Nursing Knowledge

Prior to the administration of medications, know the following facts for each drug:

1. Action.
2. Side effects.
3. Toxic effects.
4. Usual dosage.
5. Nomenclature.
6. Idiosyncratic and allergic reactions.
7. Interactions with other drugs.
8. Contraindications.

B. Drug Administration

Assure the following:

1. Right patient—Check identification bracelet and call patient by name before giving medications.
2. Right drug—Check the physician's order against the Kardex, medication sheet or card. Give medications that you alone or pharmacy has prepared. Read the label on the container before and after removing the medication. If a patient questions his/her medication, recheck the order.
3. Right dose—Calculate dosages carefully. If unsure, check with another nurse. If unusually small or large amounts of pills or volume must be given, recheck the dosage order and your calculations. Clarify order with physician if dosage ordered deviates from recommended dose in the *Physician's Desk Reference*.

4. Right route—Make sure the patient can tolerate prescribed route and that oral medications are swallowed.

5. Right time—Schedule medications so as to maximize therapeutic effects and minimize side effects. Check to see if medications should be withheld (i.e., diagnostic procedures).

6. Ascertain whether the patient has any allergies to medications. Ask the patient and check the chart.

C. Errors

Report all medication errors to the physician and nursing supervisor.

D. Documentation

Record time and location of IM medications. Document patient response to therapy, such as PRN medications or adverse reactions.

E. Patient Education

Prior to discharge, teach patient and family the following: Proper administration techniques, prescribed times, action of drug, and importance of reporting adverse reactions to the physician.

II. PATIENT SAFETY

A. Orientation

Orient patient and/or significant others to all aspects of the hospital room on admission.

B. Identibands

Check for accuracy of spelling and patient number. Identification bands must be worn at all times.

C. Nurse Call Buttons

Place within the patient's reach at all times. Orient patient and family to emergency call buttons.

D. Activity Orders

Instruct the patient regarding activity orders and when NOT to attempt to get out of bed, i.e., after narcotic or hypnotic medications, postoperatively, etc.

E. Restraints

Document usage per hospital policy when necessary for the patient's safety. Observe restricted areas for discoloration, coldness, and irritation.

F. Beds

Keep in low position except when doing patient care. Keep brakes on at all times. Keep side-rails up per hospital policy and after analgesic or hypnotic medications, postoperatively, and if the patient is disoriented.

G. Transportation

Enter elevators and doorways with yourself at the patient's head. Transport patients on a gurney with straps fastened around patients and side-rails up at all times with extremities completely within the rails. Secure IV bottles to pole. Keep IV tubing and other tubing arranged to prevent dislodgement. Keep oxygen tanks stored under the gurney or on its side at the foot of the gurney next to the patient.

H. Bathroom Locks

Instruct patients never to lock bathroom locks.

I. Electrically-Sensitive Patient

Patients with electrodes, heart catheters, pacemakers and metal implants, electrolyte imbalances, moisture in bed or on the patient are electrically sensitive and their skin should be kept dry for protection.

J. Oxygen Therapy

Check flow rate as ordered q 8 hrs. When using a mask, flow should not be less than 6 liters/min. Document flow q 8 hrs. Check humidifier for proper functioning and water level q 8 hrs. Reposition mask or cannula q 2 hrs. Note reddened areas and prevent further pressure. Post "NO SMOKING" signs. Keep flammable materials away from oxygen tank and containers. Monitor arterial blood gas values.

K. Infections

Wash hands before and after each patient contact to prevent cross contamination (see Infection Control).

III. NURSE SAFETY

A. Breaking Ampules

Protect your fingers by covering the tip with gauze or alcohol wipe.

B. Doors and Drawers

Keep closed when not in use.

C. Gatch Handles

Turn protruding handles inward.

D. Sterilizers

Turn off steam and allow excess steam to escape before opening sterilizer.

E. Phone Orders

Read the physician orders back to the physician before proceeding.

F. Unlabeled Bottles

Do not use the contents of unlabeled bottles. Identify contents or discard.

G. Medicine Cabinet

Keep locked at all times when not in use.

H. Narcotics

Keep stored under lock and key. Sign out narcotics as you use them.

I. Body Mechanics

Follow principles of body mechanics when lifting or transferring patients or equipment.

1. Explain to the patient your intention to change his/her position.

2. Use judgment as to the size of person or object to be moved beforehand. Call for assistance if necessary.

3. Check your footing; keep legs apart for a broad base of support.

4. Get as close to person or object as possible.

5. Keep back straight with knees and hips bent.

6. Use thigh muscles to lift.

7. Divide weight between two hands.

8. Bring weight up against your body.

9. Lift smoothly; avoid jerking; count with partner.

10. When possible, push or pull and avoid lifting.

11. Shift position to turn; *never* twist your body.

IV. ENVIRONMENTAL SAFETY

A. Fire

Know the location of fire alarms, extinguishers, and escape routes. Report fires per hospital procedure. In case of fire, remove patients from involved room, isolate fire, close all doors, and turn off medical gas valves.

B. Smoking

No smoking near oxygen or nitrous oxide equipment. Visitors and hospital personnel should follow hospital smoking policies.

C. Oxygen Therapy

Post an "OXYGEN—NO SMOKING" sign where in use. Store oxygen tanks in their carriages. Do not use oil, grease, or alcohol on oxygen or nitrous oxide equipment. Check oxygen supply in tanks frequently. Open cylinders slowly. Close valve when not in use. Keep electrical equipment away from and out of oxygen tents.

D. Windows

Keep windows locked per hospital policy. Report abnormalities.

E. Spills

Report spills to housekeeping and wipe up immediately.

F. Breakage and Sharps

Dispose of broken glass and needles in appropriate containers. Do not cover knives and sharp instruments with cloths or papers; place in appropriate receptacle.

V. RADIATION SAFETY—IMPLANTS

A. Alert

Post a "RADIATION PRECAUTION" sign where in use.

B. Room

Patients receiving radiation therapy from implants should have private rooms, preferably at the farthest end of the hall and adjacent to an empty room, or near patients beyond childbearing age.

C. Pregnancy

Pregnant women should not care for these patients or be allowed in the room.

D. Time

Limit time spent in the room by nurses and visitors according to physician and hospital policy.

E. Linen and Garbage

Label all materials that the patient has had contact with as radioactive.

F. Clearance

At the end of therapy, the room should be cleared by the responsible radiology inspector.

G. Distance

Distance from the radiation source is one of the most important aspects of minimizing exposure. Limit *time* spent in close proximity to the source. When conversing with the patient, stand *away* from the source.

VI. ELECTRICAL SAFETY

A. Hazards and Warning Signs

Report and discontinue use of any equipment with these warning signs:

1. Shock.
2. Frayed cords.
3. Broken wires.
4. Cracked receptacles or plugs.
5. Loose fitting or tight plugs.
6. Unchecked equipment.

B. Cords

Do not drag cords through water or oil, over rough ground or sharp edges.

C. Electrical Noise

Report and discontinue use of equipment making unusual electrical noise.

D. Electrical Equipment

Place equipment in a secure place so it cannot be tipped or its cord tripped over.

CHARTING

The patient's chart is a tool used by all members of the health care team to plan and record patient care. The chart is also a legal tool used by the court to prove or disprove aspects pertaining to the nature and quality of patient care. It is therefore important that nurses' entries be significant and, above all, accurate. This section presents a review of charting guidelines to promote pertinent and legally sound documentation in nursing practice.

I. LEGIBILITY

For legality and clarity purposes, writing or printing legibly is a must.

II. ABBREVIATIONS

Use only those accepted by your hospital.

III. DOCUMENTATION

A. Entries

1. Use only ink (color per hospital policy).
2. Write the time and date with each entry.
3. Entries must be made per consecutive shifts and days.
4. Entries must be continuous, without blank lines between entries, and without spaces before signature. (Line through blank spaces before signatures.)
5. Document events after they have occurred. Do not document procedures to be done until they *have* been done.
6. Attempt to chart at the beginning of the shift while your memory is fresh.

B. Signature

Use your legal signature at the end of each entry: First initial, full last name, position (RN, LVN, etc.).

C. Content

1. Check uncertain spelling with a dictionary.

2. Chart obvious facts. Avoid use of "appears." Do not record conclusions or assumptions.

3. Describe behavior using descriptive terms to document observations. Chart what you see, hear, smell, and feel. Avoid labeling and use of judgmental words.

4. Document changes in the patient's condition.

5. Document follow-up interventions in response to patient's needs. Chart each step taken and all attempts to contact physicians. Document the reason a physician was phoned.

6. Document the patient's response to interventions and procedures.

7. Do not omit care given or observations made. Indicate that procedures were performed according to the hospital protocol.

8. The word "patient" is not necessary in charting.

9. Use medical terms you know the meaning of.

10. Document each time a physician visits the patient.

11. Information documented on other chart forms does not need to be repeated in the nurse's notes.

D. Errors

1. Never erase mistakes.

2. Note error by lining through it, writing "error" and initialing it.

3. Avoid errors by assuring you have the right chart before making entries.

4. Never destroy or modify notes previously written.

5. The patient's name must be on each record form.

TIME MANAGEMENT

Time is an element in great demand by nurses. Frequently, the plea is made about the lack of sufficient time needed to provide quality patient care. This section presents guidelines for time management related to hospital nursing. While not purporting to be a solution to all time-related matters in hospital nursing, they will assist the nurse in maximizing time for greater productivity.

I. BEGINNING THE SHIFT

A. Arrival

Arrive to work on time.

B. Report

Start report on time.

C. Rounds

1. When making initial rounds after report, set limits on time spent with each patient.

2. During initial rounds see those patients with the most serious conditions first along with fresh postoperative cases and proceed to the less serious.

D. Plan

1. Do not wait to make a plan. While making rounds, check the Kardex, care plan, and chart. Initiate a time chart organizational tool.

2. Use an organizational tool to plan nursing activities for the entire shift. Use the one provided (Figure 1) or adapt one. A plan should be made and written by the end of initial rounds.

3. Plan according to time. High priority times are the following: Surgery times; medication, IV, treatment, and vital sign times; and other ordered activities.

II. THROUGHOUT THE SHIFT

A. Flexibility

Be flexible. Expect the unexpected—the shift seldom goes as planned.

B. Activities

When possible, start chain reaction activities. For example, set up several self-bath patients prior to giving a complete bath to another patient.

C. Assistance

Ask for help when you need it.

D. Charting

Start charting early and keep up with it throughout the shift.

E. Free Time

Use free time wisely to do care plans, help co-workers, instruct patients.

III. ENDING THE SHIFT

Give report on time to help the next shift start on time. Report relevant information only. Avoid "chit chat" during report.

ROOM	MEDICATIONS (Hours)	TREATMENTS (Hours)	VITAL SIGNS (Hours)	IV's (Hours)

FIGURE 1

When making initial patient rounds, assess each chart or Kardex to obtain the necessary information for the organization tool. Record the time each activity is to be done. When each one is complete, cross out the time. Plan to use remaining time between these tasks for patient teaching, charting, planning patient care, etc.

Example:

ROOM	MEDICATIONS (Hours)	TREATMENTS (Hours)	VITAL SIGNS (Hours)	IV's (Hours)
321	~~9~~ ~~9~~ ~~9~~ 12 13 13 14	~~9~~ 12 14	~~8~~ 12	up 10:30
322	~~9~~ ~~10~~ 11	~~10~~ 14	~~8~~	
323	~~8~~ ~~8~~ ~~8~~ ~~8~~ ~~8~~		~~8~~	up 14:00
324	~~7:30~~ ~~8~~ ~~8~~ 13 13 13	~~8~~ 12 12	~~8~~ 12	
325		12	~~8~~	
326	~~8~~ ~~8~~ ~~8~~ 13 13	~~8~~ ~~10~~ 12	~~8~~ ~~10~~ 12 14	up 11:00

INTERVIEWING

The interviewing process in nursing care takes place daily in a variety of ways. The nurse interviews the patient on admission to obtain a profile, during rounds to obtain subjective information regarding the patient's condition and progress, at the start of patient education to determine barriers to learning and patient needs, and in any situation where meaningful communication is to take place. This section presents interviewing guidelines to assist nurses in conducting effective and meaningful interchanges with patients.

I. ATMOSPHERE

Provide an atmosphere that is quiet, without distractions or interruptions, and assures privacy.

II. COMMUNICATION

A. Interest

Encourage communication by conveying interest in the patient.

1. Introduce yourself to the patient, indicating your position.
2. State the purpose of the discussion.
3. Identify how the patient desires to be addressed.
4. Facial expressions convey your interest non-verbally.
5. Be relaxed and unhurried.
6. Sit during the interview.
7. Maintain eye contact.
8. Avoid excessive writing during the interview.

B. Clarity

Communicate so that the patient understands what you are saying.

1. Speak distinctly, clearly, and not too fast.
2. Use language and terms the patient can understand.
3. If it is necessary to repeat a question, reword it.

C. Spontaneity

Allowing the patient spontaneity will provide the most information.

1. Use open-ended questions that begin with what, where, when, why, who, and how (i.e., "What types of problems are you having?").

2. Allow patient to finish each sentence.

D. Open-ended Questions

Encourage patients having difficulty responding to open-ended questions.

1. Be silent for awhile.

2. Use nonverbal behavior such as facial expressions, posture, nodding the head, looking puzzled.

3. Use verbal responses, such as saying "Mmmmm" or "Yes," repeating what the patient has said, or ask clarifying questions (i.e., "Do you mean that . . .?").

4. Directly confront the patient by describing his/her verbal or nonverbal behavior (i.e., "You appear very uncomfortable talking about this.").

E. Nonverbal Communication

Observe the patient's nonverbal response. Does it match the verbal response?

F. Confrontation

Confront patient's behaviors to clarify their meaning.

G. Direct Questions

Use direct questions to obtain information not presented in the patient's spontaneous response.

H. Things to Avoid

1. Avoid asking personal questions before establishing a good relationship with the patient.

2. Avoid multiple choice questions.

ISOLATION AND INFECTION CONTROL

I. INTRODUCTION

A. Purpose

The purpose of isolation is to protect patients, visitors, and hospital personnel by preventing the spread of microorganisms.

B. Tips on Infection Control

1. Know how infection spreads. There are three essential elements: The source, a susceptible host, and a means of transmission for the organism.

2. There are four routes of transmission.

   a) *Contact*—direct, indirect, or droplet.

   b) *Vehicle*—contaminated food, water, drugs, or blood.

   c) *Airborne*—droplets or dust.

   d) *Vectorborne*—e.g., mosquito, tick, etc.

3. Handwashing is the most effective means of preventing the spread of pathogens.

4. Wash hands:

   a) Before and after each patient contact.

   b) After handling excretions (urine, feces).

   c) After handling secretions (wounds, respiratory, etc).

   d) Before invasive procedures.

5. When instituting isolation, remember that the pathogen is isolated, not the patient.

6. Explain the purpose and technique of specified isolation to the patient and family.

II. TYPES OF ISOLATION AND SPECIFICATIONS

(Source: *Guidelines for Prevention and Control of Nosocomial Infections,* U.S. Department of Health and Human Services, Public Health Service Centers for Disease Control July/August 1983.)

TYPES OF ISOLATION
AND SPECIFICATIONS

SPECIFICATIONS	ISOLATION TYPE						
	Strict	Contact	Respiratory	Tuberculosis (AFB)	Enteric	Drainage/Secretion	Blood/Body Fluid
Private Room with Door Closed*	X	X	X				
Private Room with Door Closed and Special Ventilation*				X			
Private Room if Hygiene is Poor*					X		X
Masks When Entering Room	X						
Masks When Close Patient Contact		X	X				
Masks if Patient is Coughing without Covering Mouth				X			
Gowns When Entering Room	X						

	1	2	3	4	5	6	7
Gowns if Soiling Likely		X			X	X	X
Gowns to Prevent Cross-Contamination by Clothing				X			
Gloves When Entering Room	X						
Gloves for Touching Infective Material		X			X	X	
Gloves for Touching Blood or Body Fluids							X
Articles Contaminated with Infective material to be Discarded or Bagged, Labeled, and Sent for Decontamination	X	X	X	X	X	X	X

For all types of isolation, hands must be washed before and after patient contact and contact with infective material and before next patient contact.

*Generally, patients with the same organism may share a room.

A. Diseases Requiring Strict Isolation

1. Pharyngeal diphtheria
2. Lassa fever and other viral hemorrhagic fever
3. Marburg virus
4. Pneumonic plague
5. Smallpox
6. Varicella (chicken pox)
7. Zoster (disseminated or localized in immunocompromised patients)

B. Diseases Requiring Contact Isolation

1. Acute respiratory infections in infants, children, and young children (e.g., croup, colds, bronchitis, bronchiolitis due to respiratory syncytial virus, adenovirus, coronavirus, influenza viruses, parainfluenza viruses, rhinovirus)
2. Gonococcal conjunctivitis in newborns
3. Cutaneous diphtheria
4. Endometritis, Group A Streptococcus
5. Furunculosis, staphylococcal in newborns
6. Disseminated herpes simplex, severe primary or neonatal
7. Impetigo
8. Influenza, in infants and young children
9. Multiply-resistant bacteria, infection, or colonization with any of the following:
   a) Gram-negative bacilli resistant to all aminoglycosides
   b) *Staphylococcus aureus* resistant to methicillin, nafcillin or oxacillin
   c) Pneumococcus resistant to penicillin
   d) *Hemophilus influenzae* resistant to ampicillin and chloramphenicol
   e) Other resistant bacteria of epidemiological significance
10. Pediculosis
11. Pharyngitis, infectious in infants and young children
12. Viral pneumonia in infants and young children

13. Pneumonia, *Staphylococcus aureus,* or Group A Streptococcus

14. Rabies

15. Rubella, congenital or other

16. Scabies

17. Scalded skin syndrome, staphylococcal (Ritter's disease)

18. Major skin, wound, or burn infection

19. Vaccinia

C. Diseases Requiring Respiratory Isolation

1. Epiglottis, *Hemophilus influenza*

2. Erythema infectiosum

3. Measles

4. Meningitis:

   —*Hemophilus influenza*

   —Meningococcal

5. Meningococcal pneumonia

6. Meningococcemia

7. Mumps

8. Pertussis

9. Pneumonia, *Hemophilus influenzae* in children

D. Tuberculosis (AFB) Isolation

This type of isolation is to be used for *pulmonary* tuberculosis and *laryngeal* tuberculosis.

E. Diseases Requiring Enteric Precautions

1. Amebic dysentery

2. Cholera

3. Coxsackievirus disease

4. Diarrhea (suspected infectious etiology with acute illness)

5. Echovirus

6. Encephalitis caused by enteroviruses

7. Enterocolitis caused by *Clostridium difficile* or *Staphylococcus aureus*

8. Enteroviral infection

9. Gastroenteritis caused by the following:

   a) *Campylobacter species*

   b) *Cryptosporidium species*

   c) *Dientamoeba fragilis*

   d) *Escherichia coli* (enterotoxic, enteropathogenic or enteroinvasive)

   e) *Giardia lamblia*

   f) *Salmonella species*

   g) *Shigella species*

   h) Vibrio

   i) Viruses

   j) *Yersinia enterocolitica*

   k) Presumed infectious agent with unknown etiology

   l) Hand, foot, and mouth disease

   m) Viral hepatitis, Type A

   n) Herpangina

   o) Viral meningitis caused by enteroviruses

   p) Necrotizing enterocolitis

   q) Pleurodynia

   r) Poliomyelitis

   s) Typhoid fever (*Salmonella typhi*)

   t) Viral pericarditis, myocarditis, meningitis caused by enteroviruses

F. Diseases Requiring Drainage/Secretion Precautions

Conditions in this category must *NOT* be multiply-resistant major infections or gonococcal eye infections in newborns for which contact isolation is required.

1. Minor or limited abscesses

2. Minor or limited burn infection

3. Conjunctivitis

4. Minor or limited infected decubitis ulcer

5. Minor or limited skin infection

6. Minor or limited wound infection

G. Diseases Requiring Blood/Body Fluid Precautions

1. AIDS (acquired immunodeficiency syndrome)
2. Arthropod-borne viral fevers (dengue, yellow fever, Colorado tick fever)
3. Babesiosis
4. Creutzfeldt-Jakob disease
5. Hepatitis B and HBsAg antigen carrier
6. Hepatitis, non-A, non-B
7. Leptospirosis
8. Malaria
9. Rat-bite fever
10. Relapsing fever
11. Syphilis, primary and secondary, with lesions on skin and mucous membranes

SPECIMEN COLLECTION GUIDELINES

I. GENERAL GUIDELINES

A. Data Collection

1. Check physician order for source and type of specimen to be collected.

2. Familiarize yourself with your hospital's specimen containers and collection aids.

3. Know your hospital's policies for collecting specimens without a physician's order.

4. Check with the laboratory if unsure of which culture media to use for a particular specimen.

5. Some specimens are obtained by the laboratory. Check your hospital policies.

B. Patient Communication

Always explain the procedure and reasons for obtaining specimens to the patient beforehand.

C. Infection Control

1. Use strict aseptic technique to protect the specimen, you, and the patient from contamination.

2. Use sterile containers and collection aids for all specimens to be cultured.

3. Secure container lids tightly.

4. Protect personnel handling specimens. Make sure outside of container is not contaminated. Place in clear plastic bag, if necessary, and seal.

D. Quality Assurance

1. Label all containers with patient's name, hospital number, room number, date, and time of collection.

2. Send all specimens to the laboratory *immediately* to assure accurate results.

3. Whenever possible, collect specimens *before* initiating antibiotic therapy.

4. Cultures should be done prior to gram stain unless contraindicated.

5. Assure that the laboratory has all necessary paperwork, orders, and patient information.

II. SPECIMEN COLLECTION

A. Wound Cultures

1. Use appropriate medium for aerobes and anaerobes.
2. Cleanse around wound to avoid contamination.
3. Swab wound drainage rather than pus.
4. Use sterile swab or needle and syringe.
5. Do not let specimen dry.

B. Sputum Cultures

1. Explain procedure to patient.
2. Obtain sputum, not saliva.
3. Collection may be easier in the morning or after a nebulization treatment.
4. Use suction with a sputum trap for patients unable to cooperate (comatose, intubated, lethargic, etc.).

C. Nasopharyngeal and Throat Cultures

1. Check order for site to be cultured.
2. Explain procedure to patient.
3. Have emesis basin at hand in case of gagging and vomiting.
4. Visualize throat with a light and tongue depressor. Swab the infected area while the patient says "ah."
5. Use equipment per hospital procedure to culture nasopharynx. Obtain culture by going through the nose or through the mouth and culturing above the uvula.
6. Do not allow the specimen to dry.

D. Blood Cultures

1. Follow orders for parameters, time intervals between, and number of specimens.
2. Have culture bottles on hand before withdrawing blood.

3. Cleanse injection site per hospital procedure.

4. Wear sterile gloves.

5. Ten ml of blood is usually adequate.

6. Inject 5 ml of blood into each of the aerobe and the anaerobe bottles.

7. Explain the purpose of multiple venipunctures and time intervals to the patient.

E. Urine Cultures

1. Clean-catch (midstream) urines are the easiest and safest means of collection.

2. Explain procedure to patient. Cooperation will determine the reliability of the specimen.

3. If the patient must be catheterized, obtain an order and follow strict aseptic technique.

4. If a catheter is in place, cleanse collection port and aspirate with a 10-cc syringe.

5. Latex catheters may be punctured to obtain the specimen after being cleansed. Do not puncture lumen leading to balloon.

6. Do not puncture silicone catheters.

7. Never collect urine from the bag.

8. Ileal conduits may be catheterized by physician's order.

F. Stool Cultures

1. Stool cultures need not be sterile and may be obtained from a clean bedpan.

2. The most reliable samples are obtained in the morning.

3. Use a tongue blade. For diarrhea, use a swab.

4. A sterile container is not necessary.

G. Vaginal Cultures

1. Since most vaginal cultures require a speculum to obtain, the physician will probably do the procedure.

2. Use appropriate culture media. Prepare to culture aerobic and anaerobic bacteria.

3. Prepare to do a smear if a gram stain is ordered.

4. Prepare to do a wet mount by obtaining a swab, test tube, and saline per hospital procedure.

H. Cerebrospinal Fluid

1. Prepare consent per hospital policy for lumbar puncture.

2. Strict asepsis is required in assisting the physician.

3. Most cerebrospinal fluid studies require at least three test tubes, each filled with 1–3 cc of fluid. Test Tube #1 should contain the initial fluid, and so on.

4. It is of utmost importance that these specimens get to the laboratory immediately so that pathogens do not die, and treatment may be initiated.

APPENDIX B

ANATOMICAL REFERENCES, MOVEMENTS, AND POSITIONS

I. ANATOMICAL REFERENCES

A. Superior

(Cranial)—Upper, toward the head.

B. Inferior

(Caudal)—Lower, away from the head.

C. Anterior

(Ventral)—Front.

D. Posterior

(Dorsal)—Back.

E. Medial

Toward the median plane of the body.

F. Lateral

Away from the median plane of the body.

G. Proximal

Toward the trunk of the body.

H. Distal

Away from the trunk of the body.

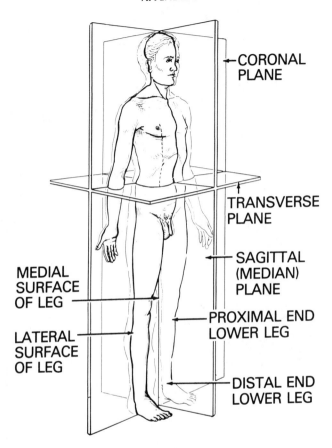

Anatomical References and Planes

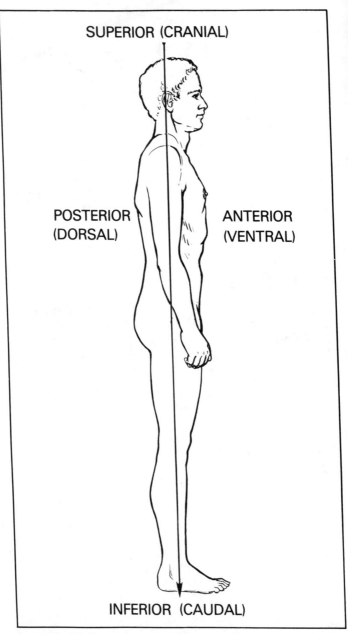

Anatomical References

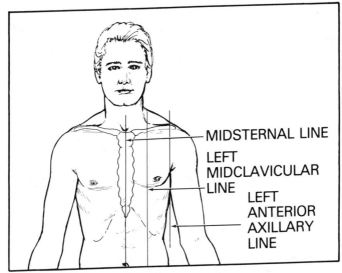

Anatomical References: Anterior

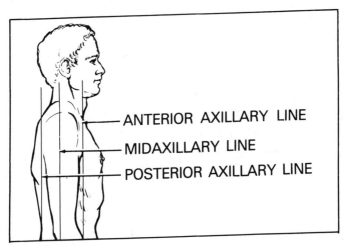

Anatomical References: Right Lateral

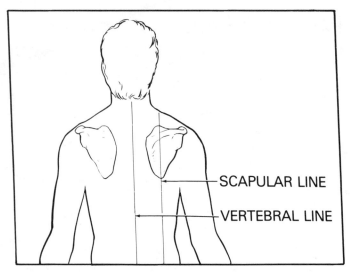

Anatomical References: Posterior

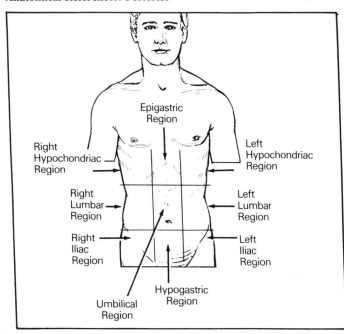

Anatomical References

II. ANATOMICAL MOVEMENTS

A. Adduction

Moving a limb or the head *toward* the median plane of the body. Moving the digits *toward* the median plane of the limb.

B. Abduction

Moving a limb or the head *away* from the median plane of the body. Moving the digits *away* from the median plane of the limb.

C. Extension

Moving a limb, the head or torso, into a straight position.

D. Hyperextension

Moving a limb, the head or torso, *beyond* the normal position of extension.

E. Flexion

The bending of any joint and the bending of the head and torso anteriorly.

F. Dorsiflexion

Bending backward. Moving the foot or hand *backward*.

G. Plantarflexion

Bending the foot *downward*, away from the head.

H. Pronation

Lying in a prone (face down) position. Turning the hand so that the palm faces downward.

I. Supination

Lying in a supine (face up) position. Turning the hand so that the palm faces up or turning the foot so that the sole faces up.

J. Rotation

Turning a body part on its axis.

K. Internal Rotation

Turning *toward* the center (inward).

L. External Rotation

Turning away from the center (outward).

III. ANATOMICAL POSITIONS

A. Erect

Standing position. Used to assess posture, body contours and the extremities.

B. Doral or Supine

Lying flat on the back with legs together and head supported. Used to assess abdomen, anterior chest, breasts, reflexes, extremities, head, neck, eyes, ears, nose, and throat.

C. Dorsal Recumbent

Lying on the back near the edge of the bed with legs separated and knees flexed and head supported. Used for rectal or vaginal examinations.

D. Lithotomy Position

Lying on the back with the buttocks near the bottom edge of the table, the knees flexed and in stirrups with the head supported. Used for digital rectal and vaginal examinations.

ABBREVIATIONS

NOTE: Each hospital varies in policy regarding approved abbreviations for charting. The following abbreviations are generally accepted; however, each hospital's policy must be observed for legality purposes.

@	at
AB	abortion
ABG	arterial blood gases
abd	abdominal, abdomen
a.c.	before meals
AD	right ear
ADA	American Diabetic Association
ad lib	as desired
AI	aortic insufficiency
am	before noon
AMA	against medical advice
amp	ampule
amt	amount
ant	anterior
AO	aorta
AP	anterior posterior
APC	aspirin, phenacitin, and caffeine citrate
approx	approximate
ARDS	adult respiratory distress syndrome
AROM	artificial rupture of membranes
AS	left ear
ASA	aspirin
ASAP	as soon as possible
ASHD	arteriosclerotic heart disease
AU	both ears
ax	axillary
Ba	barium
BE	barium enema

BFA	baby for adoption
bid	twice a day
BM	bowel movement
BOW	bag of water
BP	blood pressure
BPH	benign prostatic hypertrophy
BR	bedrest
br	bathroom
BRP	bathroom privileges
BSO	bilateral salpingo-oophorectomy
BUN	blood urea nitrogen
BX	biopsy
$\bar{c}$	with
ca	carcinoma
CAD	coronary artery disease
cal	calorie
CAN	cord around neck
caps	capsules
CAT	computerized axial tomography
cath	catheter
C/B	complete bath
CBC	complete blood count
CBG	capillary blood gas
cc	cubic centimeter
C/O	complains of
CHF	congestive heart failure
Circ	circumcision
Cl	chloride
cm	centimeter
CNS	central nervous system
COPD	chronic obstructive pulmonary disease
CPD	cephalopelvic disproportion
cpd	compound
CPR	cardiopulmonary resuscitation

C/S	Cesarean section
C&S	culture and sensitivity
CSF	cerebrospinal fluid
CVA	cerebrovascular accident
Cx	cervix
D.A.T.	diet as tolerated
D&C	dilatation and curettage
dc'd	discontinued
DOA	dead on arrival
Dr.	doctor
dr	dram
drsg	dressing
DSD	dry sterile dressing
DT's	delirium tremens
DUB	dysfunctional uterine bleeding
D/W, D5W, 5% DW	dextrose and water or glucose and water
DX	diagnosis
EBL	estimated blood loss
ECG, EKG	electrocardiogram
EEG	electroencephalogram
EFF	effacement
EMG	electromyogram
EPS	electrophysiological study
est	estimate
ext	external, extremity
f	respiratory frequency for one minute
FIO_2	Fractional concentration of oxygen of inspired gas
FB	foreign body
FBS	fasting blood sugar
F.D.	fetal distress
$FEV_{1.0}$	forced expiratory volume in one second
F.H.T.	fetal heart tones
freq	frequent

ft	foot
F.T.P.	failure to progress
fx	fracture
gal	gallon
GB	gallbladder
GI	gastrointestinal
Gm	gram
Gr	gravida
gr	grain
gtts	drops
HB	heart block
hr	hour
Hgb	hemoglobin
Hb O_2 Sat	percentage of hemoglobin saturated by oxygen
HCO_3	bicarbonate
Hct	hematocrit
hs	hour of sleep
ht	height
Hx	history
H_2O	water
H_2O_2	hydrogen peroxide
I&D	incision and drainage
IM	intramuscular
inj	injection
IOL	intraocular lens
IPPB	intermittent positive pressure breathing
IV	intravenous
IVC	inferior vena cava
IVP	intravenous pyelogram
IVPB	intravenous piggyback
K	potassium
Kg	kilogram
KO	keep open
KOR	keep open rate

KUB	kidneys, ureters and bladder
L, lt	left
L	liter
lab	laboratory
LAD	left anterior descending
lap	laparotomy
LAS	local with anesthesia standby
lat	lateral
lb, #	pound
LBBB	left bundle branch block
liq	liquid
LLE	left lower extremity
LLL	left lower lobe
LLQ	left lower quadrant
LA	left atrium
LMP	last menstrual period
LP	lumbar puncture
LUE	left upper extremity
LUL	left upper lobe
LUOQ	left upper outer quadrant
LUQ	left upper quadrant
LV	left ventricle
MBC	maximum breathing capacity
mcg	microgram
MEFR	maximum expiratory flow rate
mEq	milliequivalent
mg mgm	milligrams
M.I.	myocardial infarction
MIFR	maximum inspiratory flow rate
min	minute
ML	midline
ml	milliliter
mm	millimeter
mm Hg	millimeters of mercury

MMFR	mid-maximal expiratory flow rate
M.N.	midnight
mo	month
mod	moderate
MR × 1	may repeat one time
M.S.	morphine sulfate
MVV	maximum voluntary ventilation
NA	not applicable
Na	sodium
NaCl	sodium chloride
neg	negative
ng	nanogram
NGT	nasogastric tube
No., #	number
noc	night
NPO	nothing by mouth
N/S	normal saline
NSR	normal sinus rhythm
N/V	nausea and vomiting
NWB	non-weight bearing
NKA	no known allergies
O_2	oxygen
occ	occasional
OD	right eye
Od	overdose
ONC	oncology
OR	operating room
ortho	orthopedics
OS	left eye
OU	both eyes
oz	ounce
OOB	out of bed
P	pulse
p̄	after

Para	parity
PA	pulmonary artery
P.A.R.	post anesthesia recovery
PAC	premature atrial contractions
PAT	paroxysmal atrial tachycardia
P/B	partial bath
pc	after meal
PCN, Pen	penicillin
pCO_2	partial pressure of carbon dioxide
PCW	pulmonary capillary wedge
pH	degree of acidity or alkalinity of a solution
PID	pelvic inflammatory disease
PIP	proximal interphalangeal (joint)
PJC	premature junctional contractions
p.m.	afternoon
PMD	private medical doctor
PO	postoperative
po	by mouth
POD	postoperative day
pO_2	partial pressure of oxygen
pp	post partum
PPBS	postprandial blood sugar
PRE	progressive resistant exercise
prep	preparation
prn	as required
PT	physical therapy
pt	patient
PVC	premature ventricular contractions
q	every
qd	every day
qh	every hour
qid	four times a day
qn	every night
qns	quantity not sufficient

qs	quantity sufficient
R	respiratory
RA	right atrium
RBBB	right bundle branch block
RBC	red blood cells
RV	right ventricle
reg	regular
req	requires
RCA	right coronary artery
REUE	resistive exercise upper extremity
Resp	respiration
RLE	right lower extremity
RLL	right lower lobe
RLQ	right lower quadrant
RML	right middle lobe
R/O	rule out
ROM	range of motion
R, rt	right
R/I	reverse isolation
RUE	right upper extremity
RUL	right upper lobe
RUOQ	right upper outer quadrant
R.T.O.	return to office
Rx	treatment
s̄	without
sec	second
sg	specific gravity
S.G.	Swan-Ganz
S/I	strict isolation
sl	slight
S.L.R.	straight leg raising
S.O.	significant other
SOB	shortness of breath
sol.	solution

S/P	secretion precautions or status post
spec	specimen
S/R	side rails
SROM	spontaneous rupture of membranes
$\overline{ss}$, ss	half
SSKI	saturated solution of potassium iodide
STAT	immediately
SVC	superior vena cava
S/W	sterile water
Sx, sym	symptom
Syr	syrup
T, Temp	temperature
T&A	tonsils and adenoids, tonsillectomy and adenoidectomy
TAB	therapeutic abortion
tab	tablet
TAH	total abdominal hysterectomy
TAT	tetanus antitoxin
TB, Tbc	tuberculosis
TBA	to be absorbed
tbsp	tablespoon
tid	three times a day
tinc	tincture
TMJ	temporomandibular joint
TO, PO	telephone order
TPN	total parenteral nutrition
TPR	temperature, pulse and respiration
trans	transfer
tsp	teaspoon
TURB	transurethral resection of the bladder
TUR	transurethral resection
TURP	transurethral resection of the prostate
Tx	traction, treatment
U, u	unit
umb	umbilical

ung	ointment
URI	upper respiratory infection
V&P	vagotomy and pyloroplasty
vag	vaginal
VC	vital capacity
VCG	vectorcardiogram
VD	venereal disease
V_e	minute ventilation
VE	vaginal exam
Vit	vitamin
VO	verbal order
vol	volume
V.S.	vital signs
vs	versus
V_t	tidal volume
vtx	vertex
vg	ventral gluteal (injection site)
WBC	white blood cells
w/c	wheelchair
wh	white
WNL	within normal limits
W/S	wound and skin
wt	weight
x	times
yr	year

APPENDIX C

LABORATORY NORMS

Note: These are only general norms. Be sure to check these norms against your hospital's lab norms for any differences.

HEMATOLOGY

Bleeding Time (Duke)	1–5 mins.
Bleeding Time (Ivy)	less than 5 mins.
Clot Lysis, 37°C.	48–72 hrs.
Coagulation Time (Lee-White)	5–15 mins., glass tube 19–60 mins., siliconized tube

Coagulation Factor Assays
Factor V	60–150%
Factor VIII (antihemophiliac factor)	50–200%
Factor IX (plasma thromboplastin component)	60–140%
Factor X (Stuart factor)	60–130%
Factor XI	65–135%
Factor XII	65–150%
Factor XIII	1–2%

Erythrocyte Count
Males	4.6–6.2 million/mm^3
Females	4.2–5.4 million/mm^3

Erythrocyte Indices
MCH (mean corpuscular hemoglobin)	27–31 pg/cell
MCV (mean corpuscular volume)	80–100 micron^3
MCHC (mean corpuscular hemoglobin concentration)	32–36% hg/cell

Erythrocyte Sedimentation Rate
Male	0–9 mm/hr
Female	0–20 mm/hr
Fibrinogen	200–400 mg/100 ml
Haptoglobin	50–200 mg/100 ml

Hematocrit
  Male .... 40–54 ml/100 ml
  Female .... 37–47 ml/100 ml
Hemoglobin
  Male .... 13–18 g/100 ml
  Female .... 12–16 g/100 ml
Leukocyte Count
  Total .... 4,500–11,000 mm^3
  Band Neutrophils 3–5%
  Segmented Neutrophils 54–62%
  Lymphocytes 25–33%
  Eosinophils 1–4%
  Basophils 0–0.75%
  Monocytes 2–7%
Platelet Count .... 150,000–400,000/mm^3
Partial Thromboplastin Time
  Activated .... 20–45 sec
  Nonactivated .... 60–85 sec
Prothrombin Time .... 70–100% of control

CHEMISTRY

Acetone	0.3–2.0 mg/100 ml
Ammonia Plasma	15–120 mcg/100 ml
Amylase	15–200 units/100 ml
Ascorbic Acid	0.4–1.5 mg/100 ml
Bilirubin	
Total	0.1–1.0 mg/100 ml
Direct	0.1–0.4 mg/100 ml
Indirect	0.1–0.8 mg/100 ml
Calcium	8.5–11.0 mg/dl
	4.5–5.5 mEq/l
Chloride	95–105 mEq/l
Cholesterol	150–300 mg/100 ml
Cholesterol Esters	60–70% of total
Cholinesterase	
Serum	0.5–1.5 pH units
Red Cells	0.5–1.0 pH units
Copper	70–165 mcg/100 ml
Cortisol	
8:00 AM	5–26 mcg/100 ml
4:00 PM	2–15 mcg/100 ml
Creatine	0.2–0.8 mg/100 ml
Creatine Phosphokinase	
Male	50–325 mU/ml
Female	50–250 mU/ml
Isoenzymes	MM band present
	MB band absent
	BB band absent
Creatinine	0.7–1.5 mg/100 ml
Fatty Acids	190–420 mg/100 ml total
Fibrinogen (plasma)	200–400 mg/100 ml
Folic Acid	4–16 ng/ml
Follicle Stimulating Hormone	
Male	4–25 mU/ml
Female	4–30 mU/ml
Postmenopausal	40–250 mU/ml
Glucose	60–110 mg/100 ml fasting
Human Growth Hormone	0–10 ng/ml
Icterus Index	1–6 units
Immunoglobin A	60–333 mg/100 ml
Immunoglobin D	0.5–3.0 mg/100 ml

Immunoglobin G .... 550–1900 mg/100 ml
Immunoglobin M .... 45–145 mg/100 ml
Immunoglobin E .... less than 500 ng/ml
Insulin .... 5–25 microunits/ml
Iodine, Protein Bound .... 3.5–8.0 mcg/ml
Iron .... 75–175 mcg/100 ml
Iron Binding Capacity
   IBC .... 250–410 mcg/100 ml
   TIBC .... 250–420 mcg/100 ml
   Percent Saturation 20–50%
Lactic Acid, Whole Blood .... 9–16 mg/100 ml
Lactic Dehydrogenase (LDH) .... 100–225 mU/ml total
   Isoenzymes
      LDH-1 .... 20–35%
      LDH-2 .... 20–45%
      LDH-3 .... 20–30%
      LDH-4 .... 0–20%
      LDH-5 .... 0–25%
Lipase .... 0.2–1.5 units/ml
Lipids, Total .... 400–1,000 mg/100 ml
Lithium (Usual Maintenance Level) .... 0.5–1.0 mEq/l
Magnesium .... 1.3–2.5 mEq/l
                or 1.8–30 mg/100 ml
Manganese .... 0.08–0.26 mcg/100 ml
Non-Protein Nitrogen .... 15–35 mg/100 ml
Osmolality .... 280–300 milliosmoles/kg
Phosphatase, Acid .... 0–11 milliunits/ml total
Phosphatase, Alkaline .... 20–115 milliunits/ml
Phospholipids, Serum .... 6–12 mg/100 ml
Phosphorus .... 2.3–4.5 mg/100 ml
Potassium .... 3.5–5.0 mEq/l
Protein, Total .... 6–8 gm/100 ml
   Albumin .... 3.5–5.5 gm/100 ml
   Globulin .... 1.5–3.0 gm/100 ml
Pyruvic Acid .... 0.3–0.9 mg/100 ml
Sodium .... 135–145 mEq/l
Sulfate .... 0.5–1.5 mg/100 ml
Testosterone
   Male .... 300–800 ng/100 ml
   Female .... 25–100 ng/100 ml
T_3 Uptake 25–35%
T_3 Tri-Iodothyronine .... 75–250 ng/100 ml
T_4 Thyroxine .... 4.5–11.5 ng/100 ml

T_4 Thyroxine, Free .... 1.0–2.1 ng/100 ml
Thyroid Stimulating Hormone .... 0–10 microunits/ml
Transaminase
   (Aspartate Aminotransferase)
     (SGOT) .... 7–40 milliunits/ml
   (Alanine Aminotransferase) (SGPT) .. 10–40 milliunits/ml
Triglycerides .... 10–150 mg/100 ml
Blood Urea Nitrogen .... 10–20 mg/100 ml
Uric Acid .... 2.5–8.0 mg/100 ml
Vitamin A .... 20–220 mcg/100 ml
Vitamin B_1 (Thiamine) .... 1.6–4.0 mcg/100 ml
Vitamin B_6 (Pyridoxal Phosphate) ..... 3.6–18.0 ng/ml
Vitamin B_{12} .... 130–1,000 pg/ml
Zinc .... 50–150 mcg/100 ml

URINE CHEMISTRY

Acetone	negative
Aldosterone	3–20 mcg/24 hrs.
Alpha Amino Nitrogen	50–200 mg/24 hrs.
Ammonia Nitrogen	20–70 mEq/24 hrs.
Amylase	35–260 units/hr.
Bilirubin	negative
Calcium	less than 150 mg/24 hrs.
Catecholamines	
Total	0–275 mcg/24 hrs.
Epinephrine	10–40%
Norepinephrine	60–90%
Chlorides	70–250 mEq/24 hrs.
Chorionic Gonadotropin	
(Qualitative Pregnancy Test)	zero
Copper	0–70 mcg/24 hrs.
Creatine	0–200 mg/24 hrs.
Creatinine	15–25 mg/kg bodywt/24 hrs.
Creatinine Clearance	100–150 ml/min.
Estrogens, Total	
Female	
Onset of Menses	4–25 mcg/24 hrs.
Ovulation Peak	28–99 mcg/24 hrs.
Luteal Peak	22–105 mcg/24 hrs.
Menopause	1.4–19.6 mcg/24 hrs.
Male	5–18 mcg/24 hrs.
Glucose	negative
Hemoglobin and Myoglobin	negative
17-Hydroxycorticosteroids	2–10 mg/24 hrs.
5-Hydroxyindoleacetic Acid	negative
17-Ketosteroids, Total	
Male	10–22 mg/24 hrs.
Female	6–16 mg/24 hrs.
Lead	up to 150 mcg/24 hrs.
Lipase	0.1–0.75 units/ml
pH	4.6–8.5
Phosphorus, Inorganic	0.8–1.3 gm/24 hrs.
Pituitary Gonadotropin	10–50 mouse units/24 hrs.
Potassium	25–100 mEq/24 hrs.

Protein
    Qualitative .... negative
    Quantitative .... 10–150 mg/24 hrs.
Sodium .... 130–260 mEq/24 hrs.
Specific Gravity 1.003–1.030
Urea Nitrogen .... 9–16 gm/24 hrs.
Uric Acid .... 250–750 mg/24 hrs.
Urobilinogen .... up to 4 mg/24 hrs.
Uroporphyrins .... up to 50 mcg/24 hrs.
Zinc .... 0.15–1.2 mg/24 hrs.

CEREBROSPINAL FLUID

Albumin .... 15.5–32.0 mg/100 ml
Cell Count .... 0–5 mononuclear cells/mm^3
Chloride .... 100-130 mEq/l
Glucose .... 50–75 mg/100 ml
pH 7.35–7.40
Protein
  Total .... 15–456 mg/100 ml
  Lumbar .... 15–45 mg/100 ml
  Cisternal .... 15–25 mg/100 ml
  Ventricular .... 5–15 mg/100 ml
Specific Gravity 1.003–1.009

APPENDIX D

CONVERSION TABLES

TEMPERATURE

°F	°C	°C	°F
96	35.6	35.5	95.9
97	36.1	36	96.8
98	36.6	36.5	97.7
99	37.2	37	98.6
100	37.8	37.5	99.5
101	38.3	38	100.4
102	38.9	38.5	101.3
103	39.4	39	102.2
104	40.0	39.5	103.1
105	40.6	40	104.0
106	41.1	40.5	104.9

WEIGHT

Metric		Apothecary	
30	gm	1	ounce
15	gm	4	drams
10	gm	2½	drams
7.5	gm	2	drams
6	gm	90	grains
5	gm	75	grains
4	gm	60	grains
3	gm	45	grains
2	gm	30	grains
1.5	gm	22	grains
1	gm	15	grains
0.75	gm	12	grains
0.6	gm	10	grains
0.5	gm	7½	grains
0.4	gm	6	grains
0.3	gm	5	grains
0.25	gm	4	grains
0.2	gm	3	grains
0.15	gm	2½	grains
0.125	gm	2	grains
0.1	gm	1½	grains
75	mg	1¼	grains
60	mg	1	grain
50	mg	¾	grain
40	mg	⅔	grain
30	mg	½	grain
25	mg	⅜	grain
20	mg	⅓	grain
15	mg	¼	grain
12	mg	⅕	grain

10	mg		⅙	grain
8	mg		⅛	grain
6	mg		1/10	grain
5	mg		1/12	grain
4	mg		1/15	grain
3	mg		1/20	grain
2	mg		1/30	grain
1.5	mg		1/40	grain
1.2	mg		1/50	grain
1	mg		1/60	grain
0.8	mg		1/80	grain
0.6	mg		1/100	grain
0.5	mg		1/120	grain
0.4	mg		1/150	grain
0.3	mg		1/200	grain
0.25	mg		1/250	grain
0.2	mg		1/300	grain
0.15	mg		1/400	grain
0.12	mg		1/500	grain
0.1	mg		1/600	grain

VOLUME

1000	ml	1	quart
750	ml	1½	pints
500	ml	1	pint
250	ml	8	fluid ounces
200	ml	7	fluid ounces
100	ml	3½	fluid ounces
50	ml	1¾	fluid ounces
30	ml	1	fluid ounce
15	ml	4	fluid drams
10	ml	2½	fluid drams
8	ml	2	fluid drams
5	ml	1¼	fluid drams
4	ml	1	fluid dram
3	ml	45	minims
2	ml	30	minims
1	ml	15	minims
0.75	ml	12	minims
0.6	ml	10	minims
0.5	ml	8	minims
0.3	ml	5	minims
0.25	ml	4	minims
0.2	ml	3	minims
0.1	ml	1½	minims
0.06	ml	1	minim
0.05	ml	¾	minim
0.03	ml	½	minim

APPENDIX E

APPROVED NURSING DIAGNOSES

Activity intolerance
Activity intolerance, potential
Airway clearance, ineffective
Anxiety
Bowel elimination, alteration in: constipation
Bowel elimination, alteration in: diarrhea
Bowel elimination, alteration in: incontinence
Breathing pattern, ineffective
Cardiac output, alteration in: decreased
Comfort, alteration in: pain
Communication, impaired: verbal
Coping, family: potential for growth
Coping, ineffective family: compromised
Coping, ineffective family: disabling
Coping, ineffective individual
Diversional activity, deficit
Family process, alteration in (formerly Family dynamics)
Fear
Fluid volume alteration in: excess
Fluid volume deficit, actual
Fluid volume deficit, potential
Gas exchange, impaired
Grieving, anticipatory
Grieving, dysfunctional
Health maintenance, alteration in
Home maintenance management, impaired
Injury, potential for: (poisoning, potential for; suffocation, potential
    for; trauma, potential for)
Knowledge deficit (specify)
Mobility, impaired physical
Noncompliance (specify)
Nutrition, alteration in: less than body requirements
Nutrition, alteration in: more than body requirements
Nutrition, alteration in: potential for more than body requirements

Oral mucous membrane, alteration in

Parenting, alteration in: actual

Parenting, alteration in: potential

Powerlessness

Rape trauma syndrome

Self-care deficit: feeding, bathing/hygiene, dressing/grooming,
   toileting

Self-concept, disturbance in: body image, self-esteem, role
   performance, personal identity

Sensory-perceptual alteration: visual, auditory, kinesthetic, gustatory,
   tactile, olfactory

Sexual dysfunction

Skin integrity, impairment of: actual

Skin integrity: impairment of: potential

Sleep pattern disturbance

Social Isolation

Spiritual distress (distress of the human spirit)

Thought processes, alteration in

Tissue perfusion, alteration in: cerebral, cardiopulmonary, renal,
   gastrointestinal, peripheral

Urinary elimination, alteration in patterns

Violence, potential for: self-directed or directed at others

Approved at the Fifth National Conference on Classification of
Nursing Diagnosis.

Source: Kim, M.M., McFarland, G.K., and McLane, A.M., editors:
          Classifications of Nursing Diagnosis: Proceedings of the Fifth
          National Conference, St. Louis, 1984, The C.V. Mosby Co.

INDEX

INDEX